Jamie's
FOOD
REVOLUTION

Also by Jamie Oliver

The Naked Chef
The Naked Chef Takes Off
Happy Days with the Naked Chef
Jamie's Kitchen
Jamie's Dinners
Jamie's Italy
Cook with Jamie
Jamie at Home

Jamie's
FOOD
REVOLUTION

REDISCOVER HOW TO COOK SIMPLE, DELICIOUS, AFFORDABLE MEALS

JAMIE OLIVER

Photography by
David Loftus and Chris Terry

HYPERION

New York

I dedicate this book to all the
wonderful people of Huntington,
West Virginia. The food revolution
in Huntington was hard, but the
community came together and I
hope and pray they keep it going
and become a shining example of
how one community can make
inspiring changes.

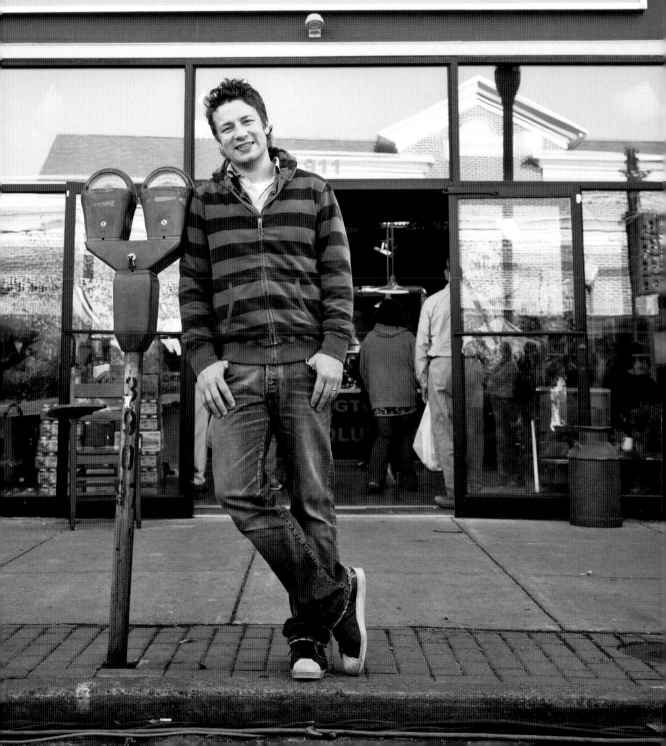

Published by arrangement with Michael Joseph / The Penguin Group

First published in the UK as *Jamie's Ministry of Food* by Penguin Books Ltd, 2008

www.penguin.com
www.jamieoliver.com

Paperback ISBN: 978-1-4013-1047-9

Hyperion books are available for special promotions and premiums. For details contact the
HarperCollins Special Markets Department in the New York office at 212-207-7528,
fax 212-207-7222, or email spsales@harpercollins.com.

First U.S. Paperback Edition

10 9 8 7 6 5 4 3 2 1

Jamie
Oliver

Contents

Introduction

Hi guys—I'd like to ask you a favor: I need your help with a food movement I've started. On the surface it's quite simply about friends teaching friends how to cook good, honest, affordable food and just generally be a bit more streetwise about cooking. But underneath that, it's about getting a really fun and important movement called *pass it on* started, which could well change the health and future of the country.

So why am I doing this?

A British cooking legend, the very lovely Marguerite Patten, inspired me to write this book. During the Second World War she was really involved with a government ministry set up to tackle the food shortages at the time. The work this "Ministry of Food" did made it possible for Brits to feed themselves well with the little food they had. Not only did it make sure there was enough food to go around, it also educated the public about food and proper nutrition so they'd be healthy and fighting fit. People started learning how to help themselves and their country, not just in Britain, but also in the United States, where the government was encouraging over twenty million Americans to plant their Victory Gardens. What I find completely inspiring is that the governments of the day didn't just watch and give lip service; they did something radical...and I like radical! The Ministry of Food went to the people, wherever they were—workplaces, factories, gentlemen's clubs, or local shopping areas. And they did this by simply mobilizing thousands of women, like Marguerite, who could cook, then sending them out across the whole country to provide support and tips to the public. Because of this, people knew how to use their food rations properly and were able to eat, and live, better.

It's such a shame, but we have a modern-day war on our hands now, and it's over the epidemic of bad health and the rise of obesity. The question is, do we wait until it's too late, or do we do something about it now? I say we do something about it now. I've been told that fewer than a third of Americans cook their dinners from scratch these days. And although 75 percent of people in the United States eat most of their meals at home, much like us Brits, over half of those dinners are fast food, delivery, or takeout! Regardless of recessions and credit crunches, we all need to know how to cook simple, nutritious, economical, tasty, and hearty food. And once we've got this knowledge, we should **pass it on** through friends, family, and the workplace to keep that cycle of knowledge alive.

So what's the plan?

I need you to get personally involved in **pass it on** by pledging to learn just one recipe from each chapter of this book. Master these in your own home first, and then **pass it on** by teaching at least two people (preferably four) how to cook them, too. Make it fun by having a bit of a cooking party where you teach your friends, family, and other guests some brilliant new skills in the comfort of your own home. Then, most importantly, you need to get your guests to promise that they'll **pass it on** to more people and then get those people to **pass it on** and on and on.... It's easy.

And don't for a minute think that your single contribution won't count, because it will. Let me share a bit of my romantic dream with you.... Let's say, for

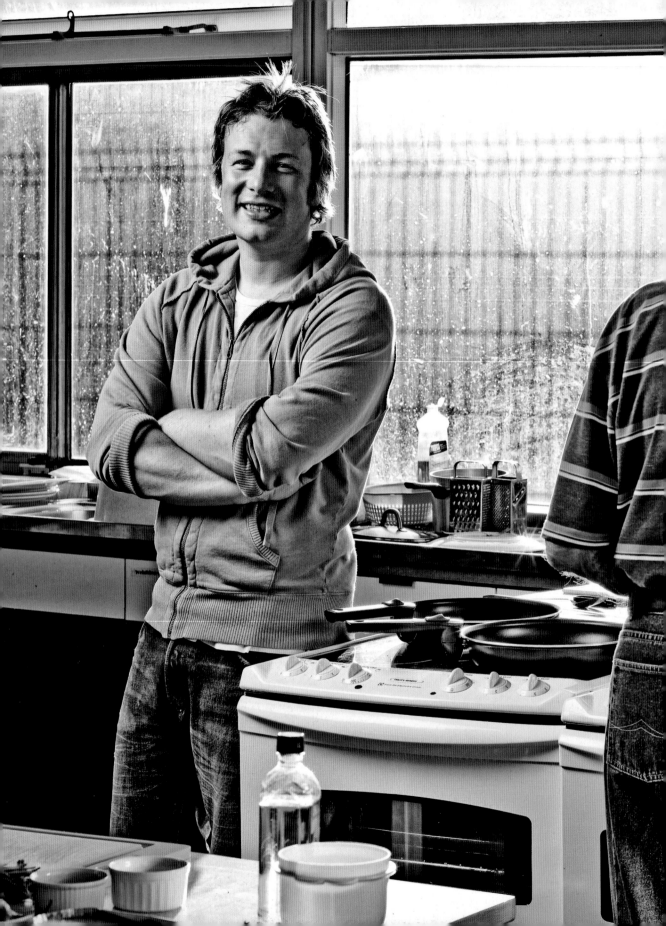

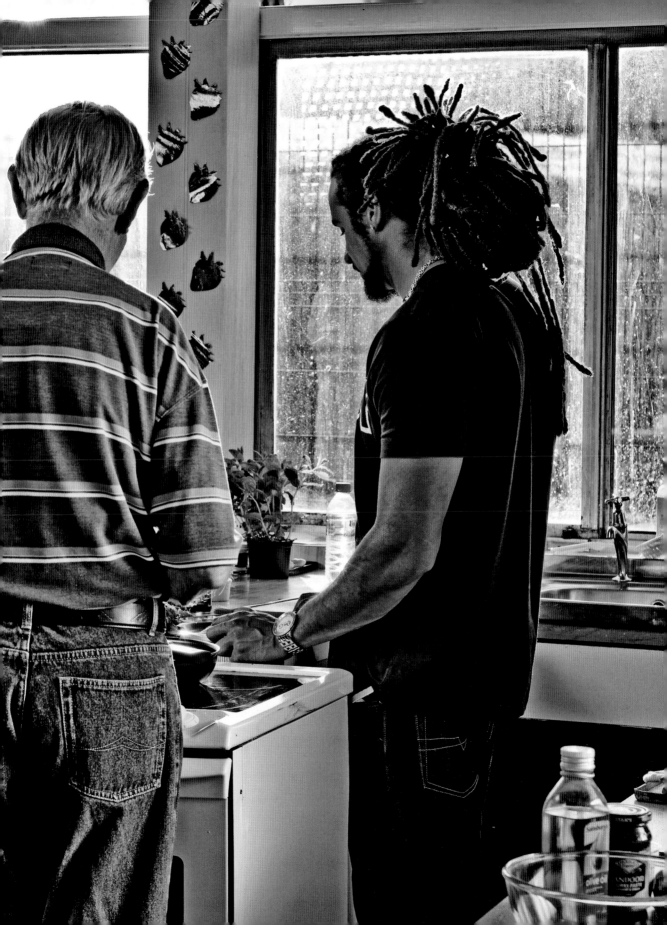

instance, that you teach four people how to make a recipe, then each of them teaches four more people, who each teach four more people....The cycle only needs to repeat itself seven times and we've packed out Yankee Stadium one-and-a-half times. Repeat it thirteen times and we've got more than the entire population of the United States cooking—high aspirations, I admit, but why the hell not? I know for a fact that there will be hundreds of thousands of you who will definitely get involved in this. Just imagine the swell of fun teaching and learning that could be going around the country! It's amazing if you think about all the social and health benefits this movement could have. I know for sure that if we do this a load of other things will start to fall into place.

This **pass it on** movement is essentially a modern-day version of the way people used to pass recipes down through generations when they weren't all at work. That dynamic is the best learning ground ever. As simple as it seems, **pass it on** could well be the most radical food movement in recent years, and you could be part of it. I wouldn't be asking for your help unless I thought it was absolutely necessary.

I decided to kick this movement off in Rotherham, in the north of England. It is a very typical industrial English town, full of hard-working, down-to-earth people who—like the rest of the country—seem to have fallen out of love with cooking. Rotherham is said to be the town that best reflects Britain's population in terms of demographic make-up. So, in a way, I figured that if I set up my own version of a Ministry of Food there and made it work, then it could work anywhere.

I also had a more personal reason for going there. A few years ago, when I campaigned for school food in British schools to be changed, some of the women who lived in the Rotherham area went down to the school gates and passed French fries and burgers through the school gates to the kids. That got the media's attention, and mine too. Julie Critchlow was one of these women, and one of my fiercest critics at the time. So I wanted to meet her and see if I could convince her to help me **pass it on**.

I brought local cooking demonstrations to the town, along with smaller cooking classes where I asked people to teach the recipes I taught them to at least two other people. The people in my cooking classes are the ones who appear—looking really pleased with themselves—in the chapter portraits. (Nice one, guys!)

While I was teaching these cooking classes, I consistently saw the most radical, inspiring, and completely emotional change happening to everyone I met, all through showing them how to cook a handful of meals. This change is so fantastic to see, and can literally happen within twenty-four hours. I know it sounds soft, but it's true. And I'm not talking about easy, cuddly individuals who thought it might be quite nice to start cooking; I'm talking about people who had never, ever wanted to cook or been interested in food for years: miners, single moms, old-age pensioners, and busy dads ... you name it!

I want this book to serve you well whether you're a complete beginner, a good cook who likes simplicity, or you're buying it for someone who needs to be dragged kicking and screaming into the kitchen. I also want it to be the catalyst for empowering millions of you to make proper home-cooked, affordable meals from scratch again. I've written the recipes in this book so they're nice and simple and anyone can follow them. I've also used copious amounts of step-by-step pictures in order to get you confident enough to understand the basics of cooking, even if you're the most reluctant cook in the world.

Why do we need to *pass it on?*

The reality is that we are in the midst of one of the worst food-related epidemics that this country has seen. And I can assure you it's not through lack of food this time, but because we're consuming far too much of the wrong stuff. According to the Institute of Food Technologists, Americans spent more money on fast food in 2007 than they did on education. We're not talking about gourmet French cheeses and expensive cuts of meat here ... we're talking about French fries, pizzas, burgers, and other food that is absolute garbage.

School lunches have been neglected for thirty years, cooking lessons at school have all but stopped, physical education has been reduced, and more and more of us are driving to work and doing office jobs. All these things are major contributors to why—unfortunately—Britain has the highest obesity levels in Europe and the United States has the highest obesity levels in the world. Much-needed urgency is required to change this.

The state of our health and cooking is a subject that's been close to my heart for many years now. I live and breathe it, it bothers me, and I think about how to do my bit every day, so this is just a small rant. If you've read this far, then I hope you're feeling where I'm coming from. Anyone can eat good food on any budget as long as they know how to cook. So come on, guys, be part of ***pass it on***.

So how will we do it?

The *pass it on* pledge

Please sign a version of this pledge online now, to help make a difference. My website, www.jamieoliver.com, will also give you a whole load of extra information: photos, videos, and tips to complement this beautiful book. If you need a little more help as you're learning, the website will have videos of me cooking a load of these recipes and they'll be free to download. There will be a whole community of people on the site who will be learning to cook too, and they'll be sharing their stories on the forums. So enjoy this book, have fun learning these recipes, and *pass it on*!

This book belongs to ....

I pledge to learn a recipe from each chapter of this book.

I will then personally teach these recipes to two or more of my friends or family, on the condition that they pledge to do the same.

Dated ....

Signed ....

Essentials

Kitchen equipment

More than ever these days, you can buy really cheap kitchen gear. This is great, because it means anyone should be able to get all the essential bits of equipment they need, no matter what their budget is. One thing I never realized until now was how big a problem bad or inappropriately sized equipment can be. I think it's probably one-third of the reason why cooking in this country is in the state it is; for me, that's a really big deal. So the fact that you can buy yourself an extra third of success in the kitchen in terms of cooking and consistency is really quite cool.

I'm giving you a list of the bare minimum items you need to have in your kitchen to be a well-rounded, efficient cook. When it comes to things like knives, food processors, and wooden chopping boards, it really is worth scrimping, saving, or borrowing money to get the best equipment you can afford. You'll be much better off with three good-quality knives, for example a 12-inch chopping knife, a 12-inch serrated carving knife, and a 6-inch paring knife, than you will be with a whole set of rubbish knives that won't last long at all and will make your chopping worse. When you're buying a knife, check that it's a good weight, the blade is nice and rigid and doesn't bend, and the handle feels good in your hand. I personally like I.O. Shen knives, Victorinox, Henckels, and Sabatiers.

When I'm buying frying pans for my home I always go for really good-quality non-stick ones. When it comes to saucepans, as long as they've got sturdy, thick bottoms, I think they're all about the same. All the other stuff on the list you can spend as little, or as much, money on as you wish.

Essential kitchen equipment

Extra-large non-stick frying pan
Large grill pan
Extra-large casserole pan or Dutch
    oven (cast iron, aluminum, or
    stainless steel)
Set of thick-bottomed saucepans
    (large, medium, and small)
Good sturdy sheet pans
Wok
Nest of mixing bowls
Metal tongs
Knives (chef's knife, serrated
    carving knife, small paring knife)

Wooden spoons
Metal whisk
Potato masher
Ladle
Slotted spoon
Slotted turner
Plastic spatula
Speed peeler
Thick, sturdy wooden chopping
    board
Small plastic chopping board
Pestle and mortar
Salad spinner

Measuring cups and weighing scales
Strainers (one coarse, one fine)
Large colander
Large measuring jug
Box grater/Microplane grater
Food processor (to this day I
    haven't found anything more
    efficient or with better
    guarantees than a Magimix)
Rolling pin
Can opener

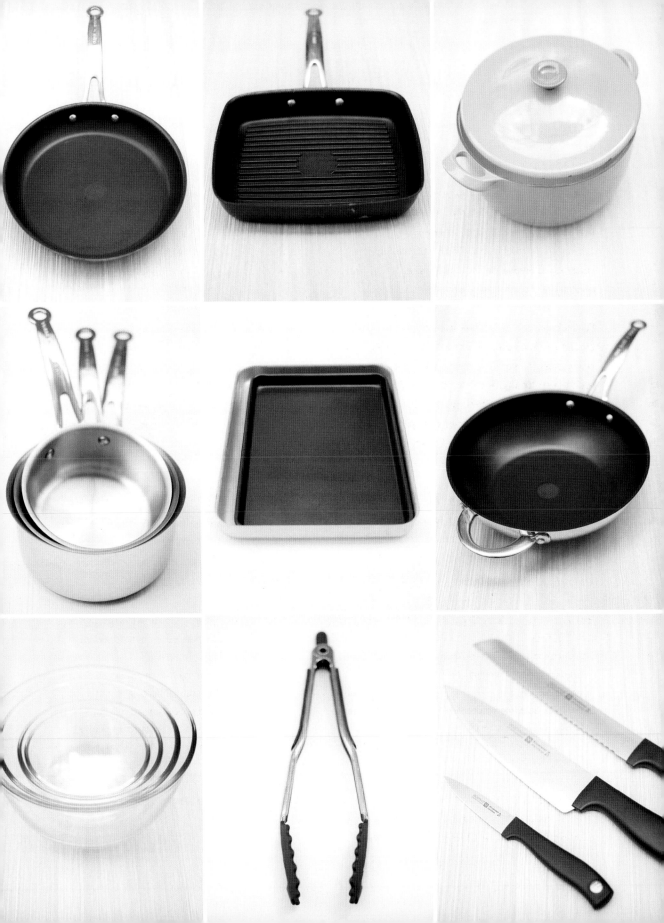

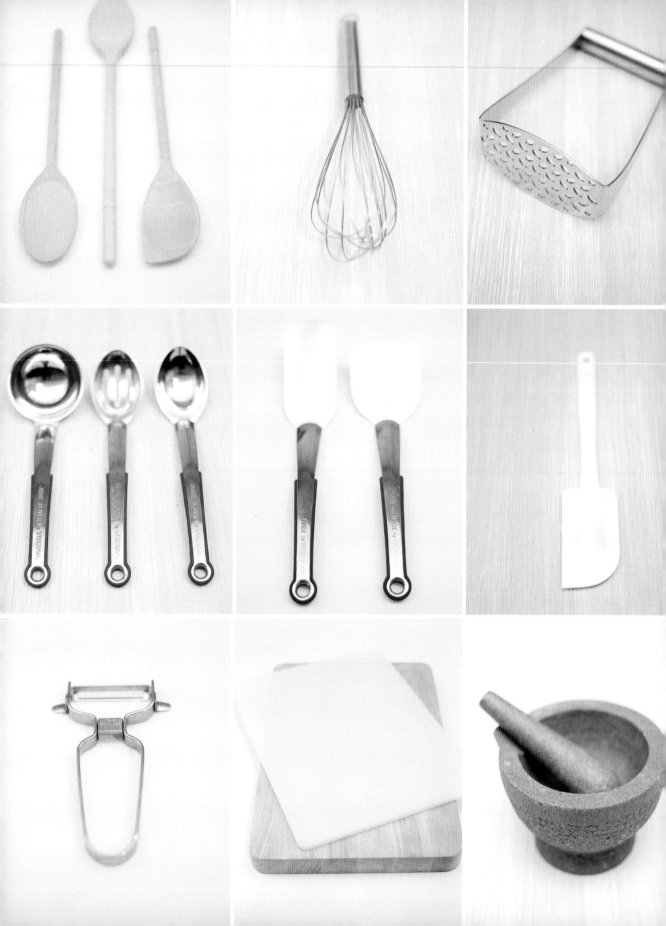

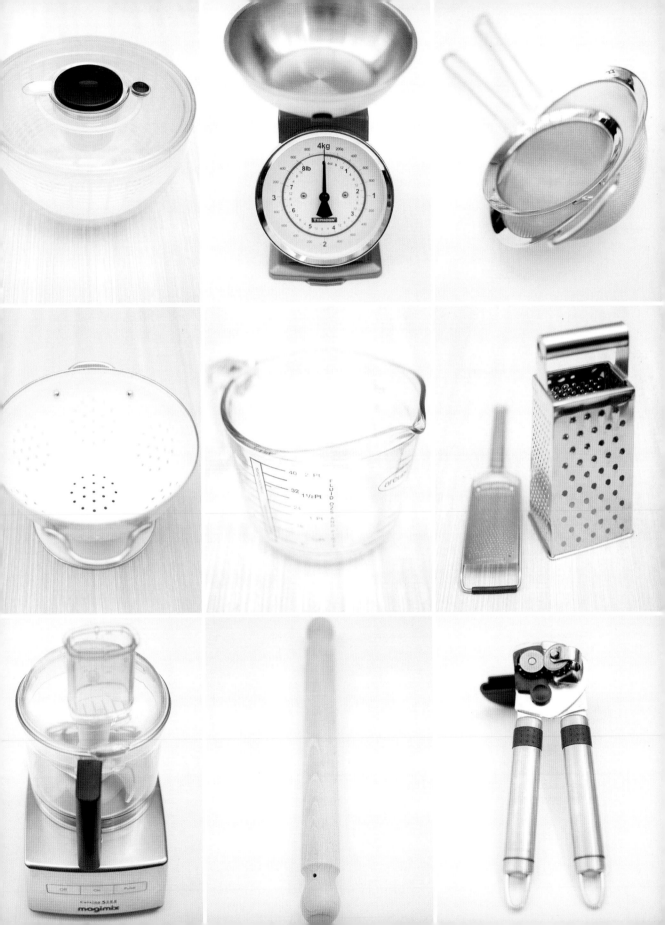

For the cupboard

As soon as you get the cooking bug you're going to want to become as good at it as you can get, and eat food that tastes as good as you can make it, as quickly as possible.

To do that you'll need the right kitchen equipment, plenty of practice, and cupboards full of good, basic ingredients. All that non-perishable stuff that sits in your cupboard, waiting for you to come home and cook, is really important, because that's what's going to help make your food taste great.

If you buy yourself a nice piece of cod, beef, or chicken, you can take it to Spain, Italy, Morocco, or China just by using certain herbs or spices from your cupboards. That's what's so exciting about cooking.

It's good to remember that there's nothing substandard about canned tomatoes, canned tuna, or frozen fruits and vegetables. Things like frozen peas are picked at their best and preserved that way until you use them. Unless you're picking them from your garden you'll have to go a long way to get a tastier and more nutritional pea than a frozen one.

The moral of the story is: use this list. Go out and buy it all. It won't cost the earth, and it's not going to go bad. It will all sit happily in your cupboard or freezer for months. Having these basics will allow you to do more exciting things with your food. The truth is: there should be enough in your stores to get you out of trouble if you get snowed in . . . so stock up!

Essential cupboard ingredients
Dijon mustard
Whole grain mustard
English mustard
Extra virgin olive oil
Olive oil
Canola or
   vegetable oil
Sesame seed oil
Peanut oil
Red wine vinegar
White wine vinegar
Balsamic vinegar
All-purpose flour
Self-rising flour
Bread flour
Whole wheat flour
Cornstarch
Baking powder
Dried yeast
Superfine sugar

Brown sugar
Confectioners' sugar
Unsweetened cocoa
   powder
Dried pasta
Egg noodles
Canned garbanzo beans
Canned cannellini beans
Canned kidney beans
Canned tomatoes
Canned tuna
Canned coconut milk
Olives (stone in)
Anchovies
Quick-cook couscous
Basmati rice
Brown rice
Oatmeal
Honey
Maple syrup
Almonds/ hazelnuts or
   mixed nuts

Mixed seeds
Cream or plain crackers
   (such as Jacob's)
Organic chicken,
   vegetable, and
   beef broth
Marmite or Vegemite
Jarred pesto
Patak's curry paste
Soy sauce
Ketchup
Tabasco sauce
HP sauce or steak sauce
Mayonnaise

Basic spices
Maldon or other sea salt
Table salt
Black peppercorns
Dried chiles
Nutmeg
Ground cinnamon

Dried oregano
Bay leaves
Fennel seeds
Coriander seeds
Cumin seeds
Chili powder
Five-spice powder
Garam masala
Curry powder
Smoked paprika

Basic frozen stuff
Peas
Fava beans
Green beans
Sweet corn
Fruits
Shrimp
Ready-made pie crust
Filo pastry
Puff pastry

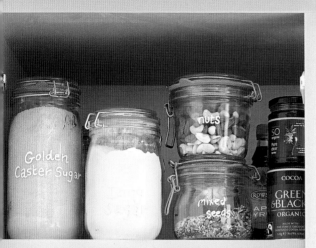
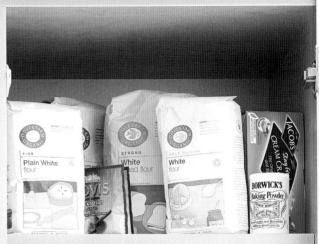
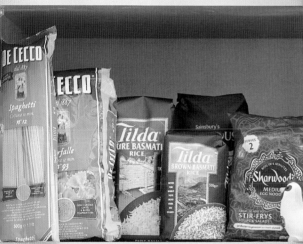
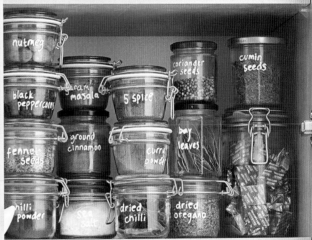
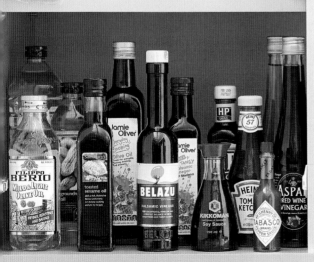
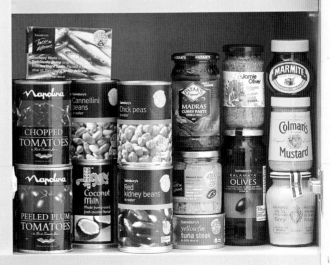

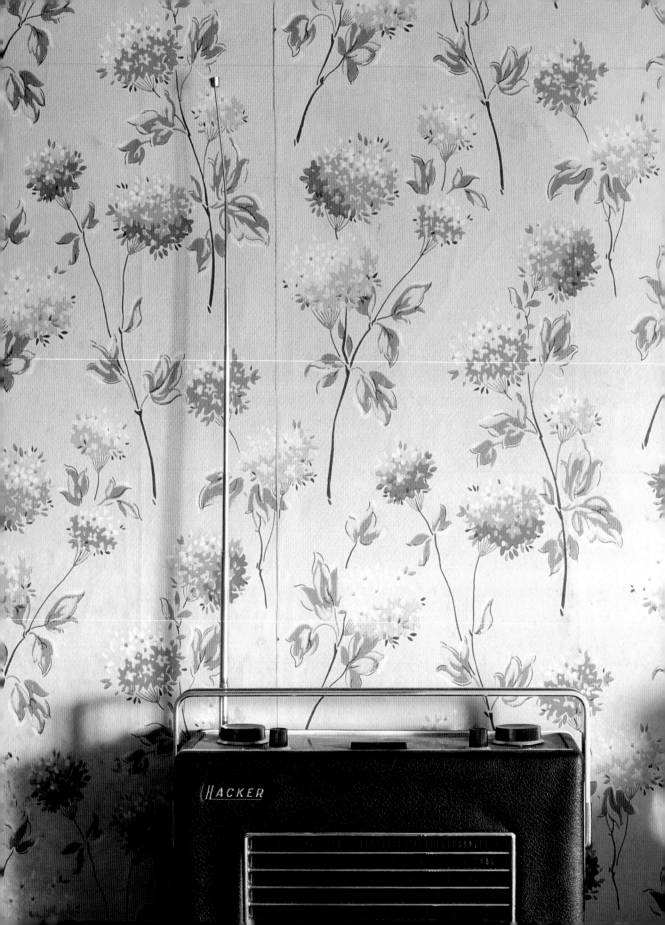

Twenty-minute meals

With a lot of people saying they're too busy and have no time to cook these days, it's not surprising that you can find a chapter on quick meals in most modern cookbooks. So here's mine! To be honest, a lot of the other recipes in this book are pretty quick anyway – have a look at the pasta, salads, or quick-cooking meat and fish chapters – but what I've tried to do with the next few recipes is make them really very quick and absolutely perfect for when you want a snack, dinner, or lunch for 1 or 2 people. They're the sort of thing I usually cook when I get home late. I always challenge myself to see how quickly I can make them. This usually happens along with some slamming of cupboard and fridge doors, but Jools doesn't seem to mind if it means we can be eating within minutes of getting through the door.

Beginner cooks should be able to make these recipes within 20 minutes. After each recipe title I've given a time for how long it should take if you're a beginner. You'll get quicker with practice.

In all types of cuisine there are always recipes that can be varied to cook in very little time. For instance, to get a fresh, tasty meal on the table really quickly, it's worth taking advantage of quality convenience ingredients like bagged salads and herbs, flatbreads, quick-cooking cuts of meat like chicken breasts or steaks, and fresh and frozen vegetables, as these will all help you achieve great results in very little time.

These recipes are certainly not hard for beginner cooks, as there isn't anything very technical going on here. But because they require lots to be happening in a short space of time, it's best to be very organized as you'll be prepping and cooking at the same time. I've written the recipes so that you can use your time well – while your pan is heating, you can be chopping and getting stuff ready, for instance.

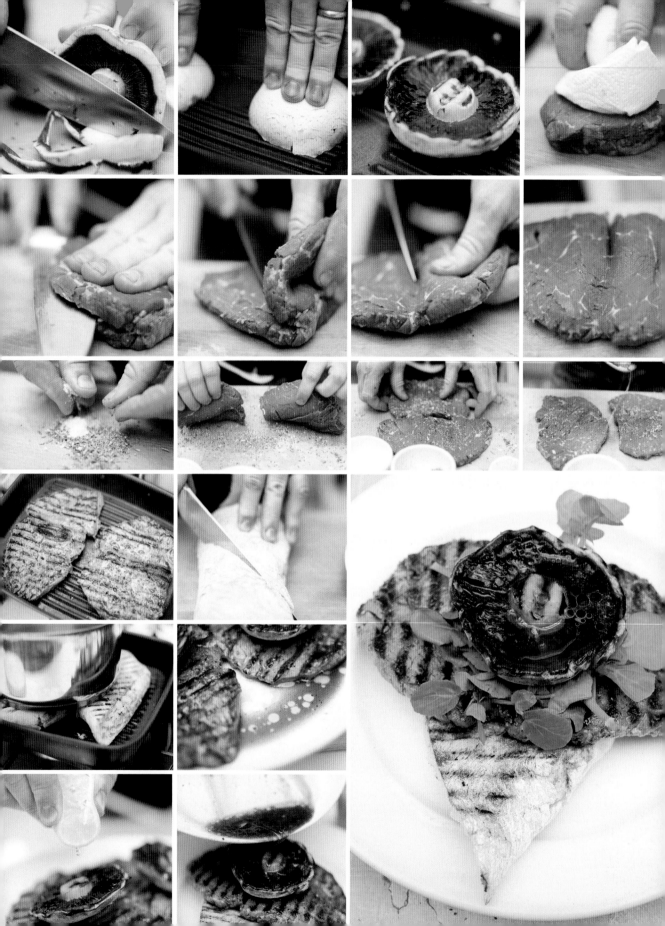

BUTTERFLIED STEAK SARNIE
(15 minutes)

"Butterflying" a steak simply means cutting it in half horizontally so that you can open it like a book. It's very simple – check out the pictures opposite.

serves 2

2 large portobello mushrooms

2 x 7-ounce filet mignon steaks

a sprig of fresh rosemary

sea salt and freshly ground black pepper

olive oil

1 ciabatta loaf

extra virgin olive oil

juice of ½ a lemon

a small handful of watercress

Dijon mustard

Place a grill pan on the highest heat • Wipe the mushrooms and slice across the bottom of each one so they sit nice and flat in your pan • While your pan is heating up, place the mushrooms on it and press down on them • Turn them over when charred –this will bring out their beautiful nutty flavor • Pat the steaks with paper towels • To butterfly your steaks, carefully slice horizontally through the middle of each one, using long, slow slicing movements, and open each one out like a book • Pick the rosemary leaves off the woody stalks and finely chop • Sprinkle the rosemary and a good pinch of salt and pepper on a chopping board and place your open steaks on top, patting them down so that the flavors and seasoning stick to the meat • Give them a little drizzle with olive oil, then turn them over and do the same with the other side

Remove the cooked mushrooms from the grill pan to a plate • Put the pan back on the heat and place the steaks in it, pressing them down • Cook for about 4 minutes in total for a medium steak, turning every minute • When done, remove the steaks from the pan to a plate to rest • Halve the ciabatta at an angle and place in the grill pan with a weight, such as another pan, on top so you get lovely charred marks on the bread • Toast for a minute or two on each side • Lightly drizzle the steaks and mushrooms with extra virgin olive oil • Squeeze over a little lemon juice and a pinch of salt and pepper • Top each piece of toasted ciabatta with a steak, a little watercress and a mushroom, then drizzle over some of the delicious juices from the meat so they soak into the bread • Drizzle with a little more extra virgin olive oil and serve with a jar of Dijon mustard on the table

SPICY MOROCCAN STEWED FISH WITH COUSCOUS (18 minutes)

You can make this recipe using any white fish or salmon fillets. It's incredibly quick to cook, and a really good thing to give the kids for dinner. I like to use a mixture of beans and peas, but if you find it easier to just use one of those that's fine – it will still be beautiful. Make sure that when you buy your fish, you ask the fishmonger to scale, fillet, and remove all the little bones from it for you. If not, you can have a go at removing the bones yourself – this is called pin-boning.

serves 2

1 cup quick-cook couscous
olive oil
2 lemons
sea salt and freshly ground black pepper
2 cloves of garlic
1 fresh red or green chile
a bunch of fresh basil
1 teaspoon whole cumin seeds

½ teaspoon ground cinnamon
2 x 6-ounce white fish fillets, skin off and bones removed
½ pound large shrimp, raw, peeled
1 x 14-ounce can of diced tomatoes
2 handfuls of fresh or frozen peas, fava beans, or green beans (or use a mixture)

Put the couscous into a bowl and add a couple of tablespoons of olive oil • Halve the lemons and squeeze in the juice from two of the halves • Add a pinch of salt and pepper • Pour in just enough boiling water to cover the couscous, then cover the bowl with a plate or plastic wrap • Let the couscous soak up the water for 10 minutes

Get a large saucepan on a medium heat • Peel and finely slice your garlic • Finely slice your chile • Pick the basil leaves off the stalks • Put the smaller ones to one side and roughly chop the larger ones • Add a couple of lugs of olive oil to the hot pan • Add the garlic, chile, basil, cumin seeds, and cinnamon • Give it all a stir and put the fish fillets on top • Scatter over the shrimp • Add the canned tomatoes and the peas and beans • Squeeze in the juice from the two remaining lemon halves • Put a lid on the pan • Bring to a boil, then turn the heat down to a simmer and cook for about 8 minutes, or until the fish is cooked through and flakes easily • Taste, and season with salt and pepper

By the time the fish is cooked, the couscous should have sucked up all the water and be ready to serve • Spoon the couscous into a large serving bowl and give it a stir with a fork to help it fluff up • Top with the fish, vegetables, and juices from the pan, sprinkle with the reserved basil leaves, and tuck in!

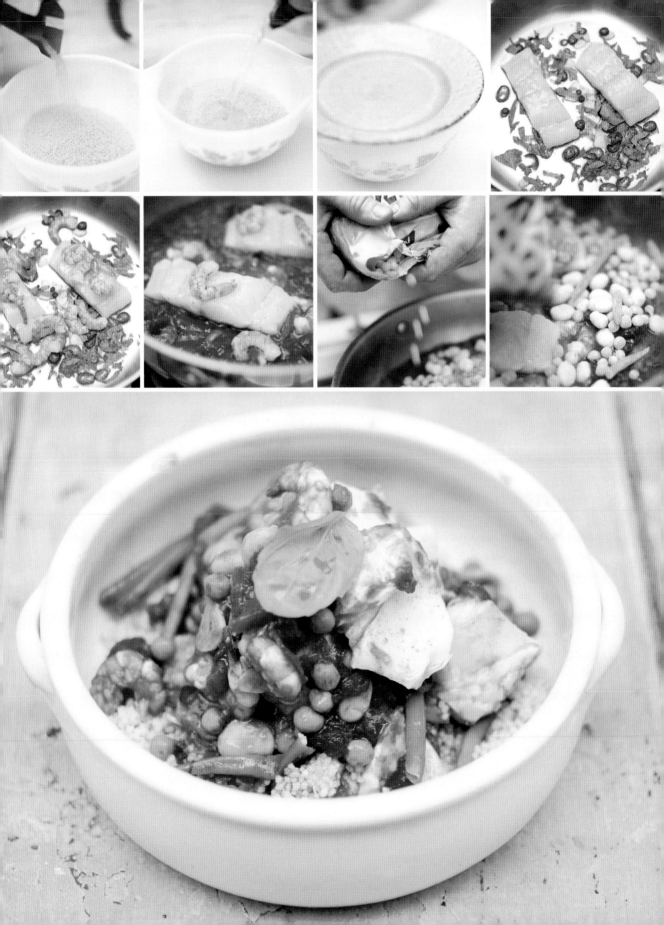

QUICK SALMON TIKKA WITH CUCUMBER YOGURT (17 minutes)

I love this dish. If you're a fan of chicken tikka masala, give this one a go. You might think it odd to use robust spice pastes on fish, but it's very common in southern India. When buying your fish, ask the fishmonger to scale it for you. You'll be amazed at how quickly these cook.

serves 2

2 naan breads or flatbreads

1 fresh red or green chile

½ a cucumber

1 lemon

¼ cup natural yogurt

sea salt and freshly ground black pepper

a few sprigs of fresh cilantro

2 x 7-ounce salmon fillets, skin on, scaled, and bones removed

1 heaped tablespoon tandoori, or mild curry paste, such as Patak's

olive oil

Preheat your oven to 225°F • Pop your naan breads into the oven to warm through • Halve, seed, and finely chop your chile • Peel and halve your cucumber lengthways, then use a spoon to scoop out and discard the seeds • Roughly chop the cucumber and put most of it into a bowl • Halve your lemon and squeeze the juice from one half into the bowl • Add the yogurt, a pinch of salt and pepper, and half the chopped chile • Pick the cilantro leaves and put to one side

Slice each salmon fillet across lengthways into three ½-inch-wide slices • Spoon the heaped tablespoon of tandoori paste into a small dish and use a pastry brush or the back of a spoon to smear the paste all over each piece (don't dip your pastry brush into the jar!) • Heat a large frying pan over a high heat • Once hot, add a lug of olive oil, put the salmon into the pan, and cook for about 1½ minutes on each side, until cooked through

Place a warmed naan bread on each plate • Top each one with a good dollop of cucumber yogurt and 3 pieces of salmon • Scatter over a little of the reserved cucumber, chile, and cilantro leaves and finish with a squeeze of lemon juice

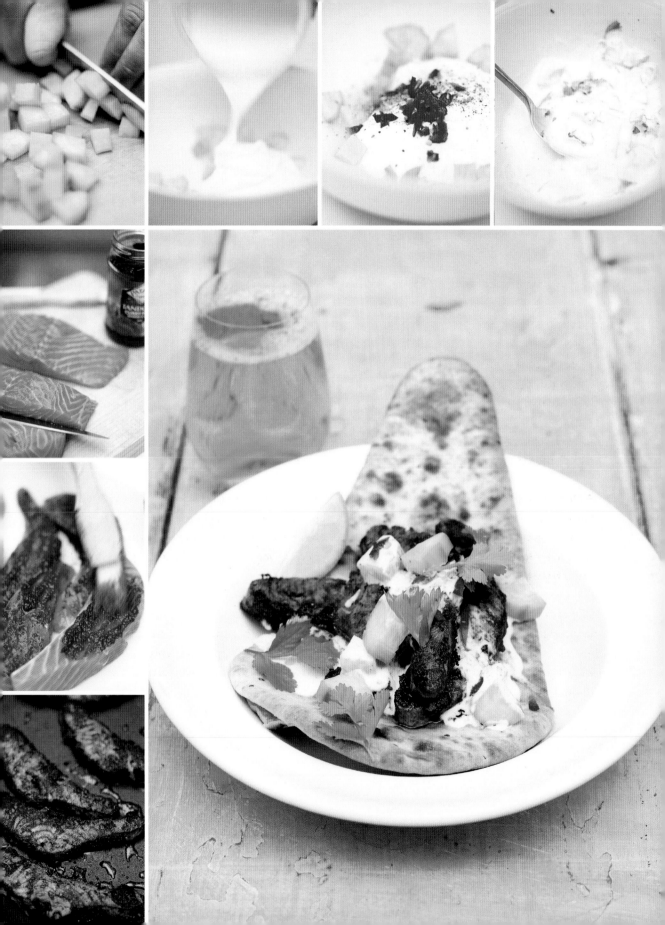

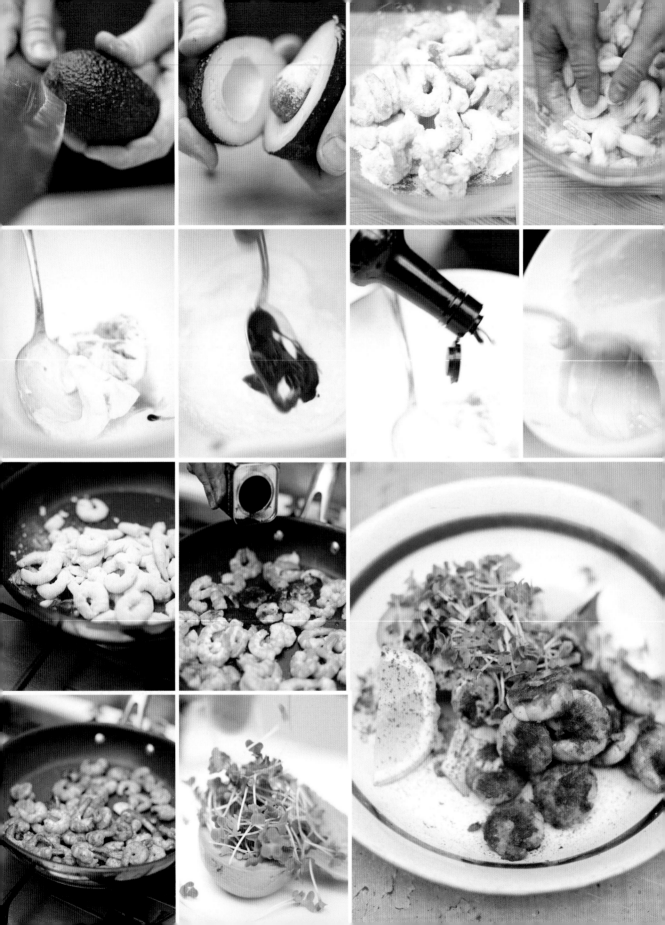

SHRIMP AND AVOCADO WITH AN OLD-SCHOOL MARIE ROSE SAUCE (12 minutes)

I grew up surrounded by shrimp cocktails in my parents' pub, so the taste of this dish reminds me of my childhood! It's simple, quick, and quite a retro little dish that makes a great, light supper. I've added unpeeled garlic cloves to the pan because they give a wonderful flavor to the shrimp.

serves 2

1 or 2 ripe avocados
1 or 2 large handfuls of sprouted cress or alfalfa
all-purpose flour
½ pound large shrimp, peeled and cleaned
olive oil
2 cloves of garlic
1 heaped teaspoon paprika
extra virgin olive oil

For the Marie Rose sauce
¼ cup mayonnaise
2 teaspoons tomato ketchup
1 teaspoon Worcestershire sauce
1 teaspoon whiskey
1 lemon
sea salt and freshly ground black pepper

Carefully cut into your avocado until you hit the pit, then run the knife around it to halve it • Gently twist the two halves and pull them apart • Carefully remove the pit and discard, then peel the skin off and discard that too • Cut the cress or alfalfa • Put a handful or two of flour into a bowl • Drop your shrimp into the bowl of flour and toss until they're completely coated • To make your sauce, put your mayonnaise into a bowl with the ketchup, a small splash of Worcestershire sauce, and the booze • Halve the lemon and squeeze in the juice from one of the halves • Cut the remaining half into wedges for serving • Add a pinch of salt and pepper and mix well • Give it a taste and add a touch more salt, pepper, and lemon juice if you think it needs it

Get yourself a large frying pan and place it on a high heat • When the pan is hot, pour in 2 good lugs of olive oil • Bash and break up your garlic cloves with your hand and add these to the pan, immediately followed by your flour-dusted shrimp • Toss them well to coat them in the hot oil • Count to ten, then add a pinch of salt and pepper, and the paprika for flavor and color • Keep tossing your shrimp, trying to keep them in a single layer in the pan so they cook evenly, for about 3 to 4 minutes, until crisp and golden

Divide your avocado halves between your plates • Divide the cress or alfalfa over the avocados and place the shrimp next to them • Drizzle a few good spoonfuls of your Marie Rose sauce over the avocados • Finish with a drizzle of extra virgin olive oil and a sprinkle of paprika • Serve with wedges of lemon for squeezing over • Fantastic!

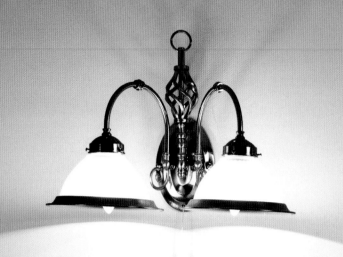

DEBBIE DENNIS

HAIR STYLIST

I felt so guilty every time I reheated a ready-prepared meal for the kids because I believed they weren't getting any goodness in their diet. Now I've had some recipes passed on to me, I'm making more of an effort. ... The ready-prepared meals have gone and everything I'm learning to make tastes delicious. Before, when I made an effort no one said, "Ooh, that was good." It was just, "Thanks for cooking. ..." Now, they're like, "Wow!!" Even I can't quite believe it's so tasty.

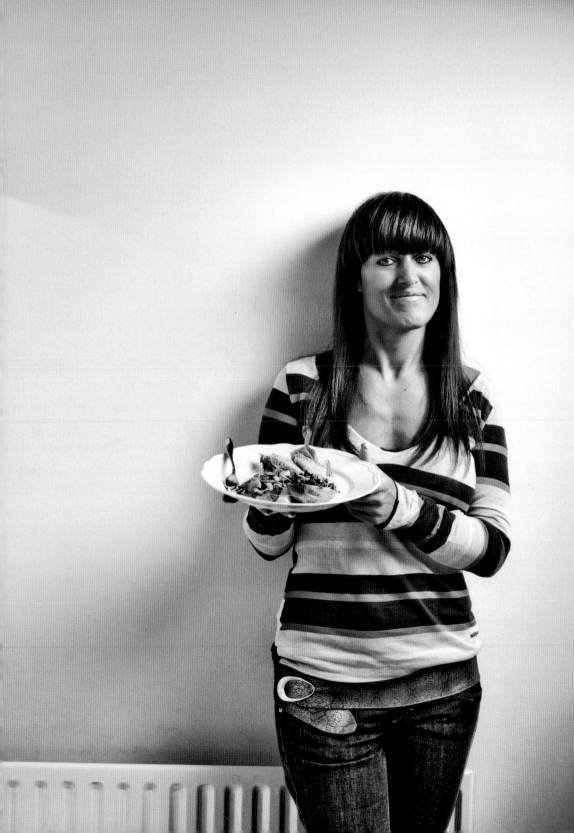

CHICKEN AND LEEK STROGANOFF (19 minutes)

This is a really tasty cross between a French fricassee and a Russian stroganoff. If you put some rice on another burner, you can quickly make the dish in another pan and by the time the rice is done everything will be ready. I like to put my mushrooms in toward the end of making the sauce, so they're nutty and firm, but if you want to add them earlier with the leeks to soften them up, that's fine.

serves 2

sea salt
¾ cup long-grain or basmati rice
1 large leek
a big handful of crimini or oyster mushrooms
2 chicken breast fillets, preferably free-range or organic
olive oil

a pat of butter
a glass of white wine
freshly ground black pepper
a bunch of fresh parsley
1¼ cups heavy cream
1 lemon

Pour boiling water from the kettle into a large pan, place on a high heat and add a pinch of salt • Add your rice, bring back to a boil, then turn the heat down slightly • Cook for the length of time given in the instructions on the package • Cut both ends off the leek, quarter lengthways, slice across thinly, then wash well under running water • Slice the mushrooms • Slice the chicken breasts into little-finger-size pieces

Put a large frying pan on a high heat and add a good lug of olive oil and a pat of butter • Add the leek to the pan with the white wine, a small glass of water, and a good pinch of salt and pepper • Let it bubble away for 5 minutes, covered loosely with a piece of aluminum foil • Meanwhile, finely chop the parsley, stalks and all • Remove the foil and add the chicken strips, most of the parsley, the cream, and the mushrooms • Stir, bring back to a boil, then turn the heat down to medium and simmer for 10 minutes • Drain your rice • Just before serving, cut your lemon in half and squeeze the juice of one half into the stroganoff • Season to taste

Spoon some rice onto each plate and top with the stroganoff • Scatter with the rest of the chopped parsley • Serve with the other lemon half, cut into wedges

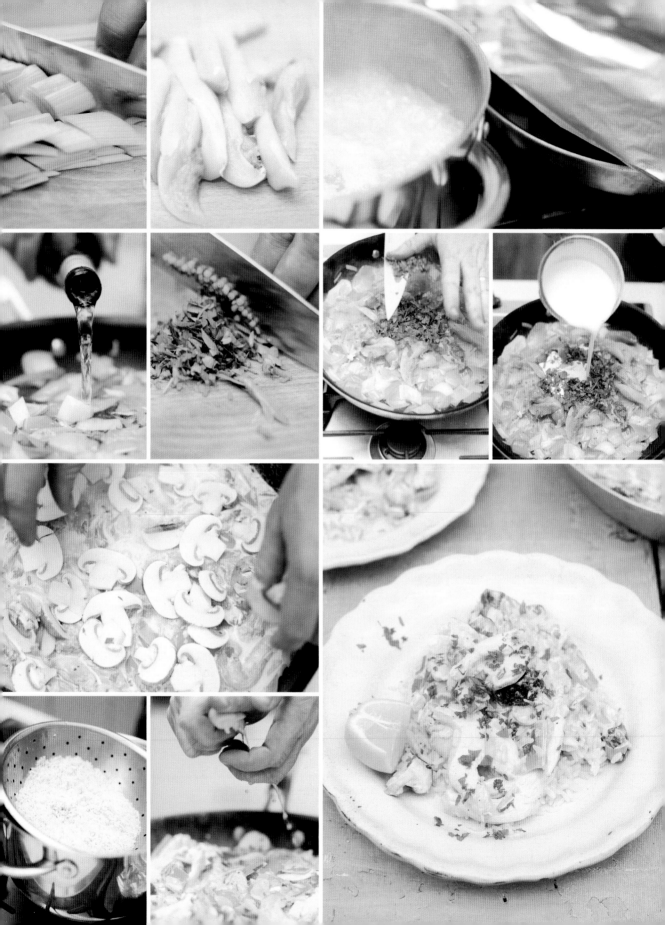

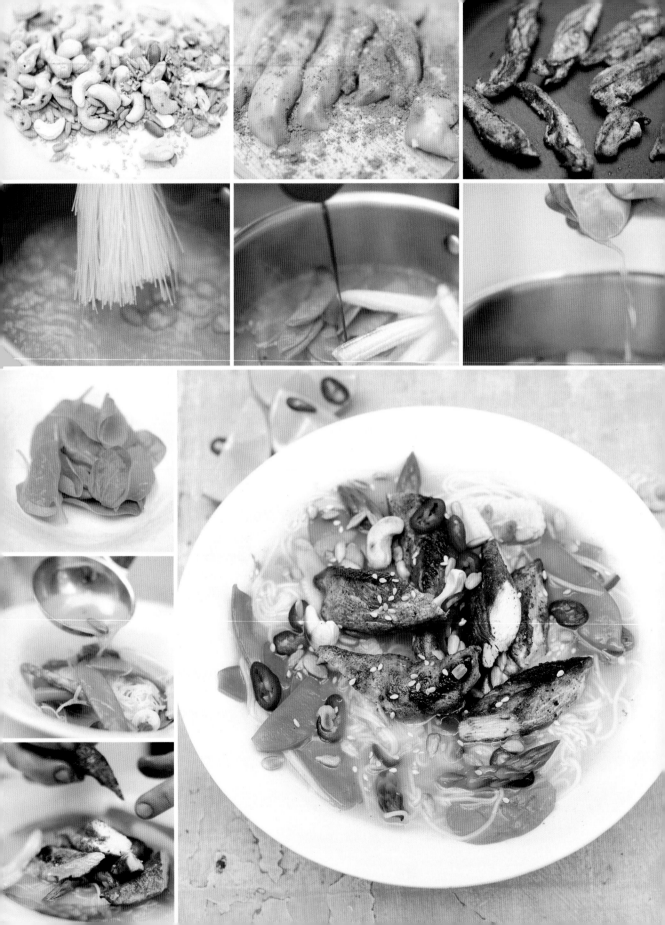

ASIAN CHICKEN NOODLE BROTH
(17 minutes)

This is a really quick dish but you're going to have to multitask, cooking your veg and noodles in one pan and your chicken in another. Read through the recipe before you start so you'll be prepared for what's going to happen. You'll be amazed at the results – just like something you can get in a posh noodle bar.

serves 2

1 tablespoon mixed seeds (pumpkin, sesame, poppy, sunflower)

a small handful of raw cashew nuts

1 quart chicken broth, preferably organic

2 skinless chicken breast fillets, preferably free-range or organic

2 teaspoons five-spice powder

sea salt and freshly ground black pepper

olive oil

a thumb-sized piece of fresh root ginger

½–1 fresh red or green chile, to your taste

4 ounces rice sticks or vermicelli

a handful of snow peas

6 thin asparagus spears or 4 regular-sized spears

6 fresh baby corn or ½ cup fresh corn kernels

soy sauce

juice of 1 lime

a small handful of spinach leaves

Put a medium frying pan or wok on a high heat and add the seeds and cashew nuts to it straight away, while it's heating up • Put a large saucepan on a high heat • Fill the saucepan with the chicken broth, heat until very hot, and put a lid on it • Toss the seeds and nuts around until heated through nicely – this will take a couple of minutes • While this is happening, slice your chicken breasts lengthways into 3 pieces and put them into a bowl • Sprinkle the chicken with the five-spice powder and a good pinch of salt and pepper and stir • When the seeds and nuts are done, transfer them to a plate • Put the empty pan back on a high heat • Add a little olive oil to your hot pan with your slices of chicken and cook for 5 minutes, until golden, tossing and turning every now and again

While the chicken's cooking, peel and finely slice your ginger and slice your chile • Take the lid off the pan with the chicken broth and add half the chile, all the ginger, your rice sticks (or vermicelli), snow peas, asparagus, and corn, with 2 tablespoons of soy sauce • Bring to a boil and cook for 2 to 3 minutes, stirring • Halve the lime and squeeze in the juice • By the time the rice sticks (or vermicelli) and veggies are done, the chicken will be cooked • Take a piece of chicken out and slice it lengthways to check if it's cooked all the way through – when done, remove all the chicken from the pan and slice each piece in half to expose the juicy chicken inside (please don't be tempted to overcook it) • To serve, divide the spinach leaves between your bowls and pour over the broth, rice sticks (or vermicelli), and vegetables • Divide the chicken pieces over and scatter with the toasted seeds, cashews, and remaining chile

CHICKEN FAJITAS (19 minutes)

A grill pan gives the nice, charred effect you want with fajitas, but you can also use a large frying pan or wok. If you use a grill pan, keep the ingredients moving around so that nothing burns or sticks to the bottom. Normally I wouldn't recommend adding extra oil to a hot pan, but in this case it's good to give everything a drizzle now and then so the chicken and bell peppers stay nice and shiny.

serves 2

1 red bell pepper

1 medium red onion

2 skinless, boneless chicken breast fillets, preferably
  free-range or organic

1 teaspoon smoked paprika

a small pinch of ground cumin

2 limes

olive oil

sea salt and freshly ground black pepper

4 flour tortillas

½ cup sour cream or natural yogurt

1 cup guacamole

4 ounces Cheddar cheese

For the salsa

½–1 fresh red or green chile, to your taste

15 ripe grape or cherry tomatoes

a small bunch of fresh cilantro

sea salt and freshly ground black pepper

1 lime

extra virgin olive oil

Put your grill pan on a high heat • Halve and seed your bell pepper and cut it into thin strips • Peel, halve, and finely slice your onion • Slice your chicken lengthways into long strips roughly the same size as your bell pepper strips • Put the bell peppers, onion, and chicken into a bowl with the paprika and cumin • Squeeze over the juice of half a lime, drizzle over a lug of olive oil, season with a good pinch of salt and pepper and mix well • Put to one side to marinate for 5 minutes or so while you make your salsa • Finely chop your chile • Roughly chop your tomatoes and the cilantro, stalks and all • Put the chile and tomatoes into a second bowl with a good pinch of salt and pepper and the juice of 1 lime • Add a good lug of extra virgin olive oil, then stir in your chopped cilantro

Use a pair of tongs to put all the pieces of bell pepper, onion, and chicken into your preheated pan to cook for 6 to 8 minutes, until the chicken is golden and cooked through • As the pan will be really hot, keep turning the pieces of chicken and vegetables over so they don't burn – you just want them to lightly chargrill to give you a lovely flavor • Give the pan a little love and attention and you'll be laughing • Warm your tortillas up in a microwave or a warm dry frying pan

Divide your warmed tortillas between your serving plates • At the table, carefully help yourselves to the chicken and vegetables straight from the hot grill pan • Just be sure to put it down on top of something that won't burn, like a chopping board • Halve your remaining lime and squeeze the juices over the sizzling pan • Serve with bowls of sour cream and guacamole alongside your Cheddar, a grater, and your lovely fresh salsa

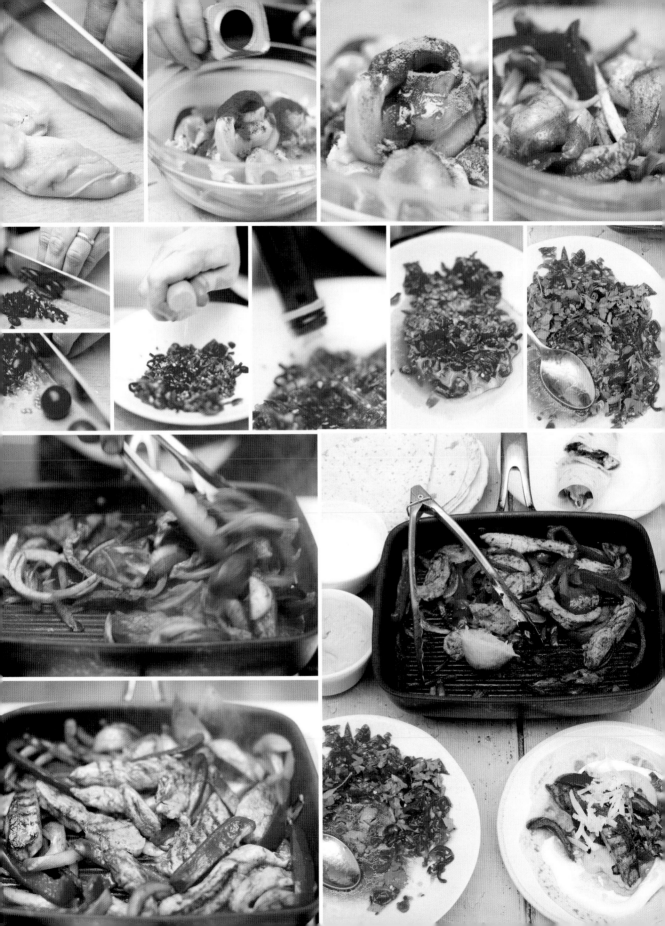

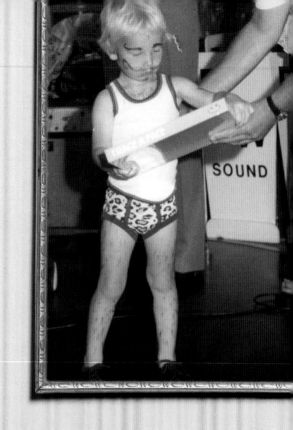

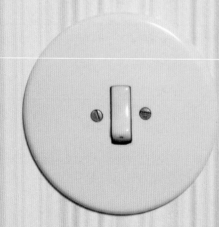

Quick pasta

I've covered a lot of pasta recipes in my other books, which kind of led me to think that if I included a chapter about pasta here it might be a bit repetitive and over the top. But then I thought, "Well, everyone loves pasta: it's quick, it's convenient, you can make great things out of non-perishable stuff in your larder or fresh, seasonal ingredients and olive oil. Variety is the spice of life, so the more recipes the merrier, I say." So what I've done with this chapter is make it completely relevant to a beginner cook by including a bundle of pasta recipes where the sauce can literally be made in the time it takes for the pasta to cook, which averages around 10 minutes. So even allowing for dressing a bagged salad and opening a bottle of wine, it's a pretty quick dinner when you've rushed back home from work.

The first thing to get right with pasta is seasoning the cooking water. If you're using table salt, you'll need 1 level teaspoon per quart. If you're using sea salt, you'll want a bit more. This may seem like a lot of salt but the pasta will only take in a little as it cooks and the rest will be drained away. Because pasta is essentially flour, eggs, and water it's important to remember this step, as it adds to the overall flavor at the end. If you don't season the water, the pasta will taste like air.

As far as I'm concerned, pasta definitely has a place in this book and in any modern-day cook's repertoire. I use dried pasta in most of the recipes in this chapter because it allows you to concentrate on the cooking of the sauce. Once you're confident with cooking this stuff, you should definitely have a look at my previous books for loads more fresh pasta recipes.

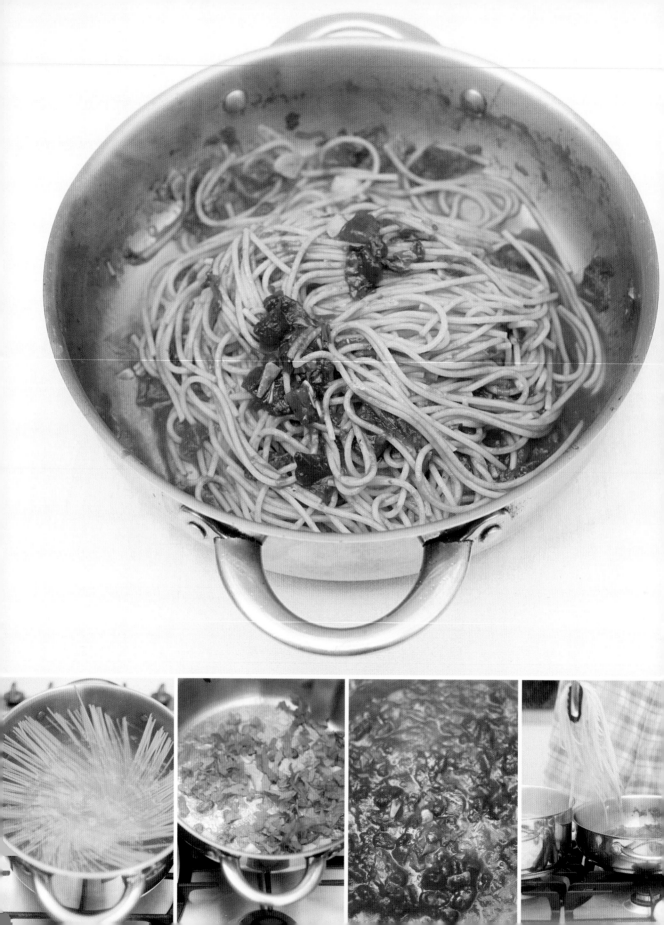

CLASSIC TOMATO SPAGHETTI

This pasta sauce takes minutes to cook. What's great about this recipe for beginner cooks is that once you've done it a few times you can add other simple ingredients to your basic tomato sauce to completely transform it. Check out the end of the recipe, where I've given you some ideas to get you started.

serves 4–6

2 cloves of garlic
1 fresh red or green chile
a small bunch of fresh basil
sea salt and freshly ground black pepper

1 pound dried spaghetti
olive oil
1 x 14-ounce can of diced tomatoes
4 ounces Parmesan cheese

To prepare your pasta

Peel and finely slice the garlic • Finely slice your chile (halve and seed it first if you don't want the sauce too hot) • Pick the basil leaves off the stalks and put to one side • Finely chop the stalks

To cook your pasta

Bring a large pan of salted water to a boil, add the spaghetti, and cook according to the package instructions • Meanwhile, put a large saucepan on a medium heat and add 2 good lugs of olive oil • Add the garlic, chile, and basil stalks and give them a stir • When the garlic begins to brown slightly, add most of the basil leaves and the canned tomatoes • Turn the heat up high and stir for a minute • Season with salt and pepper • Drain the spaghetti in a colander, then transfer it to the pan of sauce and stir well • Taste and add more salt and pepper if you think it needs it

To serve your pasta

Divide the pasta between your bowls, or put it on the table in a large serving dish and let everyone help themselves • Roughly tear over the remaining basil leaves and grate over some Parmesan

These can be added to your tomato sauce when it's finished. Just stir in and warm through:

- Add a handful of baby spinach leaves to the sauce at the same time that you add the pasta – when the leaves have wilted remove from the heat and serve with some crumbled goat's cheese on top
- A few handfuls of cooked shrimp and a handful of chopped arugula, with the juice of ½ a lemon
- A can of tuna, drained and flaked into the sauce with ½ a teaspoon of ground cinnamon, some black olives and the juice of ½ a lemon
- A handful of fresh or frozen peas and fava beans

BAKED CAMEMBERT PASTA

This recipe is so simple. All you need are a few basic ingredients and one of those little boxes of Camembert you can find in any supermarket. It cooks a treat, looks and smells wonderful, and your mates at your dinner party will just think you're the cleverest thing ever. Admittedly, pasta and runny cheese isn't the healthiest thing in the world, but it's so worth it once in a while.

serves 4–6

1 x 8-ounce box of Camembert cheese
2 cloves of garlic
1 sprig of fresh rosemary
extra virgin olive oil

sea salt and freshly ground black pepper
1 pound dried rigatoni
6 cups (approx. 6 ounces) fresh spinach leaves
4 ounces Parmesan cheese

To prepare your pasta
Preheat your oven to 350°F • Open the box of cheese and unwrap it • Place it back in the wooden container • Score a circle into the top of the skin, then lift it off and discard • Peel and finely slice the garlic • Pick the rosemary leaves off the woody stalk • Lay the garlic slices on top of the cheese, sprinkle with some pepper and drizzle with a little extra virgin olive oil • Scatter over the rosemary leaves and gently pat with your fingers to coat them in the oil • Grate the Parmesan

To cook your pasta
Place the box of cheese on a cookie sheet and put it into the preheated oven for 25 minutes, until golden and melted • Meanwhile, bring a large pan of salted water to a boil • When your cheese has 10 minutes left to cook, add the rigatoni to the pan and cook according to the package instructions • When the pasta is cooked, add the spinach to the pan – it only needs cooking for 10 seconds or so • Drain the pasta and spinach in a colander over a large bowl, reserving some of the cooking water • Return the pasta and spinach to the pan and let it wilt • Drizzle with a couple of good lugs of extra virgin olive oil and add the grated Parmesan • If the sauce is too thick for you, add a splash of the reserved cooking water to thin it out a bit • Season with salt and pepper and give it a good stir • Remove the cheese from the oven

To serve your pasta
Divide the pasta between your serving bowls • Either drizzle the melted Camembert on top or pop the box of cheese on the table and let everyone help themselves to a lovely, gooey spoonful

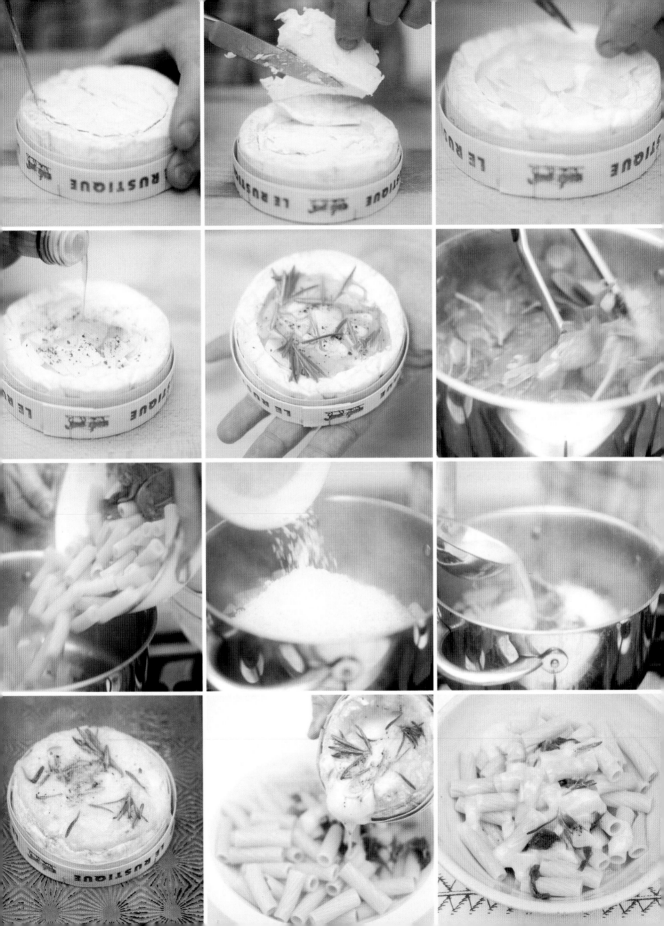

BROCCOLI AND PESTO TAGLIATELLE

This is a quick version of a classic Italian dish called tagliatelle alla Genovese. Before you decide I'm barmy for putting potato shavings into a pasta dish, I should explain that it's actually very authentic to add sliced or mashed potato to pasta. It lends a wonderful creaminess that works so well and tastes amazing – you must try it.

serves 4–6

1 medium potato
1 head of broccoli
a large bunch of fresh basil
sea salt

1 pound dried tagliatelle
¼ cup green pesto
3 ounces Parmesan cheese

To prepare your pasta
Wash and peel the potato and cut it into very thin shavings using a speed peeler • Slice the end off the broccoli stalk • Cut little broccoli florets off the head and put them to one side • Halve the thick stalk lengthways, then slice thinly • Pick the basil leaves and discard the stalks • Grate the Parmesan

To cook your pasta
Bring a large pan of salted water to a boil • Add the tagliatelle and broccoli stalks and cook according to the tagliatelle package instructions • 2 minutes before the tagliatelle is cooked, add the broccoli florets and potato slices • Drain everything in a colander over a large bowl, reserving some of the cooking water, and return to the pan • Roughly chop half your basil leaves and add to the pan with the pesto and half the Parmesan • Give it all a good stir and if the sauce is too thick for you, add a splash of the cooking water to thin it out a bit

To serve your pasta
Divide the pasta between your serving bowls • Sprinkle over the rest of the Parmesan and the remaining basil leaves • Serve with a lovely big bowl of salad

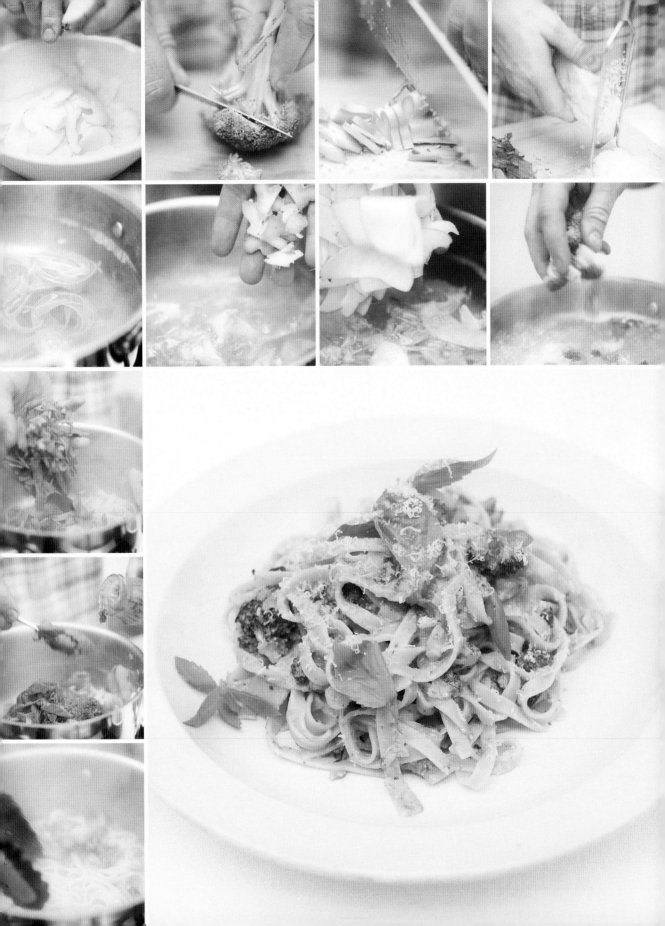

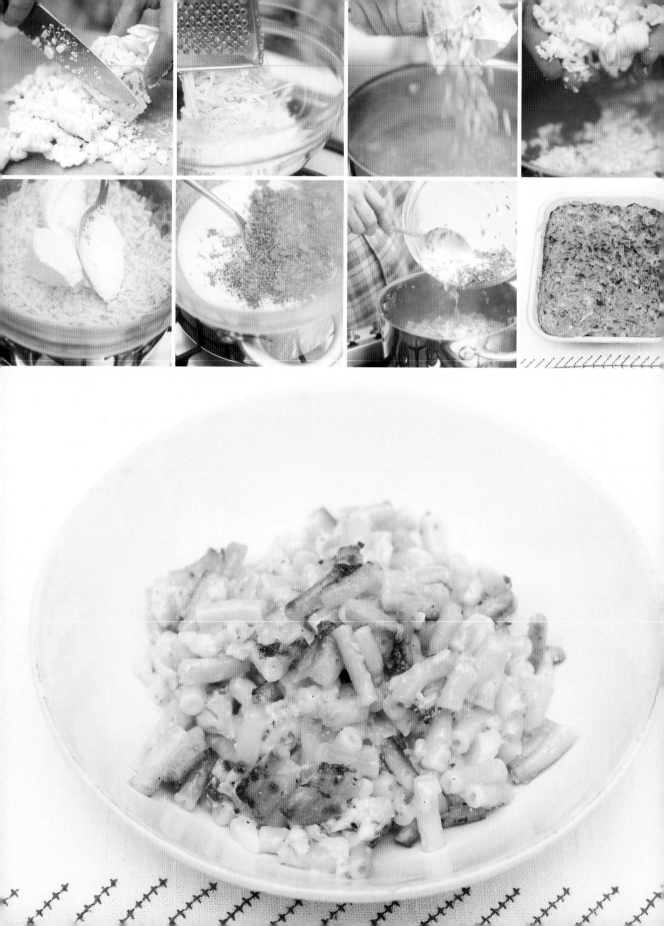

MACARONI AND CAULIFLOWER CHEESE BAKE

You can either serve this macaroni unbaked so it's loose, gooey, and silky, or bake it under the broiler for a few minutes before serving to give it a crispy, golden topping. You could even try adding a grated hard-boiled egg or cooked prawns, but I like the simple style, as here.

serves 4–6

½ a head of cauliflower

8 ounces Cheddar cheese

4 ounces Parmesan cheese

a small bunch of fresh Italian parsley

sea salt

1 pound dried macaroni (elbows)

1 cup crème fraîche or sour cream

To prepare your pasta

Remove the outer green leaves from the cauliflower and discard • Slice the end off the cauliflower stalk • Cut the head into small florets • Halve the thick stalk lengthways, then slice thinly • Grate the Cheddar and Parmesan into a large heatproof bowl • Finely chop the parsley stalks and leaves

To cook your pasta

Bring a large pan of salted water to a boil • Add the macaroni and all your cauliflower and cook according to the macaroni package instructions • Place the bowl of cheese over the saucepan and add the crème fraîche • Carefully stir every so often until the cheese is smooth and melted • If the water boils up beneath the bowl, just turn the heat down slightly • Add all the chopped parsley to the melted cheese and season with a pinch of salt and pepper • Carefully remove the bowl of cheese using a towel or oven gloves and put aside • Drain the macaroni in a colander over a bowl, reserving the cooking water • Return the pasta to the pan, pour in the melted cheese and stir • It should have a lovely, silky consistency, but if it's too thick for you, add a splash of your cooking water to thin it out a bit • At this point you can either serve the macaroni as is, or finish it under the broiler to make it crispy and golden on top • To do this, preheat your broiler to a medium to high heat • Add ⅔ cup of the reserved cooking water to the macaroni, stir in, then transfer to a baking dish • Place under the broiler until golden and bubbling

To serve your pasta

Divide the pasta between plates or bowls, or place the baking dish in the middle of the table next to a nice green salad and let everyone help themselves

PASTA AL PANGRATTATO

This is a fantastic way of using up stale bread. Pangrattato is a mix of crispy breadcrumbs, garlic, and herbs and it gives your pasta a lovely crunch. For Brits, it's a very different way to serve pasta, as it's about creating crunch and flavor rather than a cream or tomato sauce. In Italy, pasta is often served this way – simply tossed with a mixture of oil, herbs, and spices. This is great as a lunchtime snack and, if you prefer, you can use a small can of tuna, chopped up, instead of the anchovies.

serves 4–6

2 cloves of garlic
1–2 dried chiles, to your taste
4 sprigs of fresh thyme
4 slices of stale bread

sea salt
1 pound dried fusilli
8 anchovies in oil
1 lemon

To prepare your pasta

Peel and finely slice the garlic • Finely chop your chiles • Pick the thyme leaves off the stalks • Slice the crusts off the bread and discard • If they're dry enough, finely grate your slices of bread – if not, break them up into small breadcrumbs with your fingers or give them a quick whiz in a food processor

To cook your pasta

Bring a large pan of salted water to a boil • Add the fusilli and cook according to the package instructions • Halfway through the cooking time, put a large frying pan on a medium heat and let it get hot • Pour about 2 tablespoons of the oil from the tin of anchovies into the pan, let it get hot, then stir in your breadcrumbs • Add the garlic, chile, thyme leaves and anchovies (but not the remaining oil in the tin) and cook for 4 to 5 minutes, stirring every so often, until the breadcrumbs are golden brown • Drain the fusilli in a colander over a bowl, reserving some of the cooking water in case you want to add a splash to loosen up the pasta • Add to the frying pan and stir well • Squeeze the juice of half the lemon over the pasta • Give the pan a shake • Have a taste, and if you think it needs a little more lemon, squeeze the other half over too

To serve your pasta

Divide the pasta between your serving bowls, or put it on the table in a large serving dish with a nice crisp salad and let everyone help themselves

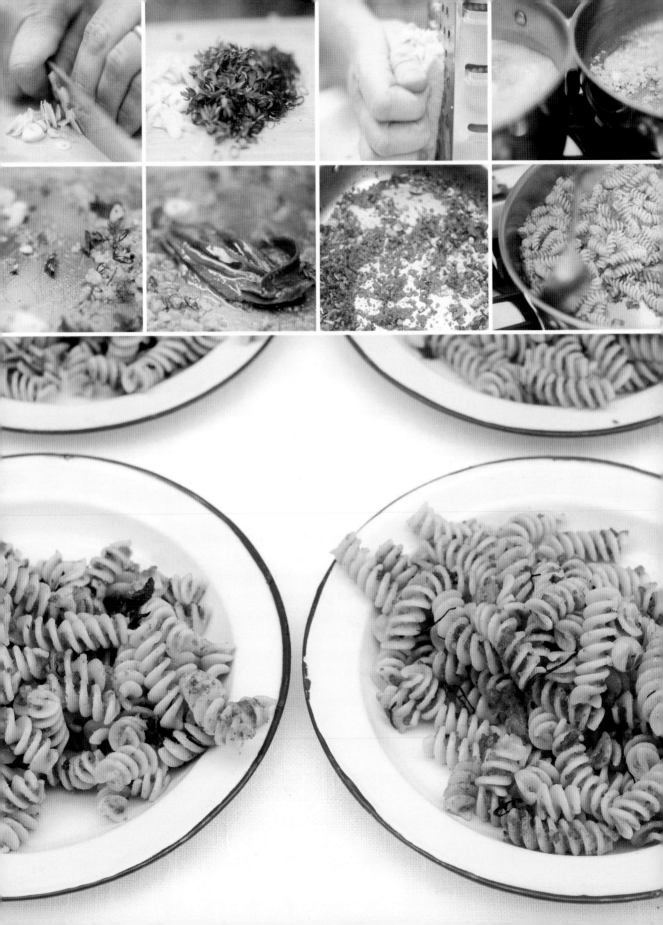

MINI SHELL PASTA WITH A CREAMY SMOKED BACON AND PEA SAUCE

This is one of the dishes I cook for my kids, but to be honest, it's so good that me and Jools always eat it too! Mini pasta shells are actually meant to be added to soups, but they're quick and easy to cook, which makes them a good thing to serve with pasta sauces. All in all this should take you no more than five and a half minutes to cook. However, if you decide to go for a bigger type of pasta, remember that it will need more time to cook than these mini shells.

serves 4–6

10 slices smoked bacon or pancetta, preferably free-range or organic

a small bunch of fresh mint

sea salt and freshly ground black pepper

1 pound dried mini shell or other type of pasta

olive oil

a pat of butter

2 cups frozen peas

2 tablespoons crème fraîche or heavy cream

1 lemon

6 ounces Parmesan cheese

To prepare your pasta

Finely slice the bacon • Pick the mint leaves and discard the stalks • Finely grate the Parmesan

To cook your pasta

Bring a large pan of salted water to a boil • Add the mini shells and cook according to the package instructions • Get a large frying pan over a medium heat and add a good lug of olive oil and the butter • Add the bacon to the pan, sprinkle a little pepper over and fry until golden and crisp • Meanwhile, finely chop your mint leaves • As soon as the bacon is golden, add your frozen peas and give the pan a good shake • After a minute or so, add the crème fraîche (or heavy cream) and chopped mint to the bacon and peas • Drain the pasta in a colander over a large bowl, reserving some of the cooking water • Add the pasta to the frying pan • Halve your lemon and squeeze the juice over the pasta • When it's all bubbling away nicely, remove from the heat • It's really important that the sauce is creamy, silky, and delicious but if it's too thick for you, add a splash of the reserved cooking water to thin it out a bit • Add the grated Parmesan and give the pan a shake to mix it in

To serve your pasta

Divide your pasta between plates or bowls, or put it on the table in a large serving dish and let everyone help themselves • Lovely with a simply dressed green salad

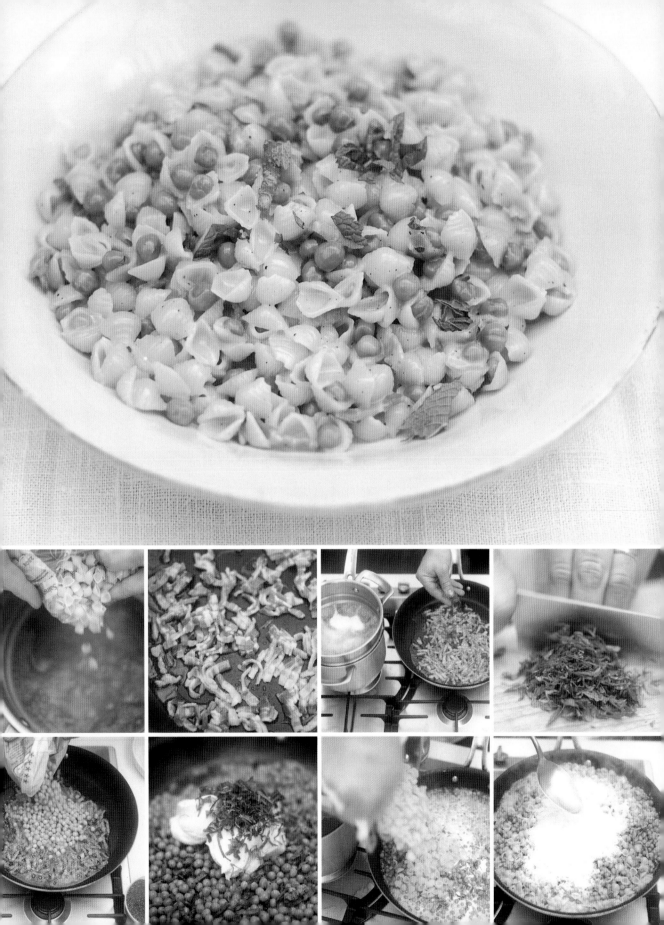

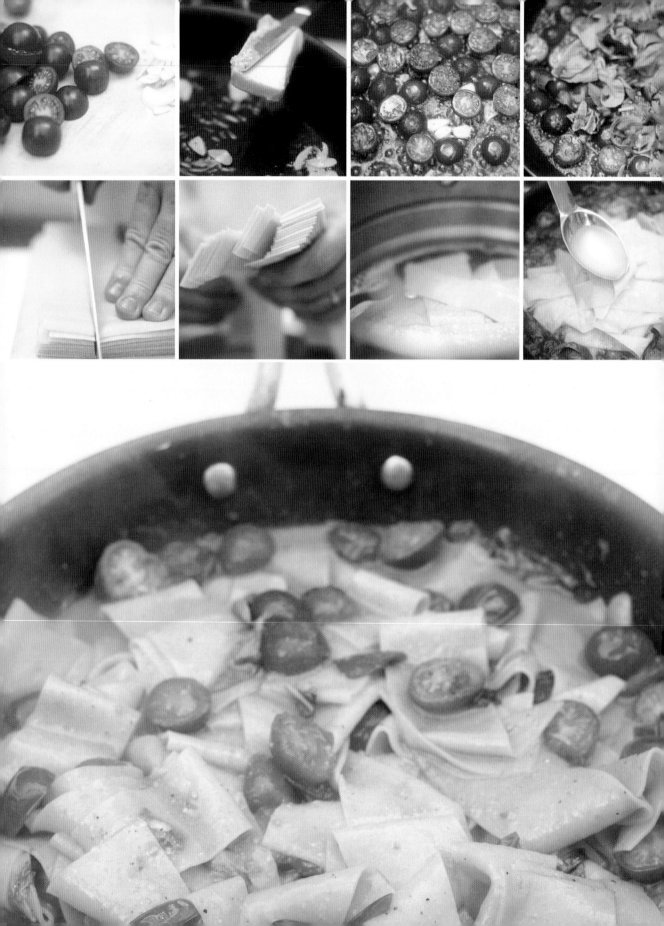

CHERRY TOMATO SAUCE WITH CHEAT'S FRESH PASTA

We've been able to buy fresh lasagne sheets in grocery stores for years and now there are also free-range and organic pastas available. The great thing about these sheets is that you can use them for more than just making lasagne: you can cut them up and use them in different ways, as I've done here. If you can't get fresh lasagne, improvise – I've made this in the past by breaking up dry sheets (but you'll need to cook them for longer). This dish is such an easy thing to make if you want to feed four people very quickly.

This is a north Italian pasta sauce, and they're more inclined than their southern neighbours to use butter in their pastas – it gives a silky texture and an extra layer of flavor.

serves 4–6

1½ pints ripe grape or cherry tomatoes	*olive oil*
4 cloves of garlic	*2 pats of butter*
a small bunch of fresh basil	*¼ cup balsamic vinegar*
1 pound fresh lasagne, defrosted if frozen	*4 ounces Parmesan cheese*
sea salt and freshly ground black pepper	

To prepare your pasta
Cut the tomatoes into halves or quarters • Peel and slice the garlic • Pick the basil leaves off the stalks and put them to one side • Finely chop the stalks • Cut the lasagne sheets into 3 or 4 long strips and put to one side • Grate the Parmesan

To cook your pasta
Bring a large pan of salted water to a boil • Put a large frying pan over a medium heat and add a couple of lugs of olive oil and the garlic • Add the butter and let it melt • When the garlic starts to brown, add the tomatoes • Give everything a good stir, then add the basil stalks and half the leaves • Add the vinegar and season with salt and pepper • Drop your fresh pasta strips into the pan of boiling water and cook for 3 minutes • Drain in a colander over a large bowl, reserving some of the cooking water • Add the pasta to the frying pan with a splash of the cooking water and half the Parmesan • Give it a good stir • Taste and add a little more salt and pepper if you think it needs it

To serve your pasta
Divide the pasta between your plates or bowls, or put the pan in the middle of the table and let everyone help themselves • Sprinkle over the rest of the Parmesan and the basil leaves, tearing any larger ones up • Lovely with a simple side salad

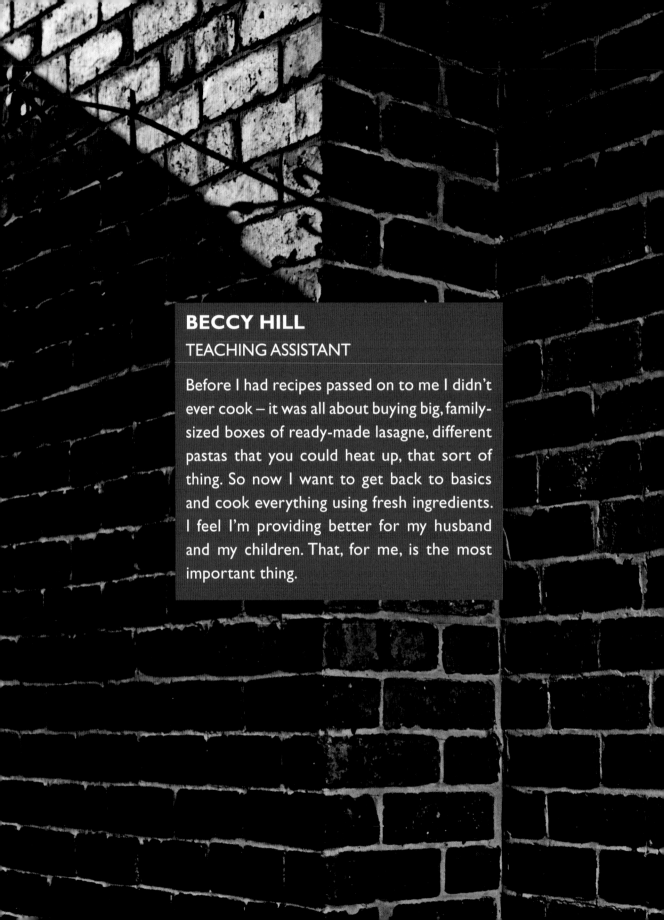

BECCY HILL
TEACHING ASSISTANT

Before I had recipes passed on to me I didn't ever cook — it was all about buying big, family-sized boxes of ready-made lasagne, different pastas that you could heat up, that sort of thing. So now I want to get back to basics and cook everything using fresh ingredients. I feel I'm providing better for my husband and my children. That, for me, is the most important thing.

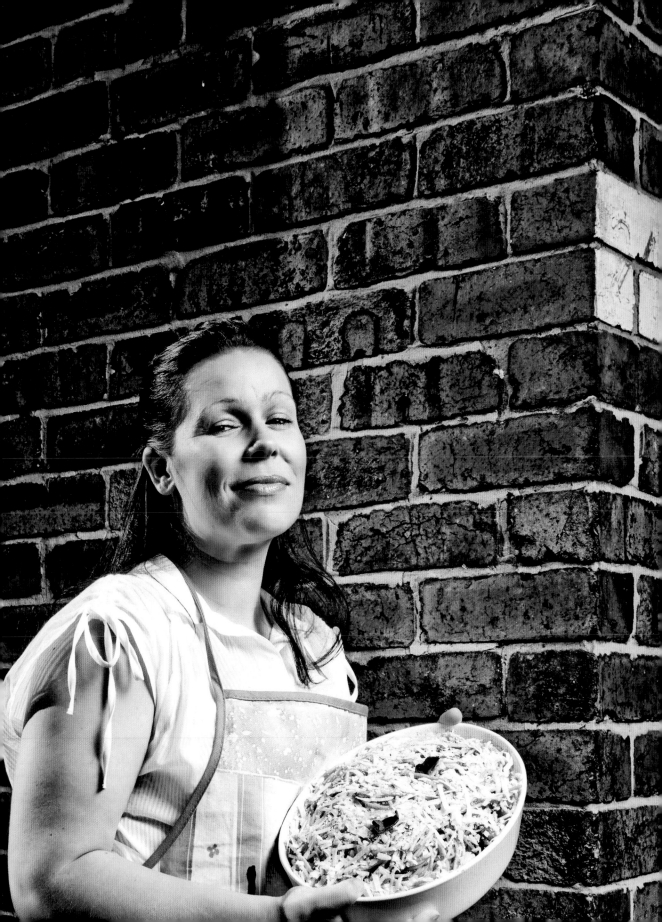

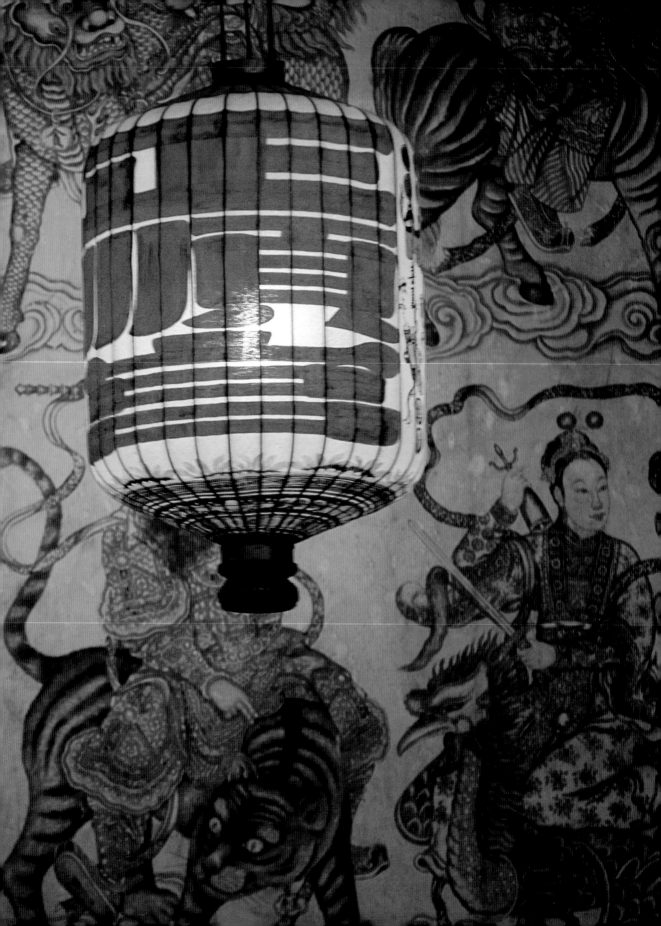

Tasty stir-fries

Everyone loves stir-fries. Even the school kids I came across in *Jamie's Dinners* loved them. I've picked a handful of the most commonly enjoyed stir-fries, the ones we tend to buy as take-out, and have given you my versions. The idea of this chapter is to get you rattling out consistently delicious stir-fries for lunch and dinner. Now this is all pretty simple, but there are a few things to bear in mind to make sure you get it right:

1. Obviously the wok is a very important cooking implement for making a stir-fry. If you haven't got one, a very large frying pan can give good results.

2. If you've got a gas stovetop, you'll be well away. If you've got an electric or induction stovetop, make sure your wok has an extra-thick bottom to retain the scorching heat.

3. I've written all the recipes to serve 2 in this chapter, because if you try to cook a larger batch, the wok will get overloaded with ingredients. If you do want to cook for 4 people, just double the ingredients and make two batches.

4. You must get your wok or pan really hot before you start cooking. And it's important that all your ingredients are ready and prepared in advance.

5. Instead of chicken or shrimp in these recipes, a delicious vegetarian alternative is diced tofu, which is made from beancurd.

Although stir-frying is a simple method of cooking, it does require you to be vigilant and hands-on — it might take only 3 or 4 minutes to cook a stir-fry, but if you don't keep tossing it and moving it around, parts will catch and burn. But don't let me scare you off, because it's exciting and alive and real cooking.

CHICKEN CHOW MEIN

This dish makes use of a tender, juicy Asian cabbage called bok choy, which is simple to cook and really tasty. You should be able to find bok choy (also know as pak choy, Chinese white cabbage, or hakusai) in your local grocery store, but, if not, a nice heart of romaine (halved) or a handful or two of baby spinach thrown into the wok for the last 2 or 3 minutes of cooking will do the trick.

serves 2

a thumb-sized piece of fresh root ginger
2 cloves of garlic
½–1 fresh red or green chile, to your taste
*1 large skinless chicken breast fillet, preferably
   free-range or organic*
sea salt and freshly ground black pepper
2 scallions
a small bunch of fresh cilantro

1 baby bok choy
optional: 4 shiitake mushrooms
4 ounces (2 bundles) chow mein noodles
peanut or vegetable oil
1 heaped teaspoon cornstarch
1 x 8-ounce can of water chestnuts
2–3 tablespoons soy sauce
1 small lime

To prepare your stir-fry
Put a large pan of water on to boil • Peel and finely slice the ginger and garlic • Finely slice the chile • Slice the chicken into finger-sized strips and lightly season with salt and pepper • Cut the ends off your scallions and finely slice • Pick the cilantro leaves and put to one side, and finely chop the cilantro stalks • Halve the bok choy lengthways • If using the mushrooms, either tear into pieces or leave whole

To cook your stir-fry
Preheat a wok or large frying pan on a high heat and once it's very, very hot add a good lug of peanut oil and swirl it around • Stir in the chicken strips and cook for a couple of minutes, until the chicken browns slightly • Add the ginger, garlic, chile, cilantro stalks, mushrooms (if using), and half the scallions • Stir-fry for 30 seconds, keeping everything moving around the wok quickly • Add your noodles and bok choy to the boiling water and cook for 2 to 3 minutes, no longer • Meanwhile, add the cornstarch, water chestnuts, and their water to the wok and give it another good shake to make sure nothing sticks to the bottom • Remove from the heat and stir in 2 tablespoons of soy sauce • Halve the lime, squeeze the juice of one half into the pan, and mix well • Drain the noodles and bok choy in a colander over a bowl, reserving a little of the cooking water • Stir in the noodles and bok choy, with a little of the cooking water to loosen if necessary, and mix well • Have a taste and season with more soy sauce if needed

To serve your stir-fry
Use tongs to divide everything between two bowls or plates, or to lift on to one large serving platter • Spoon any juices over the top and sprinkle with the rest of the scallions and the cilantro leaves • Serve with lime wedges

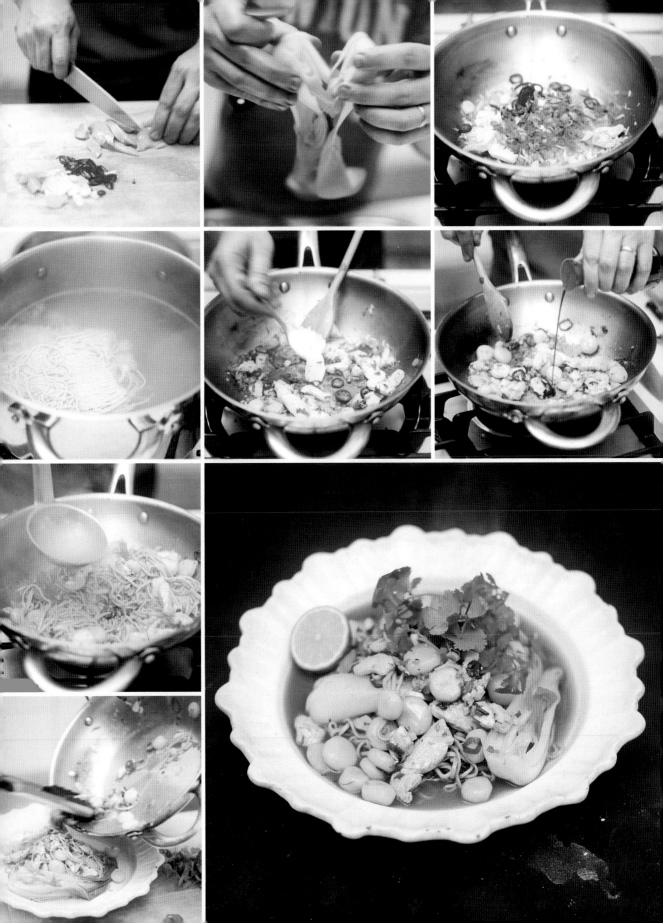

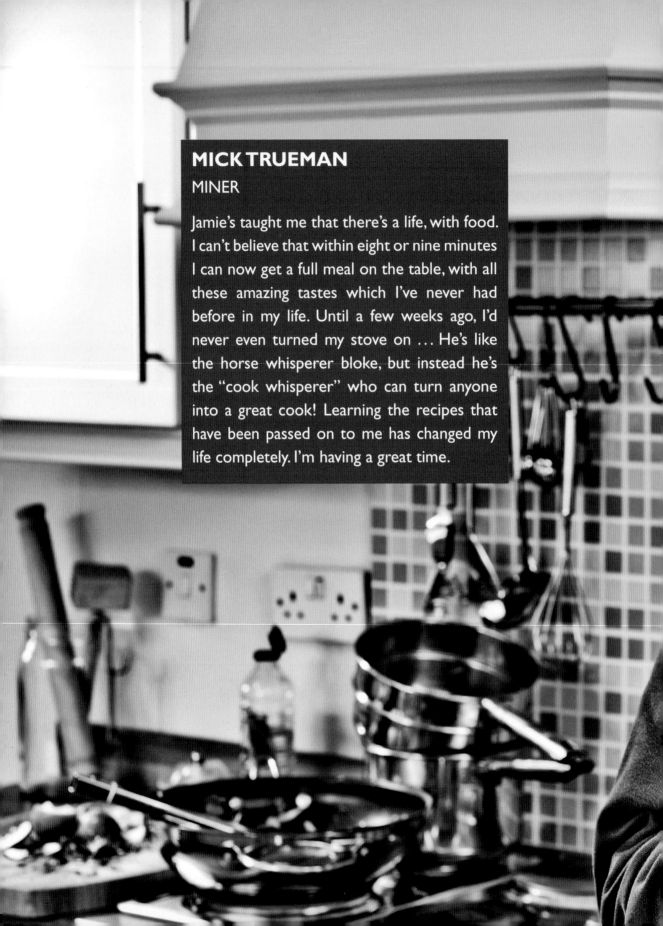

MICK TRUEMAN
MINER

Jamie's taught me that there's a life, with food. I can't believe that within eight or nine minutes I can now get a full meal on the table, with all these amazing tastes which I've never had before in my life. Until a few weeks ago, I'd never even turned my stove on ... He's like the horse whisperer bloke, but instead he's the "cook whisperer" who can turn anyone into a great cook! Learning the recipes that have been passed on to me has changed my life completely. I'm having a great time.

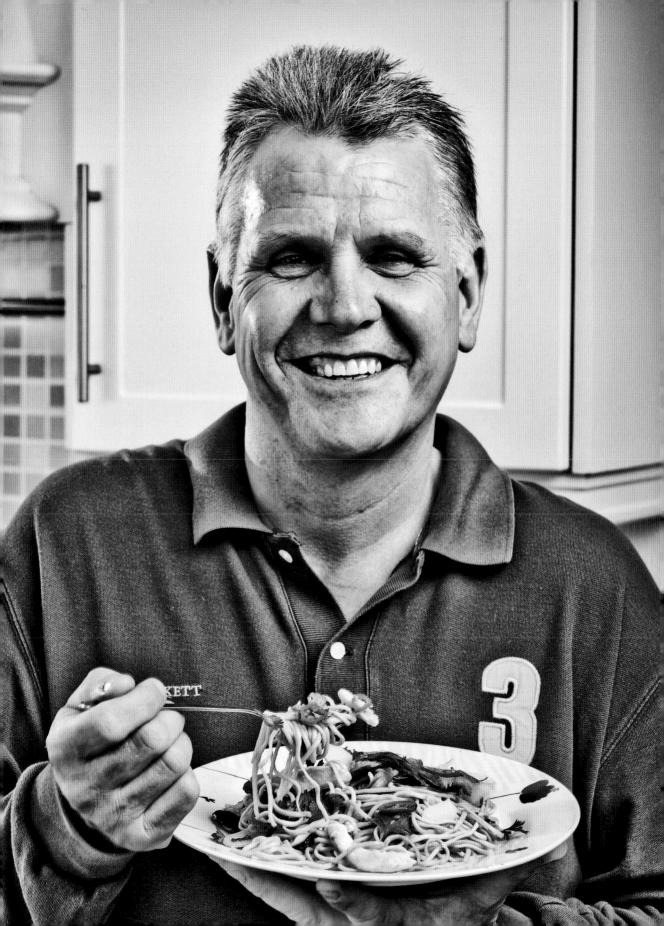

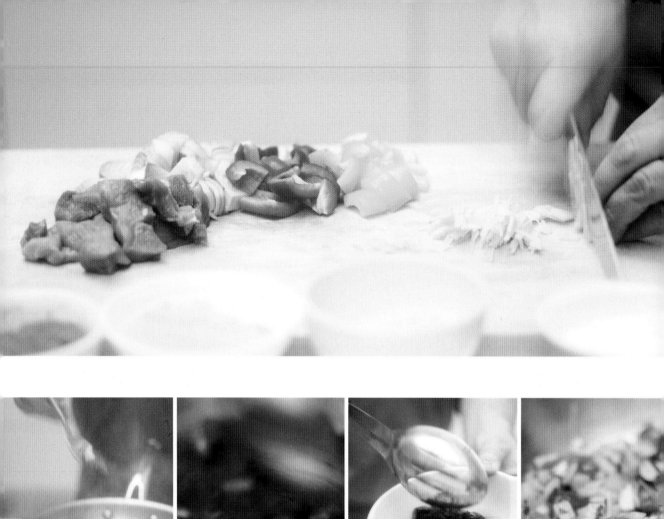
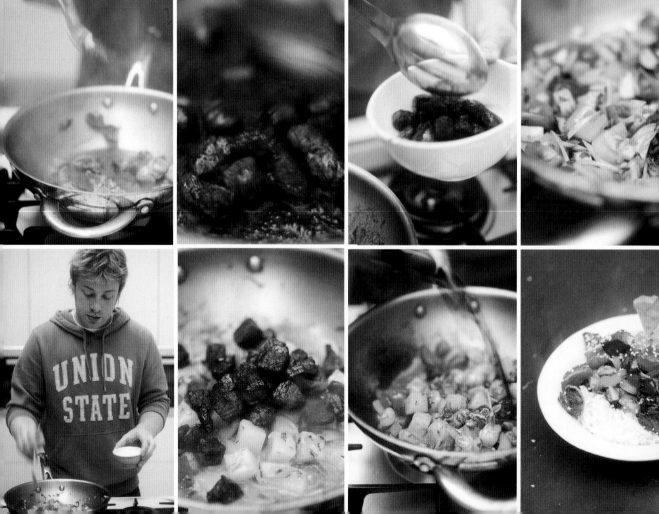

MY SWEET AND SOUR PORK

OK, this is easy but it's a quick one, so you'll have to concentrate and stay on the ball. Sweet and sour pork is an absolute classic and was one of the first Chinese-style dishes introduced to Britain. I've tried to make it fresh, light, and full of wonderful crunch, sweetness, and flavor. I've also brightened it up by introducing some lettuce leaves, which add texture and freshness. It's best to cook this for two – perfect, fast, one-pan cooking for nights in.

serves 2

sea salt and freshly ground black pepper

1 cup long-grain or basmati rice

½ pound pork tenderloin, preferably free-range or organic

1 small red onion

1 red or yellow bell pepper (or ½ of each)

a thumb-sized piece of fresh root ginger

2 cloves of garlic

½–1 fresh red or green chile, to your taste

a small bunch of fresh cilantro

peanut or vegetable oil

1 heaped teaspoon five-spice powder

1 teaspoon cornstarch

2–3 tablespoons soy sauce

1 x 8-ounce can of pineapple chunks

2 tablespoons balsamic vinegar

1 small heart of romaine or ½ a butterhead lettuce

2 teaspoons sesame seeds

To prepare your stir-fry

Bring a pan of salted water to a boil and add the rice • Cook according to the package instructions • Drain the rice in a strainer, put back into the pan, and cover with aluminum foil to keep warm until needed • Halve the pork tenderloin and cut into ¾-inch cubes • Peel and halve the red onion, then dice into ¾-inch cubes • Halve the bell pepper, seed, and cut into ¾-inch cubes • Peel and finely slice the ginger and garlic • Finely slice the chile • Pick the cilantro leaves and put them to one side • Finely chop the cilantro stalks

To cook your stir-fry

Preheat a wok or large frying pan on a high heat and once it's very, very hot add a good lug of peanut oil and swirl it around • Add the pork and the five-spice powder and toss or stir them around • Cook for a few minutes until browned, then transfer to a bowl using a slotted spoon • Carefully give the wok or pan a quick wipe with a ball of paper towels and return to the heat • When it's really hot, add 2 good lugs of peanut oil and all the chopped ingredients • Toss or stir everything together and cook for 2 minutes • Stir in the cornstarch and 2 tablespoons of soy sauce • Let everything cook for 30 to 40 seconds, then add the pineapple chunks with their juice, the browned pork and balsamic vinegar • Season with black pepper and a little more soy sauce, if needed • Break open a piece of pork, check it's cooked through, and remove from the heat • Reduce the sauce to a gravy-like consistency by cooking for a few minutes more

To serve your stir-fry

Divide the rice and lettuce between two bowls or plates • Spoon the pork, veggies, and sauce over the top and sprinkle with the sesame seeds and reserved cilantro leaves

HARDLY-ANY-PREP SHRIMP STIR-FRY

This is the kind of recipe where you can swing by the grocery store on your way home from work, pick up a few bits, and have a great meal on the table within ten minutes of arriving in your kitchen. Just get all your stuff ready for this one – when you start cooking, it all kicks off! Good luck.

serves 2

a thumb-sized piece of fresh ginger
2 cloves of garlic
1 fresh red or green chile
a small bunch of fresh cilantro
peanut or vegetable oil
½ pound large shrimp, raw, peeled
1 heaped teaspoon five-spice powder
1 teaspoon cornstarch
6 fresh baby corn or ½ cup fresh corn kernels

a small handful of snow peas
2 tablespoons soy sauce
juice of 1 lime
½ teaspoon honey
1 teaspoon sesame oil
a handful of frozen peas
7 ounces rice sticks or vermicelli
a small handful of beansprouts

To prepare your stir-fry
Put a large pan of water on to boil • Peel and finely slice the ginger and garlic • Finely slice the chile • Pick the cilantro leaves from the stalks and put to one side, then roughly chop the stalks

To cook your stir-fry
Preheat a wok or large frying pan on a high heat and once it's very, very hot add a good lug of peanut oil and swirl it around • Stir in the cilantro stalks, ginger, garlic, chile, shrimp, and five-spice powder, and fry for a minute • Add the cornstarch, baby corn, and snow peas and give them a good toss or stir for another minute • Stir in the soy sauce, lime juice, honey, sesame oil, and frozen peas • Add the rice sticks (or vermicelli) to the pan of boiling water and use a wooden spoon to break them up a bit • Cook for just 2 minutes, no longer • Drain the rice sticks (or vermicelli) in a colander over a bowl, reserving the cooking water • Add a large spoonful or ladleful of the cooking water to the wok and cook for a further minute or two

To serve your stir-fry
Use tongs to divide the rice sticks (or vermicelli) between your serving bowls, or to lift them on to one large serving platter • Spoon the shrimp, veggies, and any juices over the top and sprinkle with the beansprouts and cilantro leaves

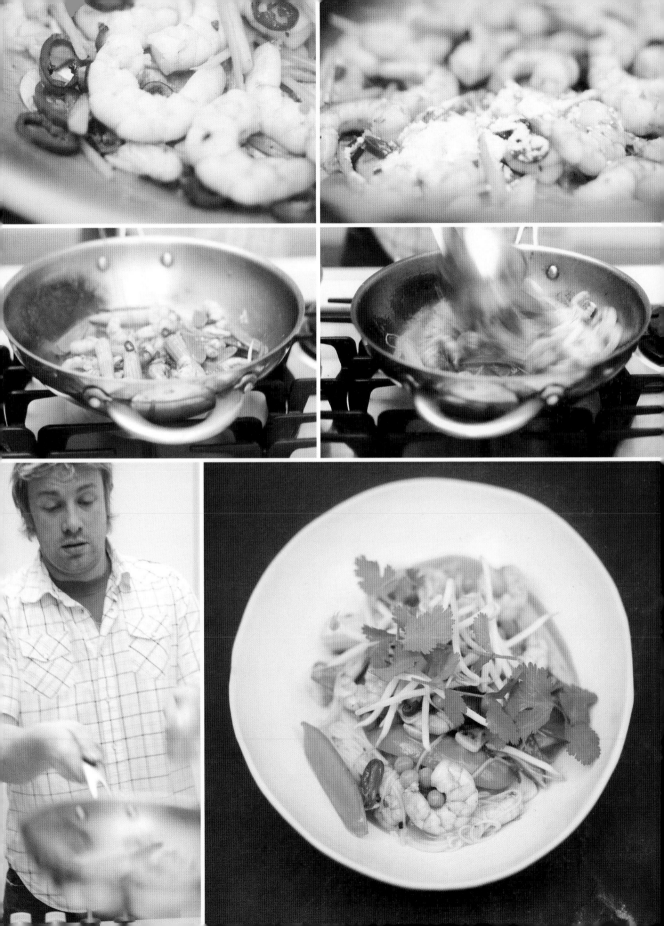

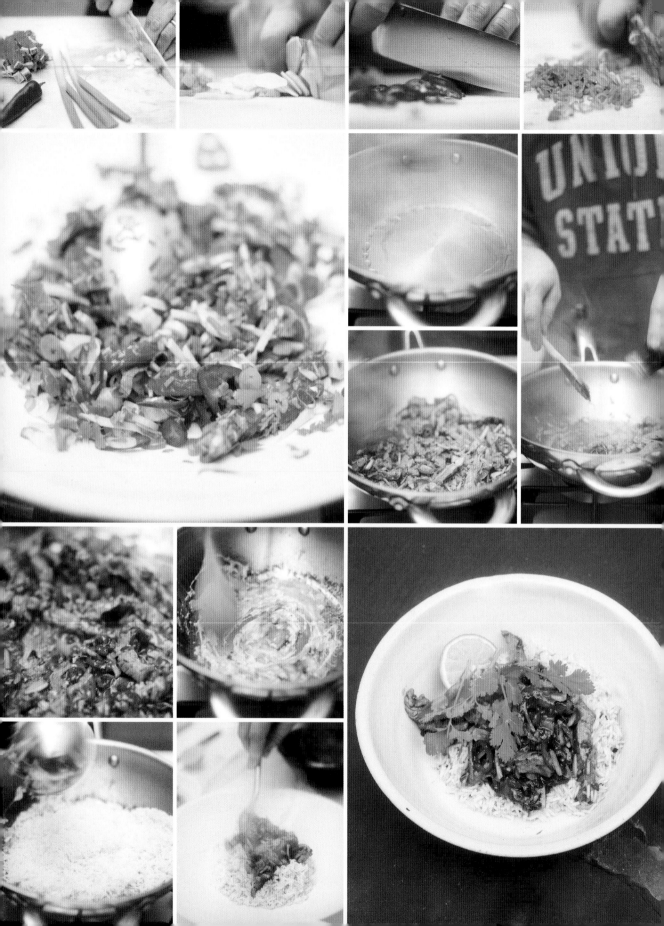

SIZZLING BEEF WITH SCALLIONS AND BLACK BEAN SAUCE

This works best with rice that has completely chilled down or, better yet, has been made earlier and kept in the refrigerator. But if you can't prepare rice for this dish in advance, you can still cook it and pop it into the refrigerator while you're cooking the rest.

serves 2

sea salt and freshly ground black pepper

1 cup long-grain or basmati rice

1 x ½-pound top loin or sirloin

a thumb-sized piece of fresh ginger

2 cloves of garlic

½ a fresh red or green chile

2 scallions

a small bunch of fresh cilantro

2 tablespoons sesame oil

peanut or vegetable oil

2 tablespoons of good-quality black bean sauce

2–3 tablespoons soy sauce

2 limes

1 egg, preferably free-range or organic

To prepare your stir-fry

Bring a pan of salted water to a boil, add the rice and cook according to the package instructions • Drain the rice in a strainer, run it under a cold tap to cool, then allow to dry out in the fridge • Trim any excess fat from your steak and slice the meat into finger-sized strips • Peel and finely slice the ginger and garlic • Finely slice the chile • Cut the ends off your scallions and finely slice • Pick the cilantro leaves and put to one side, and finely chop the cilantro stalks • Get yourself a big bowl and put in the ginger, garlic, chile, scallions, cilantro stalks, and steak strips • Add the sesame oil and mix everything together

To cook your stir-fry

Preheat a wok or large frying pan on a high heat and once it's very, very hot add a good lug of peanut oil and swirl it around • Add all your chopped ingredients from the bowl • Give the pan a really good shake to mix everything around quickly • Stir-fry for 2 minutes, taking care to keep everything moving so it doesn't burn • Add the black bean sauce, and stir in 1 tablespoon of soy sauce and the juice of half a lime • Keep tossing • Taste and season with black pepper and a little more soy sauce • Remove the pan from the heat, transfer everything to a bowl, and cover with aluminum foil • Give the pan a quick wipe with a ball of paper towels and put back on the heat • Add a lug of peanut oil and swirl it around • Crack in your egg and add a tablespoon of soy sauce – the egg will cook very quickly, so keep stirring • Once it's scrambled, stir in your chilled rice, scraping the sides and the bottom of the pan as you go • Keep mixing for a few minutes until the rice is steaming hot, then taste and season with a little soy sauce

To serve your stir-fry

Divide the rice between two bowls or plates • Spoon over the meat and black bean sauce and sprinkle over the cilantro leaves • Serve with wedges of lime – great!

SUPER-QUICK SALMON STIR-FRY

This is one of the fastest suppers ever! It only takes about five minutes from start to finish and is lovely served with rice or noodles. Just make sure you get the rice on before you start the salmon, or your stir-fry will be cold by the time it's ready. I've used tandoori curry paste in this recipe, but you can use any type of curry paste.

serves 2

sea salt and freshly ground black pepper
1 cup basmati or wild rice
¾ pound salmon fillet, skin off and bones removed
a handful of raw shelled peanuts
1 clove of garlic
a thumb-sized piece of fresh root ginger
1 fresh red or green chile
a small bunch of fresh cilantro

peanut or vegetable oil
1 heaped tablespoon tandoori or mild curry paste, such as Patak's
a handful of snow peas
½ a 14-ounce can of coconut milk
a handful of beansprouts
1 lime

To prepare your stir-fry
Bring a pan of salted water to a boil, add the rice, and cook according to the package instructions • While that's cooking away, chop the salmon into even-sized 1-inch chunks • Crush the peanuts up in a pestle and mortar, or else put them into a kitchen towel or plastic sandwich bag and use a rolling pin to bash them up • Peel and finely chop your garlic and ginger • Halve, seed, and finely slice your chile • Pick the cilantro leaves from the stalks, finely chop the stalks, and put the leaves to one side

To cook your stir-fry
Put a wok on a high heat and add 2 lugs of peanut oil • Add the garlic, ginger, most of the chopped chile, and the cilantro stalks • Stir for 30 seconds, then add the curry paste and stir for another 30 seconds • Add the salmon, cook for a minute or so, then add the snow peas and coconut milk • Let everything cook for another minute • Taste and season with a little salt and pepper if you think it needs it

To serve your stir-fry
Drain your cooked rice and divide it between your serving bowls • Spoon over the salmon and sprinkle over the beansprouts and crushed peanuts • Halve your lime and squeeze over the juice • Sprinkle with the remaining chile and the cilantro leaves

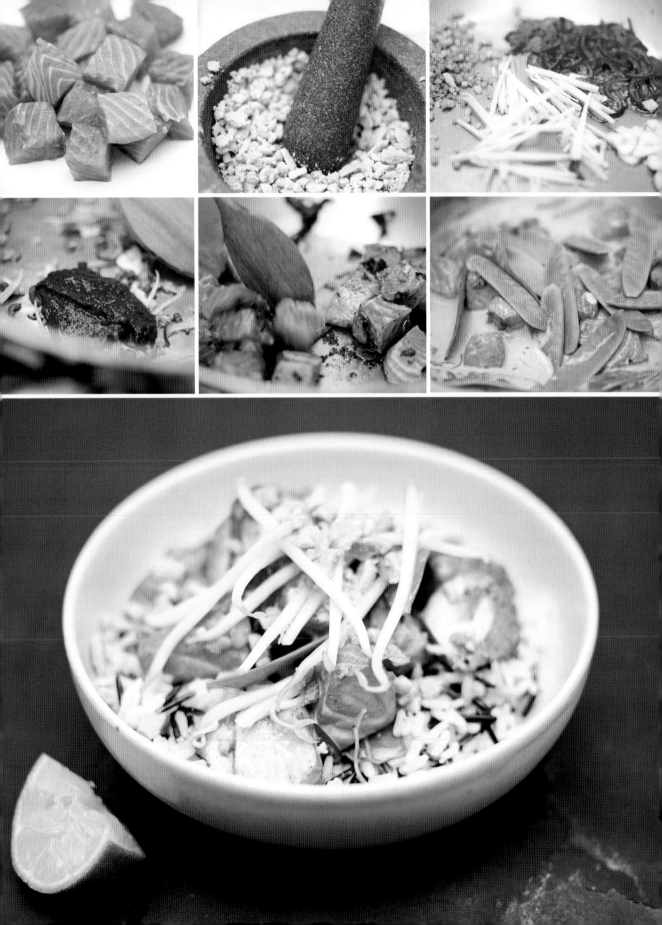

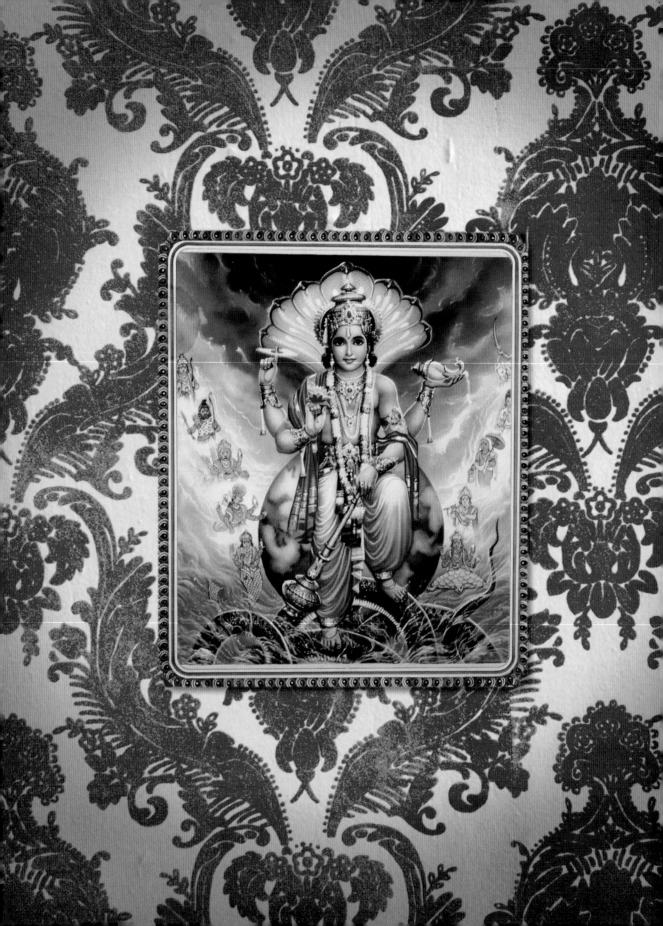

Easy curries

I've decided to dedicate a whole chapter to curries, as over in the UK we love our curries. Most Brits need to get their weekly fix, and I'm no different! So, when putting this chapter together, I started to think about the most common and best-loved curries, the ones we buy every week, whether from restaurants or ready-prepared from the grocery store. After I'd finished writing the recipes, though, I realized that the sheer complexity of the spice combinations and the instructions for how to grind and toast them were way too advanced for this book and beginner cooks. So I was going to remove the chapter completely. But then I came across a product that completely changed my thinking. Instead of jarred curry sauces, I found these fragrant curry pastes which are available in many grocery stores and on-line at www.qualityspices.com and which are made by a British company called Patak's. I've named the brand specifically in each recipe because I think they are one of the highest-quality curry pastes around (and I say that completely independently) – they are made up of a carefully balanced combination of all sorts of spices, herbs, and fragrant ingredients. So I've kept a reworked version of the curry chapter in this book. The recipes are easy and give consistently great results and flavors. You're going to love them. You can also tweak them by using beef, lamb, chicken, or vegetables in any of them.

Once you've got the hang of using the pastes, you might want to have a go at making up your own curry pastes instead, in which case you can turn to page 99, where I've given you alternative homemade versions for when you've got a bit more confidence and time to spend on making a curry from scratch.

I've also given you a couple of simple vegetable side dishes and some really reliable rice recipes, which I'm sure will have you buying ready-prepared and take-out curries far less often. Combine a curry with maybe a veg dish and some rice, with a pack of pappadams and a nice lemony green salad, a little jar of mango chutney, some natural yogurt, and a load of beers at the table. Brilliant, I'm coming round!

CHICKEN KORMA

This is a much-loved curry. It's got a slightly milder, creamier taste than the other curries in this chapter, which makes it a great one for kids to try. Because I love fresh chiles I've added one here, but if you want to keep the flavors nice and mild feel free to leave it out. Kormas are also delicious made with shrimp.

serves 4–6

1¾ pounds skinless chicken breasts, preferably
   free-range or organic
2 medium onions
optional: 1 fresh green chile
a thumb-sized piece of fresh root ginger
a small bunch of fresh cilantro
1 x 15-ounce can of garbanzo beans
peanut or vegetable oil
a pat of butter

½ cup korma or mild curry paste, such as Patak's, or
   my korma paste (see page 99)
1 x 14-ounce can of coconut milk
a small handful of sliced almonds, plus extra for
   serving
2 heaped tablespoons unsweetened shredded coconut
sea salt and freshly ground black pepper
1 cup natural yogurt
1 lemon

To prepare your curry

Cut the chicken into approximately 1-inch pieces • Peel, halve, and finely slice your onions • Halve, seed, and finely slice the chile if you're using it • Peel and finely chop the ginger • Pick the cilantro leaves and finely chop the stalks • Drain the garbanzo beans

To make your curry

Put a large casserole-type pan on a high heat and add a couple of lugs of oil • Add the onions, chile, ginger, and cilantro stalks with the butter • Keep stirring it enough so it doesn't catch and burn but turns evenly golden • Cook for around 10 minutes • Add the curry paste, coconut milk, half your sliced almonds, the drained garbanzo beans, unsweetened shredded coconut, and sliced chicken breasts • Half fill the empty can with water, pour it into the pan, and stir again • Bring to a boil, then turn the heat down and simmer for 30 minutes with the lid on • Check the curry regularly to make sure it's not drying out, and add extra water if necessary • When the chicken is tender and cooked, taste and season with salt and pepper – please season carefully

To serve your curry

Feel free to serve this with any of my fluffy rice recipes (see pages 95–96) • Add a few spoonfuls of natural yogurt dolloped on top, and sprinkle over the rest of the sliced almonds • Finish by scattering over the cilantro leaves, and serve with lemon wedges for squeezing over

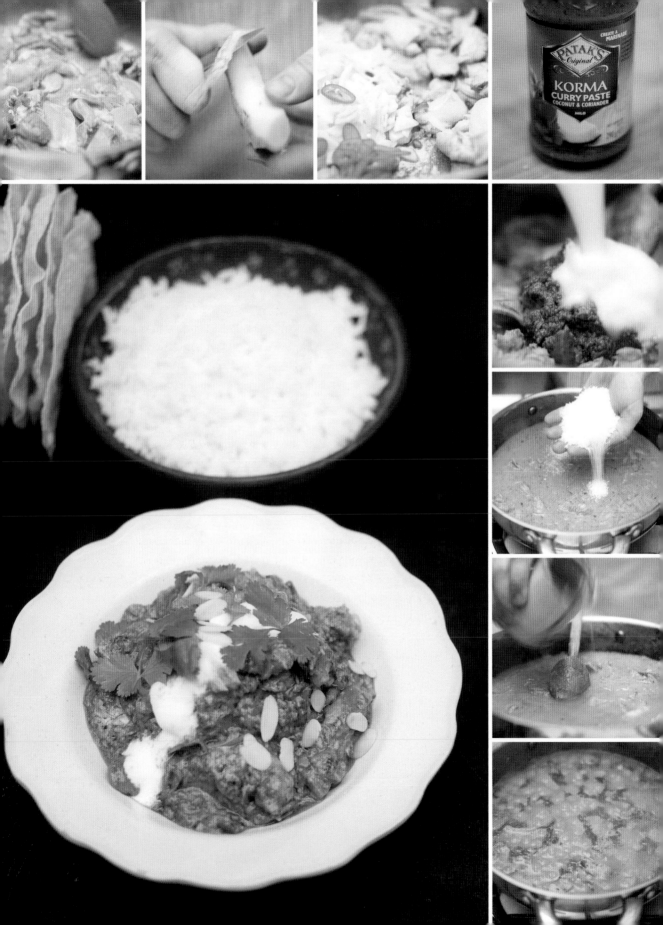

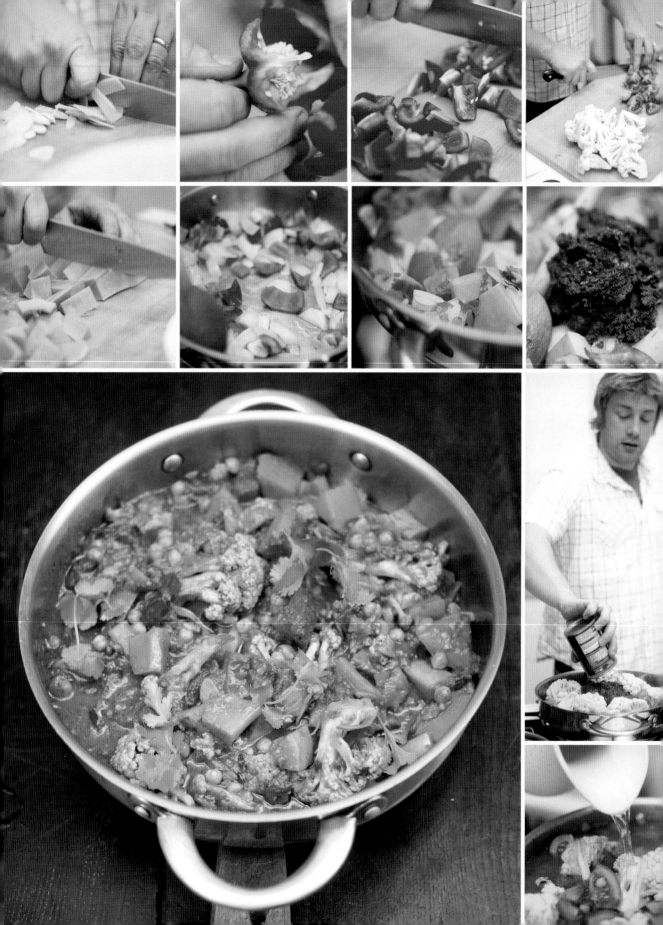

VEGETABLE JALFREZI

The great thing about this curry is the slightly sweet and sour flavor from the bell peppers. Do experiment with other combinations of vegetables such as zucchini, eggplant, or potatoes once you've mastered this version – bigger, chunkier veggies need longer cooking times, so add them at the start, and delicate veggies like peas and spinach need only minutes, so they can go in right at the end. This will serve 8 people – just halve the recipe if your pan isn't large enough, or else freeze any leftovers.

serves 8

1 medium onion
1 fresh red or green chile
a thumb-sized piece of fresh root ginger
2 cloves of garlic
a small bunch of fresh cilantro
2 red bell peppers
1 cauliflower
3 ripe tomatoes
1 small butternut squash
1 x 15-ounce can of garbanzo beans

peanut or vegetable oil
a pat of butter
½ cup of jalfrezi or medium curry paste, such as Patak's, or my jalfrezi paste (see page 99)
2 x 14-ounce cans of diced tomatoes
¼ cup balsamic vinegar
sea salt and freshly ground black pepper
2 lemons
1 cup natural yogurt

To prepare your curry

Peel, halve, and roughly chop your onion • Finely slice the chile • Peel and finely slice the ginger and garlic • Pick the cilantro leaves and finely chop the stalks • Halve, seed, and roughly chop the bell peppers • Break the green leaves off the cauliflower and discard • Break the cauliflower into florets and roughly chop the stalk • Quarter the tomatoes • Carefully halve the butternut squash, then scoop out the seeds with a spoon and discard • Slice the squash into inch-size wedges, leaving the peel on but removing any thick skin, then roughly chop into smaller pieces • Drain the garbanzo beans

To cook your curry

Put a large casserole-type pan on a medium to high heat and add a couple of lugs of oil and the butter • Add the onions, chile, ginger, garlic, and cilantro stalks and cook for 10 minutes, until softened and golden • Add the peppers, butternut squash, drained garbanzo beans, and jalfrezi curry paste • Stir well to coat everything with the paste • Add the cauliflower, the fresh and canned tomatoes, and the vinegar • Fill 1 empty can with water, pour into the pan, and stir again • Bring to a boil, then turn the heat down and simmer for 45 minutes with the lid on • Check the curry after 30 minutes and, if it still looks a bit liquidy after this time, leave the lid off for the remaining 15 minutes • When the veggies are tender, taste and add salt and pepper – please season carefully – and a squeeze of lemon juice

To serve your curry

Delicious with pappadams or any of my fluffy rice recipes (see pages 95–96) and with a few spoonfuls of natural yogurt, a sprinkle of cilantro leaves, and a few lemon wedges for squeezing over

LEFTOVER CURRY BIRIANI

This is a delicious dish that can be made using any type of leftover homemade curry. If you don't have any leftovers to use up, it's well worth making a curry especially for the recipe. Don't use take-out curries to make this, as you don't know how many times they've been reheated. Unlike the other curries in this chapter, this is a baked dish, made by layering rice, meat, and onions – think of it as a sort of Indian lasagne! It gives you a slightly drier dish with loads of flavor and a gorgeous, crispy texture.

serves 4–6

sea salt and freshly ground black pepper
1½ cups basmati rice
around 4 cups of leftover curry
2 tablespoons butter
2 teaspoons ground turmeric
2 medium onions

peanut or vegetable oil
4 whole cloves
a large handful of sliced almonds
1 cup natural yogurt
1 lemon

To prepare your biriani

Preheat the oven to 450°F • Get yourself a large pan of salted water and bring to a boil • Cook the rice according to the package instructions • When done, drain in a colander and put to one side to cool down • Remove your leftover curry from the fridge • Rub all around the inside of a baking dish with one of the tablespoons of butter • Sprinkle over the turmeric and give it a good shake around the dish so it sticks to the butter • Peel, halve, and finely slice the onions

To cook your biriani

Place a frying pan on a high heat and add a good lug of oil • Add the onion, the cloves, and a pinch of salt and pepper • Stir the onions, cooking them for 7 to 10 minutes until golden and crispy • Place another pan on a medium heat and add your leftover curry with a little splash of water and simmer for a few minutes, stirring every now and then • Spoon a layer of rice into your ovenproof dish, followed by a layer of warmed curry and a layer of crispy onions • Scatter over a few almonds and then repeat the layers, finishing with a layer of rice • Gently press down on the top to even it out a little • Break up the remaining tablespoon of butter and dot it all over the rice • Fold a large piece of aluminum foil in half and lightly oil one side of it • Place the aluminum foil over the dish, oil-side down, then pinch it tightly around the dish to secure it • Place the dish on the very bottom of your preheated oven and bake for 50 minutes – this will give you a delicious crispy bottom and lovely golden top

To serve your biriani

Put the baking dish in the middle of the table so everyone can help themselves • Lovely served with a few spoonfuls of natural yogurt dolloped on top, and some lemon wedges for squeezing over • Big green salad, chutney – nice!

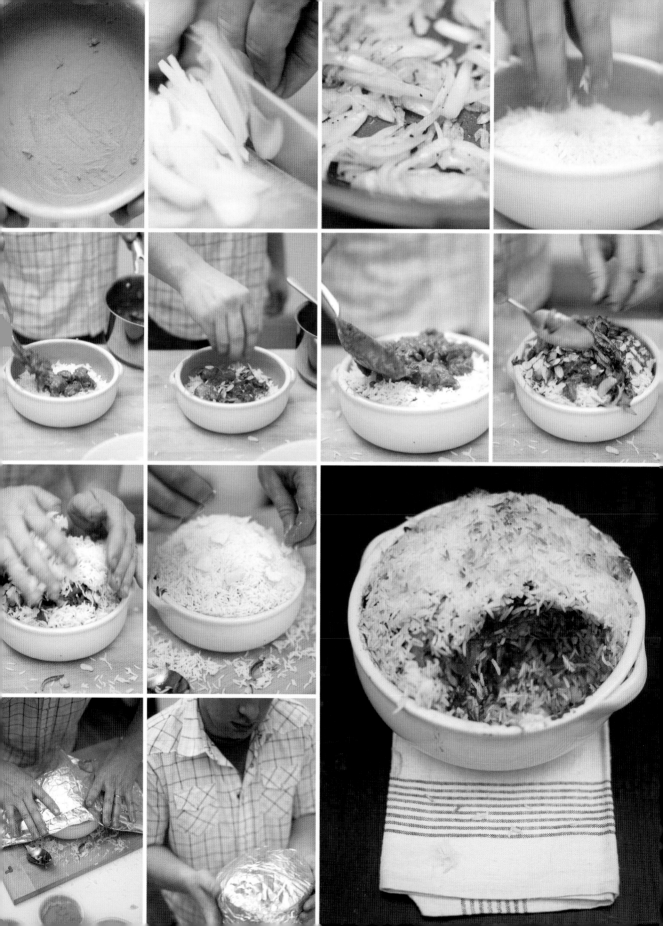

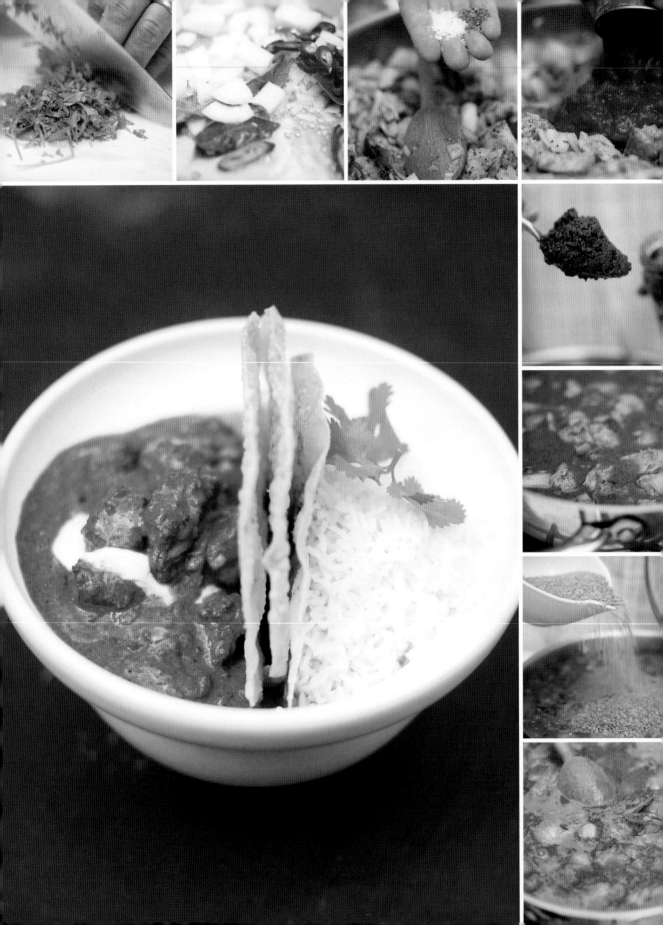

LAMB ROGAN JOSH

Get ready for an absolutely delicious curry! Rogan josh is like a hearty stew and is slightly more robust than some of the other curries commonly eaten in Britain, which have lighter, sweeter tastes. One of the nicest things about this recipe is the layers of flavor you get. It's completely different from a store-bought rogan josh. You've got to try it to taste the difference. I like making this curry with lamb, but feel free to use chicken or pork instead. The cooking time will be the same if you use other meat, just make sure you cut it into the same 1-inch cubes. For a vegetarian version, use vegetables such as squash, potatoes, and cauliflower and shorten the cooking time to 45 minutes.

serves 4–6

1¾ pounds lamb leg steaks

2 medium onions

1 fresh red or green chile

a thumb-sized piece of fresh root ginger

a small bunch of fresh cilantro

peanut or vegetable oil

a pat of butter

4 bay leaves

sea salt and freshly ground black pepper

2 tablespoons balsamic vinegar

1 x 14-ounce can of diced tomatoes

optional: 3⅓ cups chicken broth

½ cup rogan josh or medium curry paste, such as
    Patak's, or my rogan josh paste (see page 99)

2 handfuls of red lentils

1 cup natural yogurt

To prepare your curry

Cut the lamb into 1-inch cubes • Peel, halve, and finely chop your onions • Finely slice the chile • Peel and finely chop the ginger • Pick the cilantro leaves from half the bunch and put to one side for sprinkling over • Chop the remaining cilantro, including the stalks

To make your curry

Put a large casserole-type pan on a medium to high heat and add a couple of lugs of oil and the butter • Add the onions, chile, ginger, cilantro stalks, and bay leaves and cook for 10 minutes, until the onions are softened and golden • Add the lamb pieces and a little salt and pepper and cook until lightly browned • Add the balsamic vinegar and cook for 2 minutes, then add the tomatoes, stock (or 3⅓ cups of hot water), and rogan josh curry paste • Stir in the lentils • Bring to a boil, then turn the heat down and simmer with the lid on for about an hour • If your curry looks a bit liquidy after this time, simmer it for a few more minutes with the lid off • When the meat is tender and cooked, taste and add more salt and pepper only if you think it needs it

To serve your curry

This will be fantastic served with any of my fluffy rice recipes (see pages 95–96), some pappadams, and with a few spoonfuls of yogurt dolloped on top • Sprinkle over the cilantro leaves and serve with some lemon wedges for squeezing over • Don't forget a little green salad

CHICKEN TIKKA MASALA

This is one of the most widely eaten Indian dishes in Britain, probably to the bemusement of most Indians, as the regionality and diversity of their dishes is massive. To build up the popularity of just one dish would probably be seen as ludicrous in India. There's a big debate over the exact origins of this recipe – most Indians would say it's a bastardized British dish. What is certain is that you'll love the combination of the classic tikka flavors with the creamy, slightly sweet sauce. I've sprinkled my tikka masala with raw sliced almonds, but if you fancy toasting them first, simply pop them into a dry pan on the heat for a few minutes.

serves 4–6

*4 skinless chicken breast fillets, preferably free-range
  or organic*
2 medium onions
1 fresh red chile
a thumb-sized piece of fresh root ginger
a small bunch of fresh cilantro
peanut or vegetable oil
a pat of butter

*½ cup tikka masala or mild curry paste, such as
  Patak's, or my tikka masala paste (see page 99)*
sea salt and freshly ground black pepper
1 x 14-ounce can of diced tomatoes
1 x 14-ounce can of coconut milk
1 cup natural yogurt
a small handful of sliced almonds
1 lemon

To prepare your curry
Slice the chicken breasts lengthways into ¾-inch-thick strips • Peel, halve, and finely slice the onions • Finely slice your chile • Peel and finely slice the ginger • Pick the cilantro leaves and put to one side, then finely chop the stalks

To make your curry
Put a large casserole-type pan on a medium to high heat and add a couple of lugs of oil and the butter • Add the onions, chile, ginger, and coriander stalks and cook for 10 minutes, until softened and golden • Add the curry paste and the strips of chicken • Stir well to coat everything with the paste and season with salt and pepper • Add the tomatoes and the coconut milk • Bring to a boil, then turn the heat down and simmer for 15 minutes with the lid on • Take the lid off and cook for another 5 minutes, stirring occasionally • When the meat is tender and cooked, taste and add a bit more salt and pepper – please season carefully

To serve your curry
This will be fantastic served with any of my fluffy rice recipes (see pages 95–96) and with a few spoonfuls of yogurt dolloped on top • Sprinkle over the almonds and cilantro leaves and serve with some lemon wedges for squeezing over • And a little lemon-dressed green salad would round it off

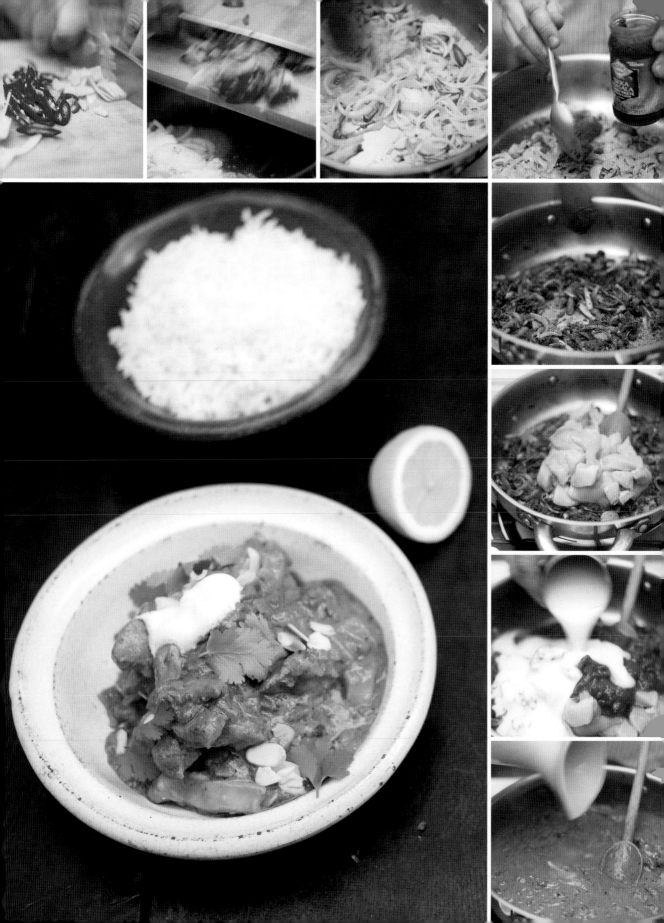

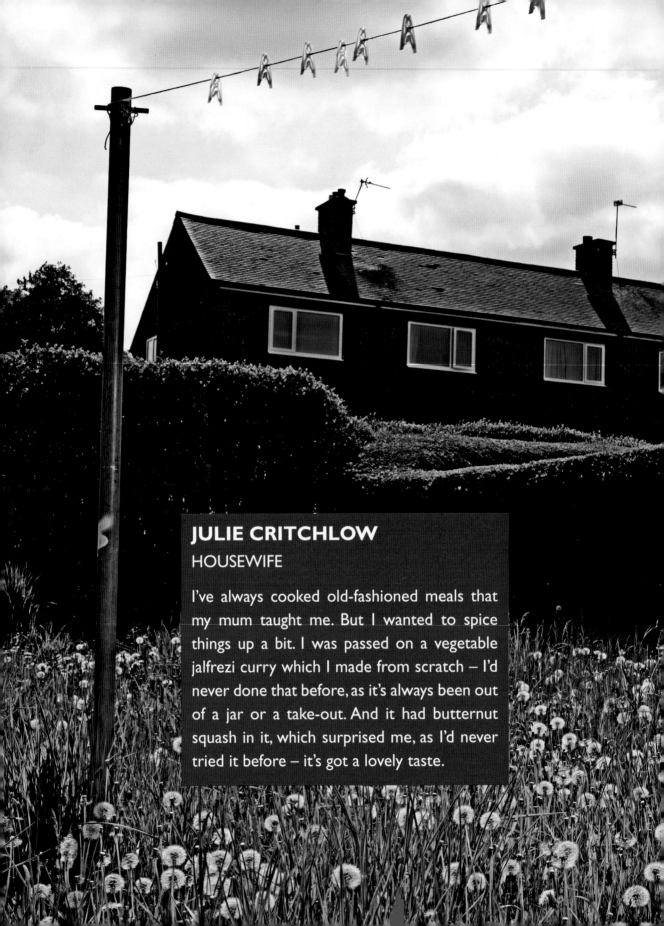

JULIE CRITCHLOW
HOUSEWIFE

I've always cooked old-fashioned meals that my mum taught me. But I wanted to spice things up a bit. I was passed on a vegetable jalfrezi curry which I made from scratch – I'd never done that before, as it's always been out of a jar or a take-out. And it had butternut squash in it, which surprised me, as I'd never tried it before – it's got a lovely taste.

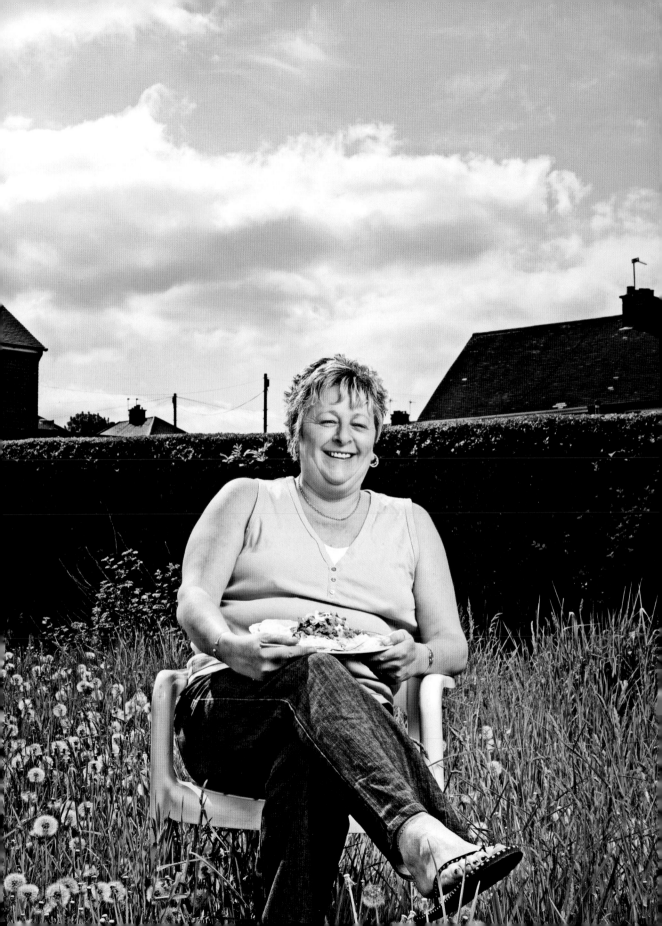

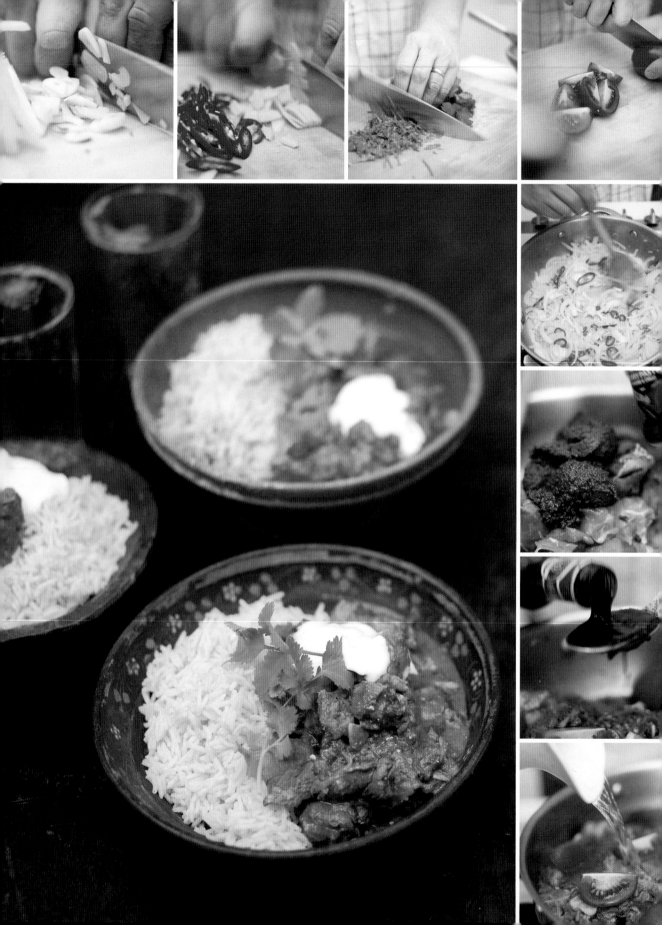

VINDALOO

Now we're talking! I've loved eating vindaloo ever since I was a kid, and it's where my passion for eating chiles first started. This type of curry is the beautiful result of European and Indian cooking coming together. The word "vindaloo" means "vinegar and garlic." Thanks to Portuguese settlers bringing their original recipe to Goa, this dish got the Indian treatment, which added plenty of wonderful spices to the mix. I'm using pork here, but it will work just as well with chicken or lamb. A word of warning, though — this is a hot curry and not for the faint-hearted, but you can always remove the chile.

serves 4–6

2 medium onions

4 cloves of garlic

1–2 fresh red or green chiles, to your taste

a thumb-sized piece of fresh root ginger

a small bunch of fresh cilantro

4 ripe tomatoes

peanut or vegetable oil

a pat of butter

1¾ pounds diced pork shoulder, preferably free-range
or organic

½ cup vindaloo or hot curry paste, such as Patak's, or
my vindaloo paste (see page 99)

sea salt and freshly ground black pepper

⅓ cup balsamic vinegar

1 tablespoon honey

1 cup natural yogurt

1 lemon

To prepare your curry

Peel, halve, and finely slice your onions • Peel and finely slice the garlic • Finely slice the chile • Peel and finely slice the ginger • Pick the cilantro leaves and finely chop the stalks • Cut the tomatoes into quarters

To cook your curry

Get a large casserole-type pan on a medium to high heat and add a couple of lugs of peanut oil and the butter • Add the onions, garlic, chile, ginger, and cilantro stalks and cook for 10 minutes, until softened and golden • Add the pork and the curry paste • Stir well to coat everything with the paste and season with salt and pepper • Add the tomatoes, balsamic vinegar, honey, and about 1⅔ cups of water, enough to cover everything, and stir again • Bring to a boil, then turn the heat down and simmer for 45 minutes with the lid on • Check the curry regularly to make sure it's not sticking to the pan, and add extra water if necessary • Only when the meat is tender and cooked, taste and season with salt and pepper – please season carefully

To serve your curry

Feel free to serve with any of my fluffy rice recipes (see pages 95–96) and with a few spoonfuls of natural yogurt dolloped on top • Sprinkle over the cilantro leaves and serve with some lemon wedges for squeezing over

ALOO GOBHI

I often think of this as a vegetable side dish but it's actually a curry in its own right. It's a really delicious combination of potato and cauliflower with spices, and it gets its gorgeous yellow color from the turmeric that is used to flavor it.

serves 4

1 medium onion	*a pat of butter*
2–3 fresh green chiles, to your taste	*1 tablespoon black mustard seeds*
a thumb-sized piece of fresh root ginger	*1 teaspoon ground turmeric*
a small bunch of fresh cilantro	*1 level teaspoon ground cumin*
½ a cauliflower	*2 tablespoons unsweetened shredded coconut*
1 pound potatoes	*sea salt and freshly ground black pepper*
peanut or vegetable oil	*1 lemon*

To prepare your curry
Preheat the oven to 425°F • Peel, halve, and finely chop the onion • Finely slice your chiles • Peel and finely chop the ginger • Pick the cilantro leaves and finely chop the stalks • Discard the outer green leaves of the cauliflower, break it into florets, and cut the thick middle stem into cubes • Peel the potatoes and cut them into ¾-inch cubes

To make your curry
Put a large ovenproof pan on a medium to high heat and add a couple of lugs of oil and the butter • Add the onion, chiles, ginger, cilantro stalks, mustard seeds, turmeric, and cumin and cook for 7 to 10 minutes, until softened and golden • Stir in the cauliflower, potatoes, and coconut • Season with salt and pepper and add 1⅔ cups of water • Bring to a boil, then turn the heat down and simmer with the lid on until the veggies are cooked and soft • Check the curry regularly to make sure it's not drying out, and add extra water if necessary • Give it another stir, then put the pan into the preheated oven for another 20 minutes • Taste and add more salt and pepper if you think it needs it

To serve your curry
Serve with any of my fluffy rice recipes (see pages 95–96) • Sprinkle with the chopped cilantro leaves, and serve with some lemon wedges for squeezing over

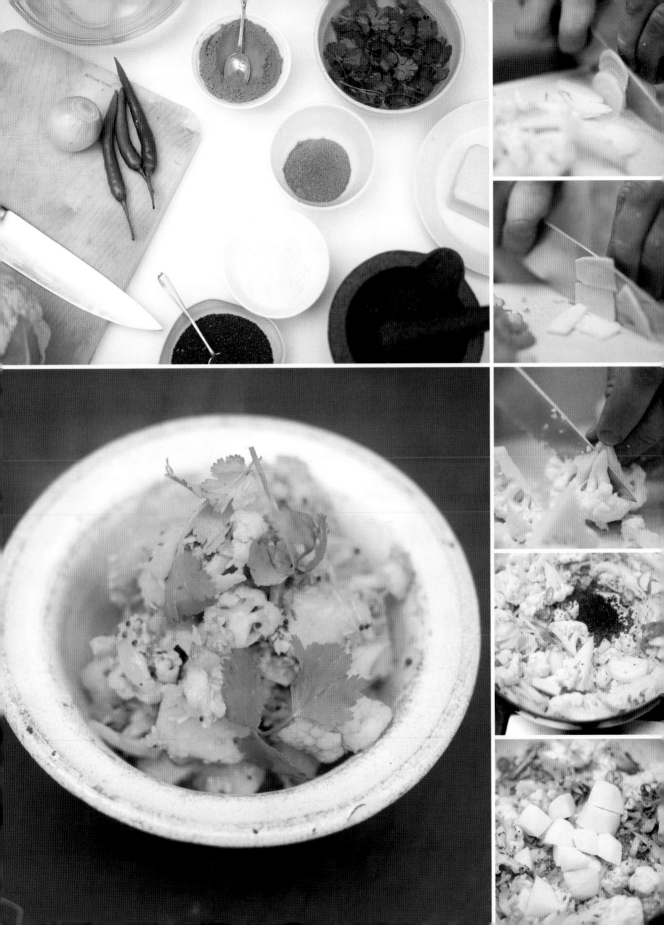

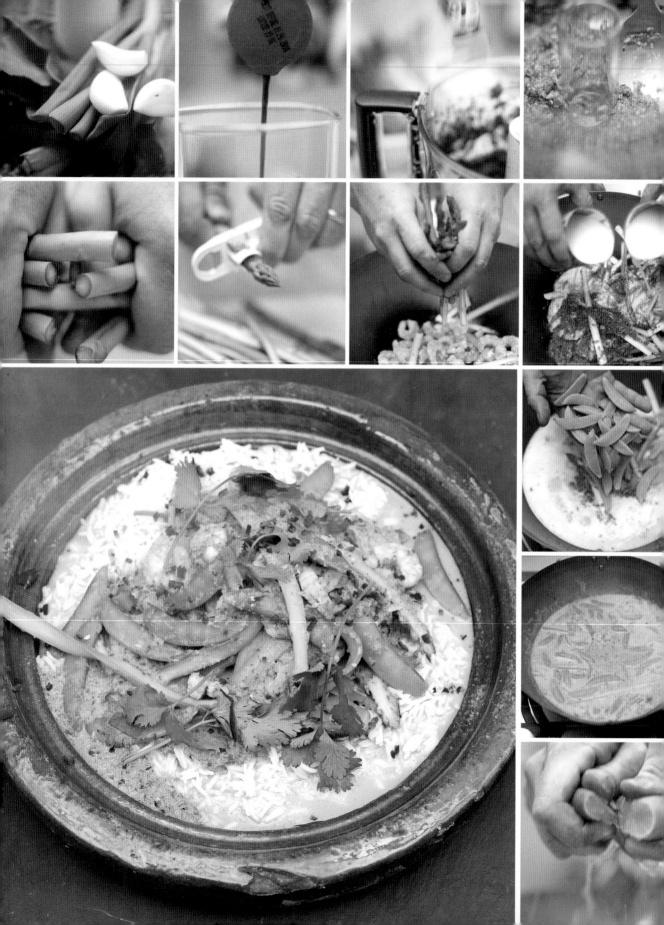

THAI GREEN CURRY

This green curry recipe is one of the best I've ever made. It's also good made with chicken instead of shrimp – just substitute 2 skinless chicken breast fillets, slice them into finger-sized strips, and stir-fry them with the paste for around 8 minutes before adding the other ingredients.

serves 2

a large bunch of asparagus
½ a fresh red or green chile
1 tablespoon peanut or vegetable oil
1 tablespoon sesame oil
1 pound large shrimp, raw, peeled
1 x 14-ounce can of coconut milk
a handful of snow peas
1 lime

For the green curry paste
2 stalks of lemongrass
4 scallions
3 fresh green chiles
4 cloves of garlic
a thumb-sized piece of fresh root ginger
a large bunch of fresh cilantro
1 teaspoon coriander seeds
optional: 8 fresh or dried kaffir lime leaves
3 tablespoons soy sauce
1 tablespoon fish sauce

To make your green curry paste

Trim the lemongrass stalks, peel back and discard the outer leaves, and crush the stalks by bashing them a few times with the heel of your hand or a rolling pin • Trim the scallions • Halve and seed the green chiles • Peel and roughly chop the garlic and ginger • Set aside a few sprigs of fresh cilantro, and whiz the rest in a food processor with the lemongrass stalks, scallions, chiles, garlic, ginger, coriander seeds, and lime leaves (if using), until everything is finely chopped – the smell will be amazing! • While whizzing, pour in the soy sauce and fish sauce and blitz again until you have a smooth paste • If you don't have a food processor, chop everything by hand as finely as you can – it may take a while but it will be so worth it

To make your curry

Snap the woody ends off the asparagus and discard them • Run the stalks through a string bean slicer, or finely slice them lengthways with a knife • Finely chop the red chile and put to one side • Place a large frying pan or wok over a high heat • When it's really hot, add the peanut and sesame oils, swirl them around, then carefully drop in the shrimp • Add the asparagus and your green curry paste and stir-fry for about 30 seconds • Pour in the coconut milk and add the snow peas • Give it all a good stir, bring to a boil, and cook for a few minutes • Have a taste and add a bit more soy sauce if you think it needs it • Push down on the lime and roll it around to get the juices going, then cut it in half • Squeeze the juice into the pan – this will give your curry a lovely twang

To serve your curry

Pick the leaves off the remaining cilantro sprigs • Serve the curry sprinkled with the cilantro leaves and the chopped red chile, and some fluffy cilantro and lime rice (see pages 95–96)

VEGETABLE BHAJIS

Bhajis are Indian vegetable fritters and a great thing to eat with your curry (especially after a few drinks!). They should always be made fresh and be eaten immediately. They can be made using all sorts of soft veggies – always keep onions in the mixture, but try adding grated yams or sweet potatoes, finely sliced bell peppers, leeks, or even garbanzo beans instead of carrots. It's up to you whether to make your bhajis large or small. A food processor or coarse grater is very handy for this recipe. It's also so important to be incredibly careful when you're deep-frying like this. Don't move the pan or leave it alone, and don't have kids or pets running around while you're doing this.

serves 4–6

2 large carrots

a 4-inch piece of fresh root ginger

2 medium red onions

2–3 fresh red or green chiles, to your taste

a large bunch of fresh cilantro

2 teaspoons yellow mustard seeds

1 teaspoon turmeric

1 heaped teaspoon cumin seeds

2 teaspoons sea salt

1 heaped cup self-rising flour

1 quart vegetable oil

a piece of potato

juice of 1 lemon

2 limes

To prepare your bhajis

Peel and finely grate or shred the carrots, ginger, and red onions and put them into a large bowl • Finely chop the chiles and add to the bowl • Roughly chop the cilantro leaves and stalks • Add the mustard seeds, turmeric, cumin seeds, salt, and chopped cilantro to the bowl • Then add the flour and ½ cup of cold water and scrunch together well, using your hands, until you have a nice thick mixture

To cook your bhajis

It's best to make these in a deep fat fryer, or you can put a large pan on a medium to high heat and add the oil • Drop in a piece of potato – when it floats to the surface and begins to sizzle, the oil has reached the right temperature • Remove the potato using a slotted spoon • Pick up a tablespoon of bhaji mixture, press it together tightly and carefully lower it into the hot oil • Repeat until you have several on the go • Cook for 5 minutes, until crispy and golden • Remove the cooked bhajis using your slotted spoon and put them on some paper towels to drain • Sprinkle with a little salt and a squeeze of lemon juice • Lower more tablespoonfuls into the oil until you have used up all the mixture

To serve your bhajis

Cut the limes into wedges and serve them on a big platter or plate with your bhajis • Eat at once!

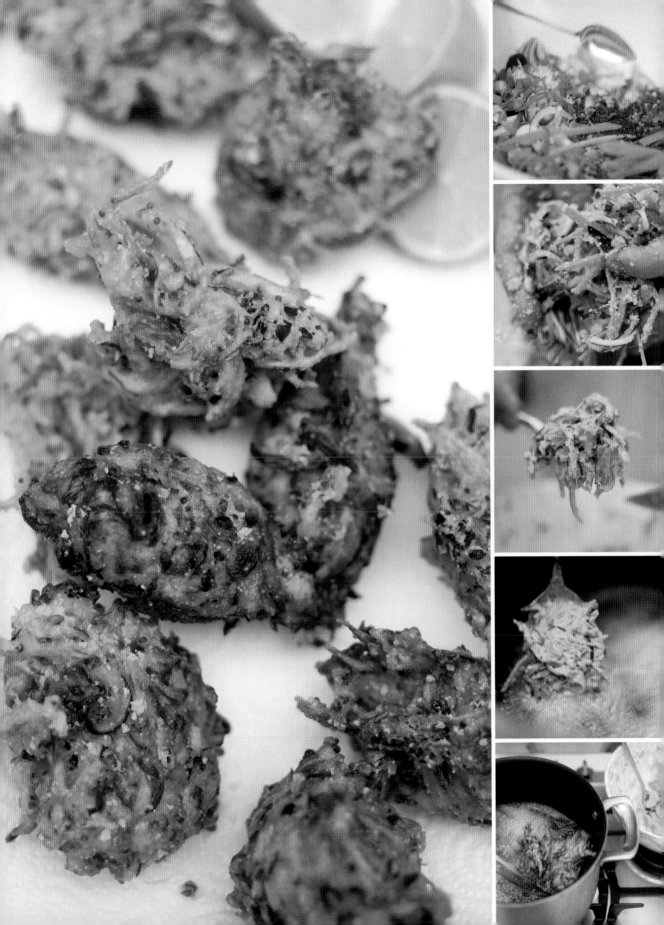

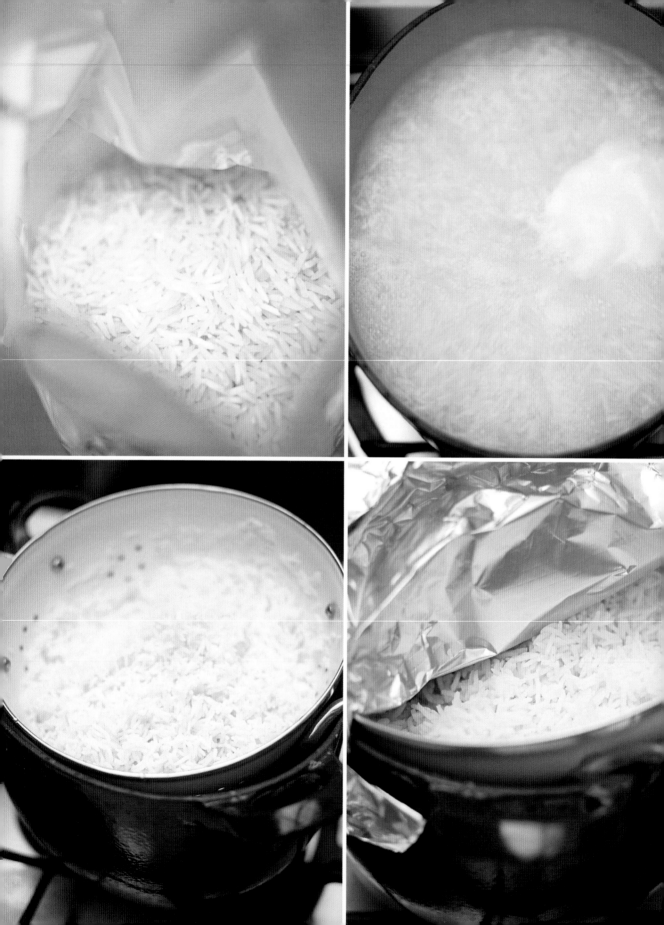

LIGHT AND FLUFFY RICE

Rice has been an important part of people's everyday diet for centuries, and it's still one of the most important foods in many different cultures. There are loads of varieties of rice available in our stores now, but in this chapter basmati is the king. I'm going to give you my basic recipe for getting perfect rice every time, as well as a few of my favorite ways to flavor it. Having said that, I want to point out that the natural nuttiness and flavor of plain rice is not to be underestimated. Have a go at mastering simple plain rice first – you'll be amazed at the light and fluffy results.

Once you've got the hang of that, you can give the other recipes a go. It's worth remembering that any flavoring you boil with the rice will infuse it with wonderful fragrances and flavors. So try boiling things like fresh herbs, a cinnamon stick, a few cardamom pods, a strip of lemon zest, or even a green tea bag in the water with the rice. Just double the recipe for 8 to 12 people.

For perfect, basic rice

serves 4–6
sea salt
1 ½ cups basmati rice

Put a large pan of salted water on a high heat and bring to a boil • Rinse the rice in a colander under running water for about 1 minute, or until the water runs clear (this will stop the grains sticking together later) • Add your rice to the boiling water and wait for the grains to start dancing around • From that point, boil for 5 minutes • Drain the rice in a colander • Pour 1 inch of water into the pan, put it back on the heat, and bring it to the boil again, then turn down to a simmer • Cover the rice in the colander with aluminum foil or a lid • Place the colander on top of the pan of simmering water and let the rice steam over it for 8 to 10 minutes • Remove from the heat and, if you're ready, serve immediately • If not, leave the aluminum foil or lid on and put aside until ready to serve – it should stay warm for about 20 minutes

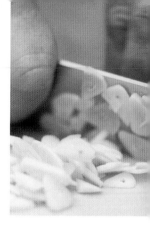

For garlic and nutmeg rice

8 cloves of garlic / ¼ of a nutmeg / olive oil / a pat of butter / sea salt and freshly ground black pepper / 1 level teaspoon ground cinnamon / 1 small lemon

Cook your rice • Peel and finely chop the garlic • Grate the nutmeg • Put a large frying pan on a low heat and add a lug of olive oil and the butter • When the butter melts add the garlic and season with salt and pepper • Cook until the garlic starts to color • Stir in the nutmeg and cinnamon • Add your cooked rice and stir thoroughly until well coated • Remove from the heat, squeeze over the lemon juice, stir well, then serve

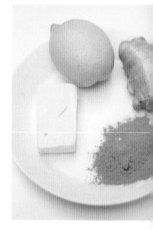

For lemon, ginger, and turmeric rice

1 lemon / 1-inch piece of fresh root ginger / olive oil / a pat of butter / 1 heaped teaspoon turmeric / sea salt and freshly ground black pepper

Cook your rice • Zest your lemon, then cut it in half • Peel and grate the ginger • Put a large frying pan on a low heat and add a lug of olive oil and the butter • When it starts to bubble gently, add the lemon zest, ginger, and turmeric and squeeze over the lemon juice • Season with salt and pepper • Stir until you have a golden paste • Spoon your cooked rice into the frying pan • Stir thoroughly and serve

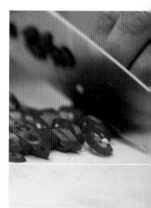

For spicy chile rice

4 cardamom pods / 1–2 fresh red or green chiles, to your taste / olive oil / 2 pats of butter / 4 whole cloves / 1 tablespoon tomato paste / sea salt and freshly ground black pepper / 1 small lemon

Cook your rice • Crack open the cardamom pods in your hands, then keep the seeds and discard the pods • Finely chop your chiles • Put a large frying pan on a low heat and add a lug of olive oil and the butter • When it starts to bubble add the cardamom seeds, chiles, cloves, and tomato paste and season with salt and pepper • Stir and cook for 2 minutes • Spoon your cooked rice into the frying pan • Stir thoroughly until well coated • Remove from the heat, squeeze over the lemon juice, stir well, and serve

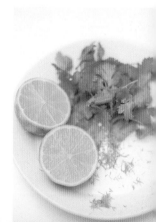

For cilantro and lime rice

a large bunch of fresh cilantro / 2 limes / extra virgin olive oil / sea salt and freshly ground black pepper

Cook your rice • Pick the cilantro leaves off the stalks and finely chop • Zest your limes and cut them in half • Mix the cilantro and lime zest into your rice, then squeeze over the lime juice • Drizzle over a good lug of extra virgin olive oil and season with salt and pepper • Stir well and serve

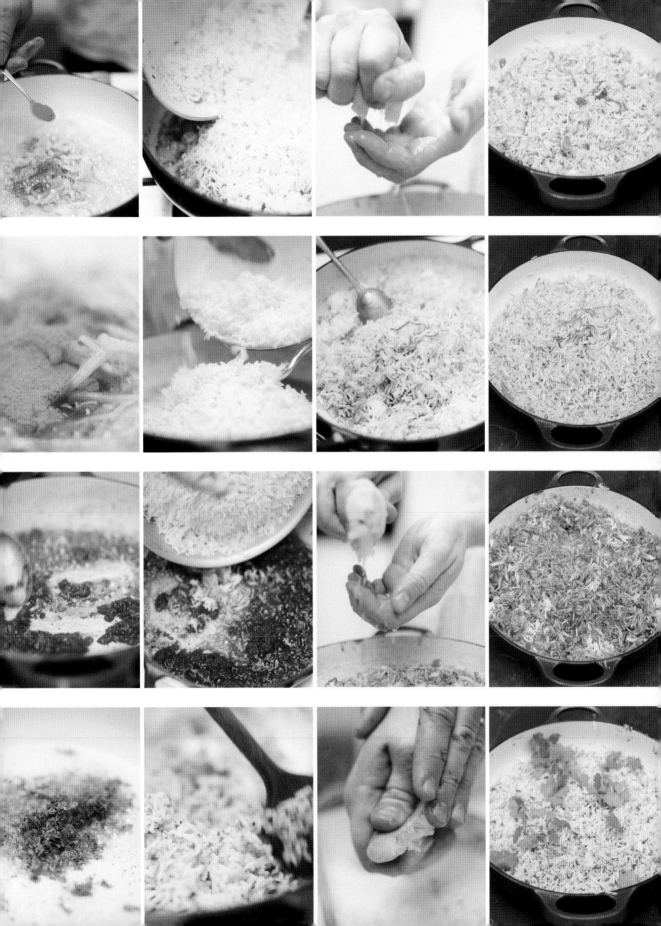

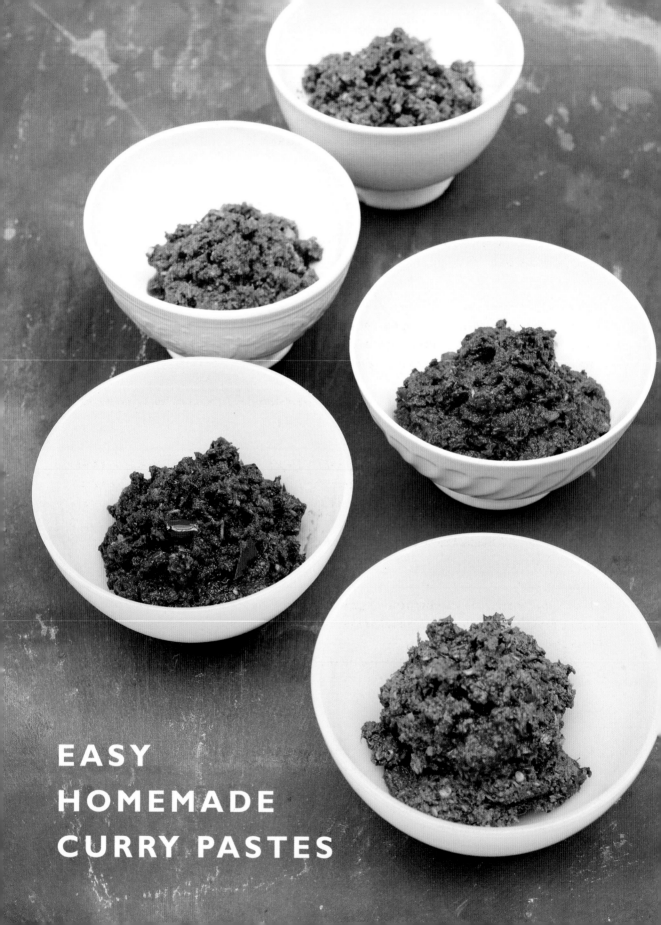

EASY
HOMEMADE
CURRY PASTES

Korma paste

2 cloves of garlic / a thumb-sized piece of fresh root ginger / ½ teaspoon cayenne pepper / 1 teaspoon garam masala / ½ teaspoon sea salt / 2 tablespoons peanut oil / 1 tablespoon tomato paste / 2 fresh green chiles / 3 tablespoons unsweetened shredded coconut / 2 tablespoons almond flour / a small bunch of fresh cilantro

Spices for toasting 2 teaspoons cumin seeds / 1 teaspoon coriander seeds

Jalfrezi paste

2 cloves of garlic / a thumb-sized piece of fresh root ginger / 1 teaspoon turmeric / ½ teaspoon sea salt / 2 tablespoons peanut oil / 2 tablespoons tomato paste / 1 fresh green chile / a small bunch of fresh cilantro

Spices for toasting 2 teaspoons cumin seeds / 1 teaspoon brown mustard seeds / 1 teaspoon fenugreek seeds / 1 teaspoon coriander seeds

Rogan josh paste

2 cloves of garlic / a thumb-sized piece of fresh root ginger / 3 ounces roasted bell peppers, from a jar or deli counter / 1 tablespoon paprika / 1 teaspoon smoked paprika / 2 teaspoons garam masala / 1 teaspoon turmeric / ½ teaspoon sea salt / 2 tablespoons peanut oil / 2 tablespoons tomato paste / 1 fresh red or green chile / a small bunch of fresh cilantro

Spices for toasting 2 teaspoons cumin seeds / 2 teaspoons coriander seeds / 1 teaspoon black peppercorns

Tikka masala paste

2 cloves of garlic / a thumb-sized piece of fresh root ginger / 1 teaspoon cayenne pepper / 1 tablespoon smoked paprika / 2 teaspoons garam masala / ½ teaspoon sea salt / 2 tablespoons peanut oil / 2 tablespoons tomato paste / 2 fresh red or green chiles / a small bunch of fresh cilantro / 1 tablespoon unsweetened shredded coconut / 2 tablespoons almond flour

Spices for toasting 1 teaspoon cumin seeds / 1 teaspoon coriander seeds

Vindaloo paste

2 cloves of garlic / a thumb-sized piece of fresh root ginger / 4 dried red chiles / 1 tablespoon turmeric / ½ teaspoon sea salt / 3 tablespoons peanut oil / 2 tablespoons tomato paste / 2 fresh red or green chiles / a small bunch of fresh cilantro

Spices for toasting 1 teaspoon black peppercorns / 4 whole cloves / 2 teaspoons coriander seeds / 2 teaspoons fennel seeds / 1 teaspoon fenugreek seeds

To make any of the above curry pastes

First peel the garlic and ginger • Put a frying pan on a medium to high heat and add the spices for toasting to the dry pan • Lightly toast them for a few minutes until golden brown and smelling delicious, then remove the pan from the heat • Add the toasted spices to a pestle and mortar and grind until fine, or put them into a food processor and whiz to a powder • Either way, when you've ground them whiz the toasted spices in a food processor with the rest of the ingredients until you have a smooth paste

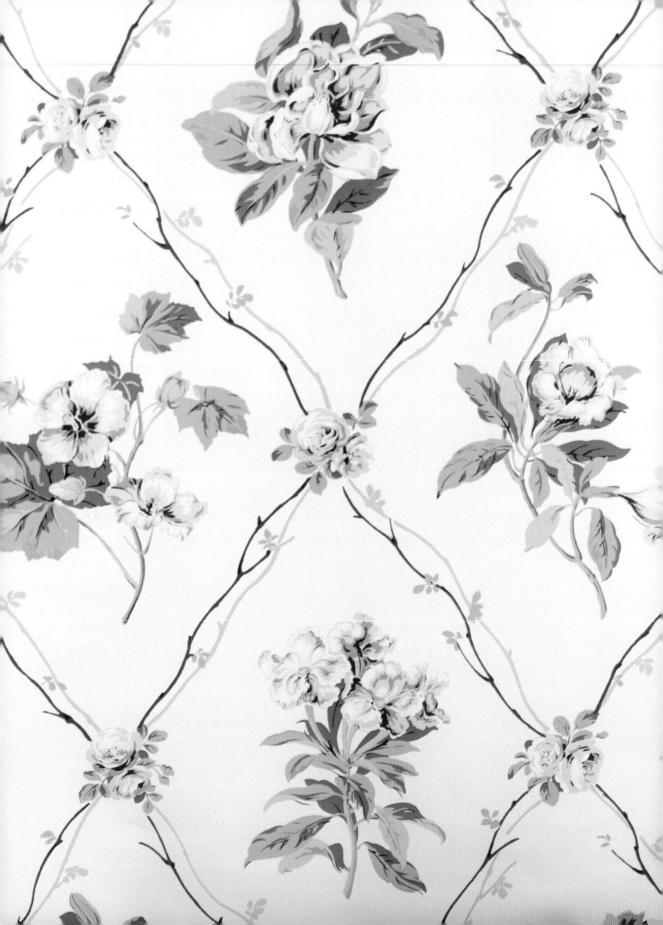

Lovin' salads

In my view, salads are a really important part of modern-day eating. Finding ways for your family to want to eat them is what it's all about. So I want to help you understand and master the key "salad skills" – how to tear or chop ingredients, how to make a simple dressing, what combinations of flavor and texture to put together in a salad. I want you to think about how a big chunk of cucumber might taste in a salad, compared to a thin sliver. Even though this isn't a chapter about "cooking," all these things are important parts of your cooking knowledge. It's important to know about dressing a salad at the last minute at the table, or to have a few large platters or bowls at your disposal specially for serving salads in so they look fantastic.

When it came to deciding which salads to include in this chapter, you'll see that I've included my versions of a couple of the biggest-selling ones from grocery stores – potato salad and rice salad – and given you my homemade equivalent. I've also tried to show, using words and pictures, how different elements of a salad can add real character. Have a look at the pick and mix salad on pages 118–19. I've given you a list of criteria, and as long as you pick one thing from each group you can't go wrong – choose a cheese, a soft lettuce, a crunchy lettuce, an herb, and a topping like croutons or pine nuts to scatter over. I promise you, you'll be making Formula One salads every time! Have a look now and it will instantly become clear.

The other thing I wanted to show you is how a simple salad can evolve very easily into something a little sexier, with a bit more dimension and interest to it than a few dressed leaves. A good salad can be made from two ingredients or twenty. The number of ingredients doesn't qualify it to be a better salad, that's for sure. Check out the different styles of "evolution salad" and I know you'll make them part of your cooking repertoire.

DRESSED GREEN SALAD

This first salad recipe may seem a bit boring and insignificant, but this page is sort of the basic foundation of salads. It will help you learn how to wash, look after, prepare, and dress your salads so you can really enjoy them.

I know salad bags are really convenient and, yes, I do use them at times, but I've also got into the habit of picking a few different lettuce heads like Romaine, butterhead lettuce, oak leaf, a little radicchio, and also sprouted seeds and herbs, to make up my own salad mix once a week. It works out a lot cheaper to do it this way – it only takes about 15 minutes to sort out.

To wash your salad leaves
When you get your lettuces home, remove the roots and any not-so-nice outside leaves first, then click or tear off the rest of the leaves and give them a good old wash in cold water • Once they're clean, give them a spin in a salad spinner or shake them dry in a kitchen towel

To store your salad leaves
If you line a salad crisper drawer in your refrigerator with a couple of clean kitchen towels and lay your leaves on top, covering them with another towel, they'll keep there happily for 4 days • Then you can simply make up your own mixed salads, dressing the leaves with one of my jam jar dressings on pages 106–7

To dress your salad leaves
Pour the dressing from a height and gently toss the leaves, using the tips of your fingers, until every single leaf is coated

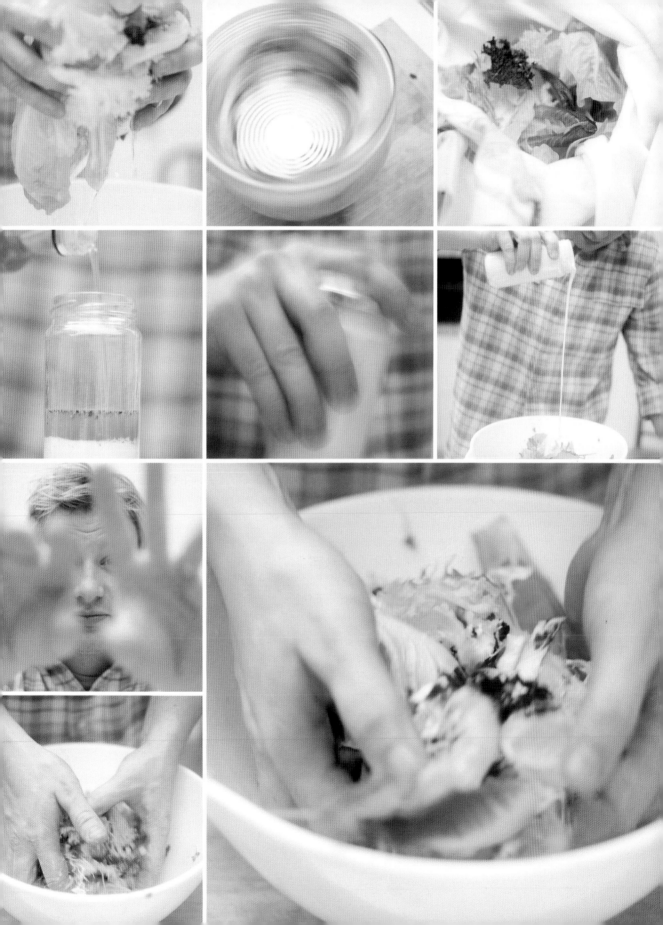

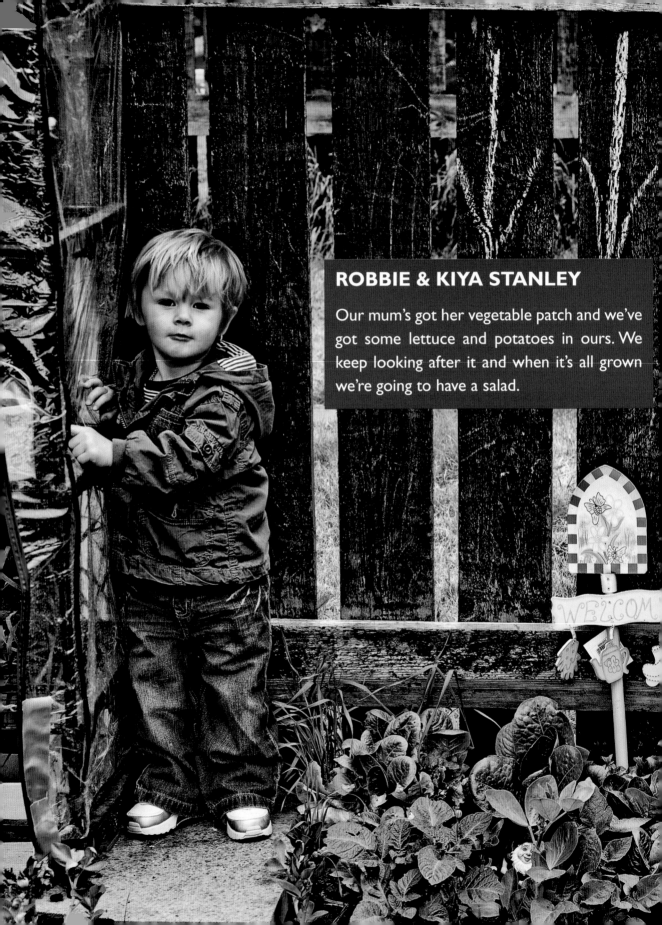

ROBBIE & KIYA STANLEY

Our mum's got her vegetable patch and we've got some lettuce and potatoes in ours. We keep looking after it and when it's all grown we're going to have a salad.

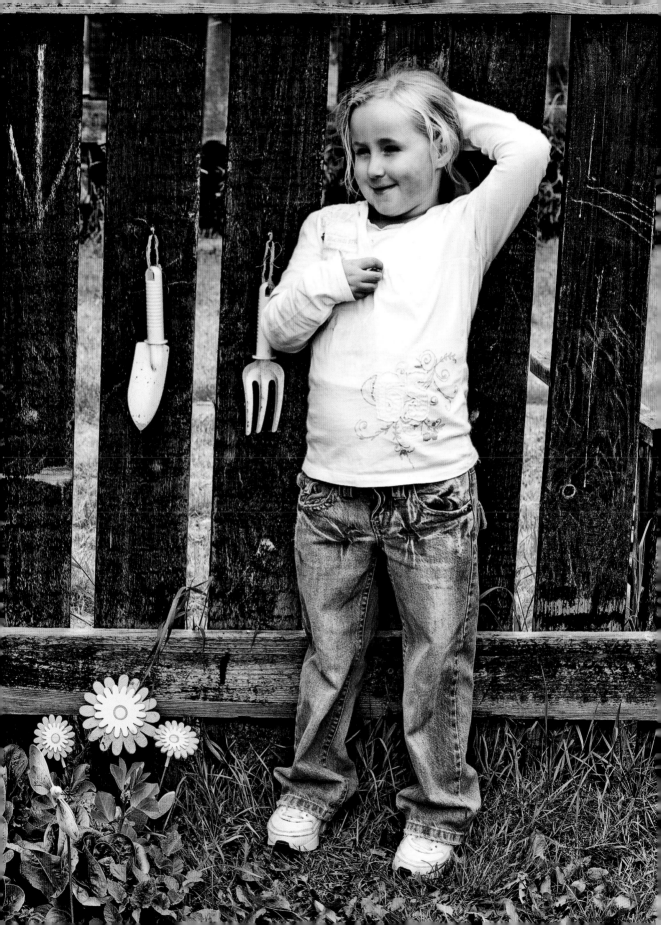

JAM JAR DRESSINGS

In my opinion, the most important part of a salad is the dressing. It's all very well saying everyone needs to eat more salad, fruit, and veggies (it's true, we do), but it should be a pleasure, not a chore! By dressing a salad you can make it delicious, meaning you want to eat it rather than feel you have to. The other good news is that your body can absorb far more of the nutrients from salads because of the presence of oil and acid in the dressing. So dressings give you the double whammy of being a healthy benefit and also delicious! Don't drown your salads in dressing, though – remember, a little goes a long way – and always dress them at the last minute before serving.

I like to make my dressings in jam jars because it's so easy to see what's going on – you can shake them up easily and any leftovers can be kept in the jars in the fridge. I'm going to give you four basic dressings that can be used with all the salads in this chapter. With the exception of the yogurt dressing, they are based on a ratio of 3 parts oil to 1 part acid (vinegar or lemon). Generally, this ratio is a really good benchmark for making any dressing, but it's always sensible to have a little taste once you've shaken it up. If the seasoning is there but you're finding it a little too acidic, you've cracked it, because once the dressing is on the salad leaves it will be perfect.

French dressing

Peel and finely chop ¼ of a clove of **garlic** • Put the garlic, 1 teaspoon of **Dijon mustard**, 2 tablespoons of **white or red wine vinegar**, and 6 tablespoons of **extra virgin olive oil** into a jam jar with a pinch of **sea salt and freshly ground black pepper** • Put the lid on the jar and shake well

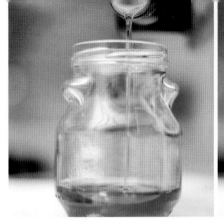
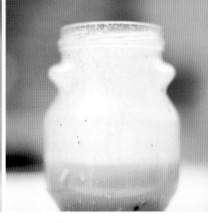

Yogurt dressing

Put ⅓ cup of **natural yogurt**, 2 tablespoons of **white or red wine vinegar**, and 1 tablespoon of **extra virgin olive oil** into a jam jar with a pinch of **sea salt and freshly ground black pepper** • Put the lid on the jar and shake well

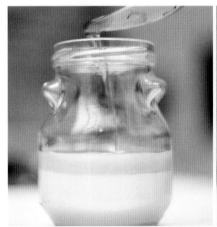
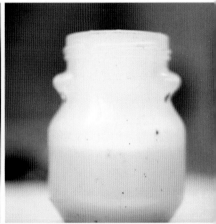

Lemon dressing

Put 6 tablespoons of **extra virgin olive oil** into a jam jar with a pinch of **sea salt and freshly ground black pepper** • Squeeze in the juice of 1 **lemon** • Put the lid on the jar and shake well

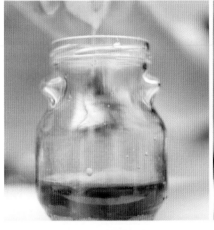
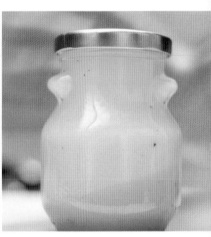

Balsamic dressing

Put 6 tablespoons of **extra virgin olive oil** and 2 tablespoons of **balsamic vinegar** into a jam jar with a pinch of **sea salt and freshly ground black pepper** • Put the lid on the jar and shake well

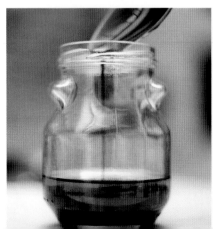
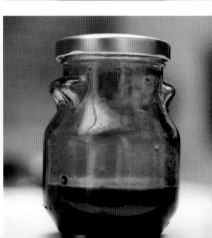

EVOLUTION GREEN SALAD

The idea behind this evolution salad is to empower you with the basic confidence to move your cooking on – to be able to see that a plain, simple salad can be absolutely fantastic if put together well. Each stage adds just one more element into the mix, evolving it into something a little more interesting each time.

serves 4

1) Get yourself 1 **butterhead lettuce** • Click the leaves off, discarding any limp or discolored outer ones • Wash the leaves and spin them dry • If ready to serve, put them into a bowl and lightly drizzle over 2 tablespoons of any of the **jam jar dressings** from pages 106–7 • If you want to add more, move on to the next steps ...

2) Heat a frying pan on a medium heat and add 4 slices of **pancetta or smoked bacon, preferably free-range or organic** • Cook for a few minutes, turning a couple of times, until sizzling and golden • If you're taking your salad further, remove the slices from the pan and put to one side so they stay crispy until ready to serve • If you're ready to tuck in, just drape the warm slices over the lettuce and serve

3) Carefully wipe the pan with a ball of paper towels and put it back on a medium heat • Add a handful of **pine nuts** and toast them for a couple of minutes, until just golden brown • Sprinkle them over the salad

4) Get a small chunk of **Parmesan cheese** and use a speed peeler to carefully shave strips of it over the salad

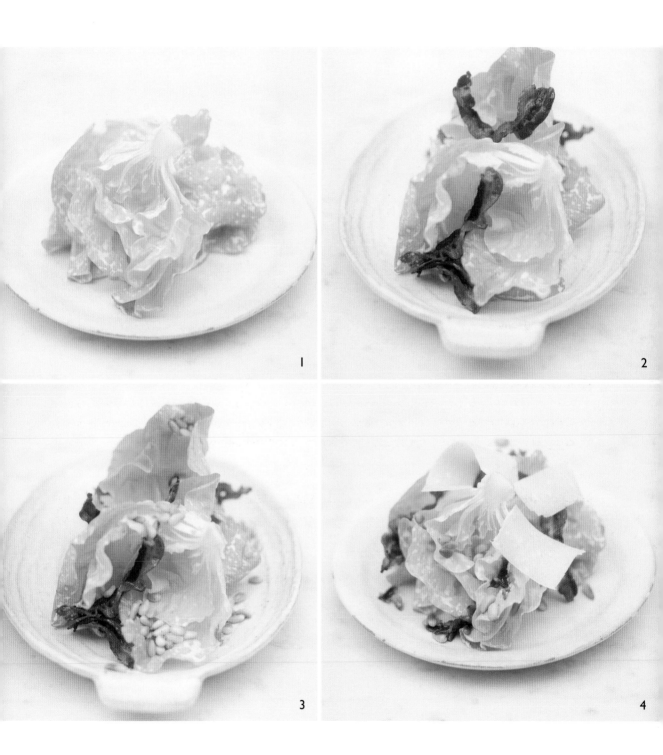

1 2 3 4

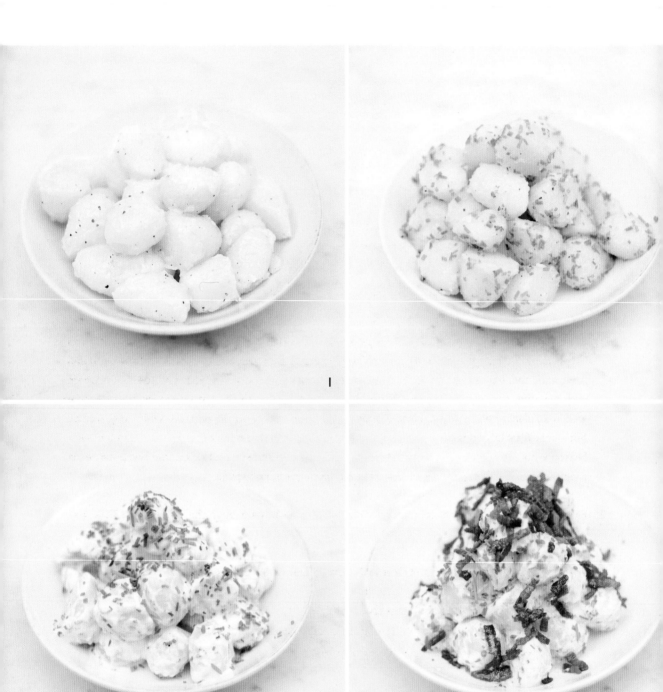

1

3

EVOLUTION POTATO SALAD

Everyone clearly loves potato salad, as we buy the ready-prepared stuff in huge amounts from our grocery stores. The sad thing is that as a result we've become used to the boring, almost stale taste of it: there's nothing remotely exciting about it and it's expensive too. Try making a fresh potato salad and you won't buy ready-prepared again! Not only will it keep for a week in your refrigerator, but you can add all sorts of things to it: from soft herbs like basil, dill, parsley, tarragon, marjoram, celery leaves, and thyme tips to lemon juice, yogurt, pieces of crispy bacon, freshly grated or jarred horseradish, chopped celery … the list goes on! Serve it alongside cold meats, cheeses, or smoked salmon. Also ideal when you're having a barbecue on a hot summer's day.

serves 4

1) Bring a pan of **salted water** to a boil • Peel 1¾ pounds of **baby potatoes** and chop any larger ones in half, leaving the smaller ones whole • When the water is boiling, add the potatoes to the pan and bring back to a boil for about 10 to 15 minutes, depending on the size of your potatoes • Test them with the point of a knife to make sure they're cooked through • As soon as they're ready, drain them well in a colander and put them into a bowl • The trick is to dress the potatoes while they are still hot – mix 6 tablespoons of **extra virgin olive oil** and 2 tablespoons of **lemon juice** in a bowl • Season with **sea salt and freshly ground black pepper** and stir well • Toss the hot potatoes in the dressing • Serve right away, as it is, or move on to the next steps …

2) Finely chop a small bunch of **fresh chives** and sprinkle them over the potatoes • Toss well before serving

3) Toss the dressed potato salad and chives with the zest of 1 **lemon** and ¼ cup of **natural yogurt**

4) Put a frying pan on the heat and add a splash of **olive oil** • Thinly cut slices of **smoked bacon or pancetta, preferably free-range or organic**, into small pieces and add to the pan • Toss and cook for 2 to 3 minutes, or until the bacon is crispy and golden • Remove from the heat • Sprinkle over your potato salad and serve

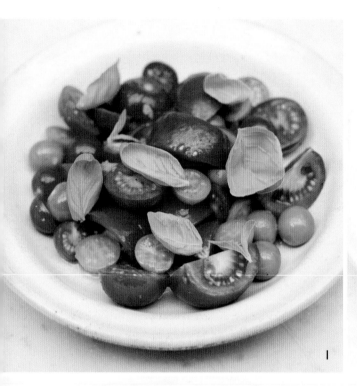

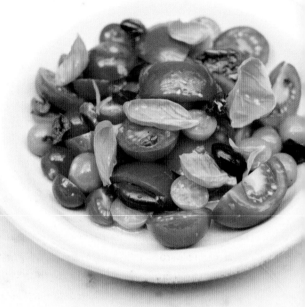

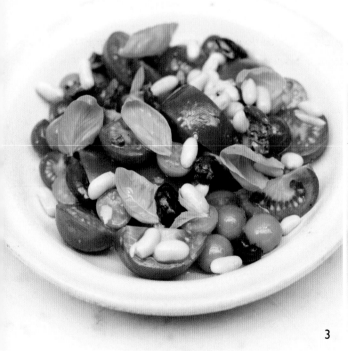

1

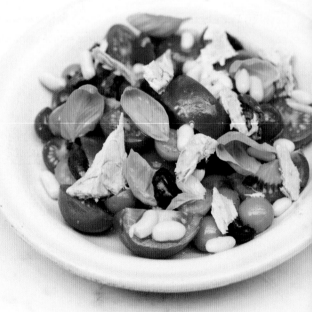

3

EVOLUTION TOMATO SALAD

For this salad, the key is to use lovely ripe tomatoes. Pick bright red ones that smell delicious and come away from the stalks easily. Choose different sizes and colors if they're available, and just chop them up, leaving any smaller ones whole.

serves 4

1) Get yourself about 1½ pounds of **ripe grape or cherry, vine, and regular tomatoes** • Cut the larger tomatoes into wedges, halve the grape or cherry tomatoes, and leave the smaller ones whole • Put them into a bowl with 6 tablespoons of **extra virgin olive oil** and 2 tablespoons of **red wine vinegar** • Toss well to coat all the tomatoes with the dressing • Pick the leaves off a few sprigs of **fresh basil** and scatter them over the salad • Season really well with **sea salt and freshly ground black pepper**

2) Put a large handful of **black olives** on a clean surface and press down on them with the palm of your hand to remove the pits • Discard the pits and add the olives to the salad • Mix up well in a bowl before serving on plates

3) Drain a 15-ounce can of **cannellini beans** in a colander and add to the tomato salad • Mix up well to coat everything in the dressing

4) Drain a small can or jar of **tuna**, break the fish into small flakes or chunks, and scatter over the salad

EVOLUTION CUCUMBER SALAD

When it comes to making any salad using cucumber, it's a really good idea to remember to peel the cucumber and scoop out the seeds first. This will make the salad less watery and much more crunchy and fresh.

serves 4–6

1) Peel 2 **cucumbers**, using a speed peeler, chop off the ends, and halve them lengthways • Use a teaspoon to gently scoop the seeds out, and discard them • Chop the cucumber into irregular bite-size chunks and place in a bowl • Season with a good pinch of **sea salt and freshly ground black pepper** • Add 6 tablespoons of **extra virgin olive oil** and 2 tablespoons of **lemon juice** and mix well • Pick some leaves off a few sprigs of **fresh mint** and roughly chop them • Add them to the salad and toss together • Serve the salad simply as it is, or let it evolve …

2) Add a large tablespoon of **natural yogurt** to the cucumber salad • Toss until well coated and serve drizzled with a little **extra virgin olive oil**

3) Put a large handful of **black olives** on a clean surface and press down on them with the palm of your hand to remove the pits • Discard the pits and add the olives to the salad • Toss together well

4) Halve 1 **fresh red or green chile** lengthways, seed, and finely chop • Scatter over your cucumber salad and serve drizzled with a little **extra virgin olive oil**

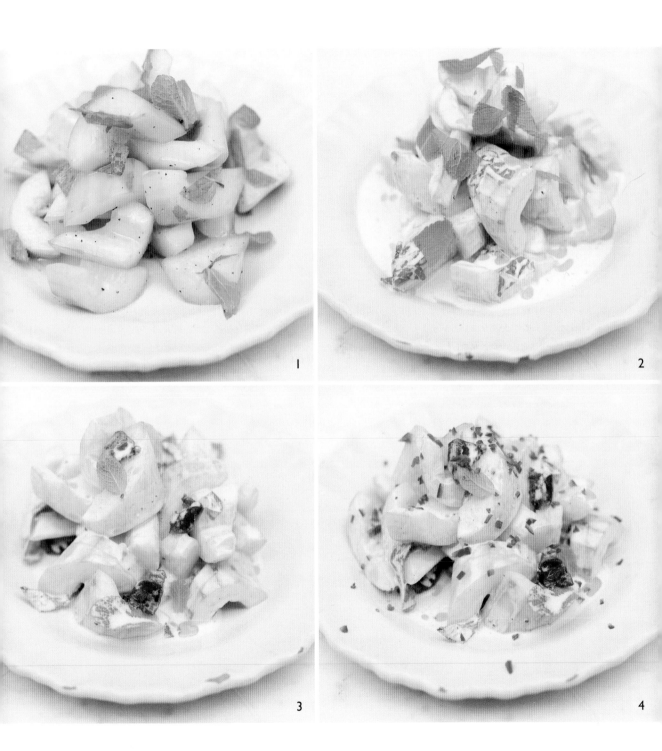

EVOLUTION CARROT SALAD

This carrot salad is so quick to make and is absolutely delicious. Look out for all the different colored carrots you can get these days: yellow, purple, even white ones can make a humble salad extra cool. Either try out my different evolution suggestions, or try a few of your own ideas – use your imagination and see where it gets you.

serves 4

1) Peel 4 or 5 large **carrots** and grate them into a bowl • Pick the leaves off a few sprigs of **fresh mint** and **cilantro** and finely chop them – you can also use **fresh chives** • Add them to the bowl and toss with the carrots • Season with a pinch of **sea salt and freshly ground black pepper** • Add 6 tablespoons of **extra virgin olive oil** and 2 tablespoons of **lemon juice** and mix well • Serve right away, as it is, or let it start evolving . . .

2) Put a good handful of **mixed seeds** into a hot, dry frying pan and toss and toast them for a minute • Once toasted, sprinkle the seeds on to your salad • Peel 2 or 3 small **clementines** and cut into nice thick slices • Either toss these slices into your salad, or lay a few slices on a serving platter and pile the carrot salad on top

3) Get yourself 1 or 2 ready-to-eat **pappadams** and break them up into small pieces • Either toss into the salad or sprinkle over the top

4) And for the full Monty, crumble over some **feta or goat's cheese** before tucking in!

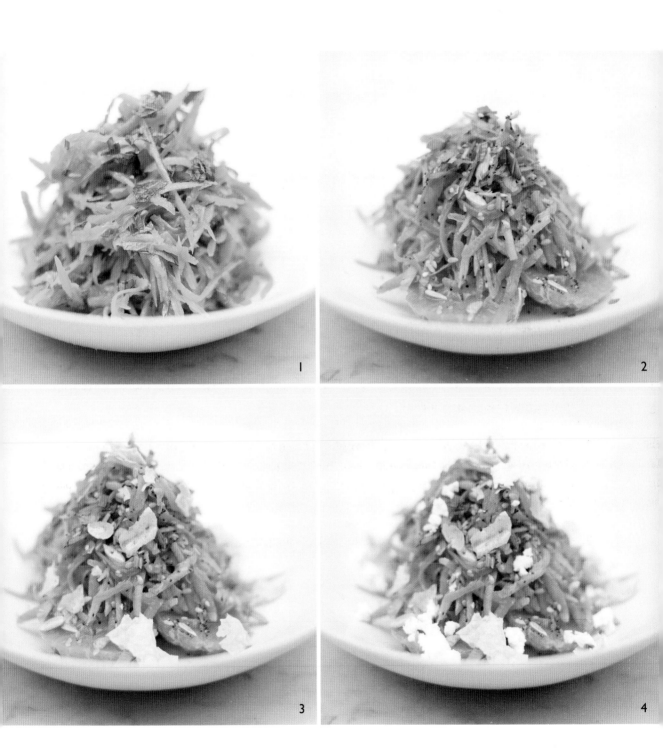

1

2

3

4

THE PHILOSOPHY OF A GREAT SALAD, PICK-AND-MIX STYLE

The idea of me presenting this salad to you like this is to give you the general philosophy behind creating a great, great salad so you can start making your own. When you go shopping and then go to make the salad, pick and mix different elements like soft and crunchy lettuce, herbs, veggies, cheese, and various toppings. Once you've done that, simply mix them together, season, and dress the salad. If you do this, the end result every time will be incredible. There are no rules, just start picking and mixing. Even using just 3 or 4 ingredients will give you a salad that rocks.

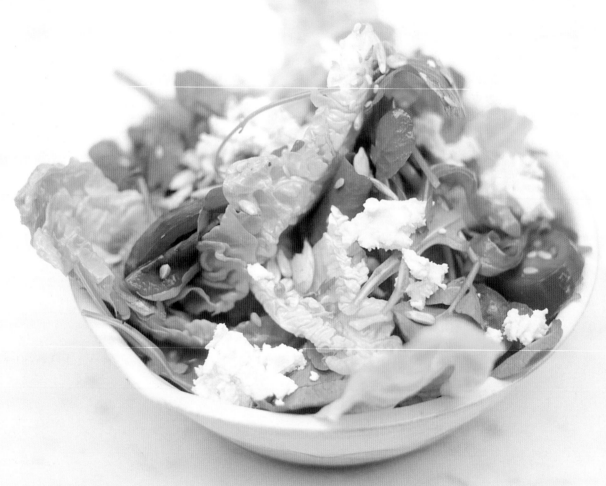

Choose an ingredient from each row on the opposite page • Wash and spin dry the soft, and crunchy leaves • Pick the herby leaves off their stalks • Finely slice or peel the veggies and shave, tear, or crumble up the cheese • Toss everything together in a large bowl • Dress simply with one of the jam jar dressings from pages 106–7 and season with a good pinch of sea salt and freshly ground black pepper if needed • Divide the salad between your serving bowls and sprinkle over your chosen topping

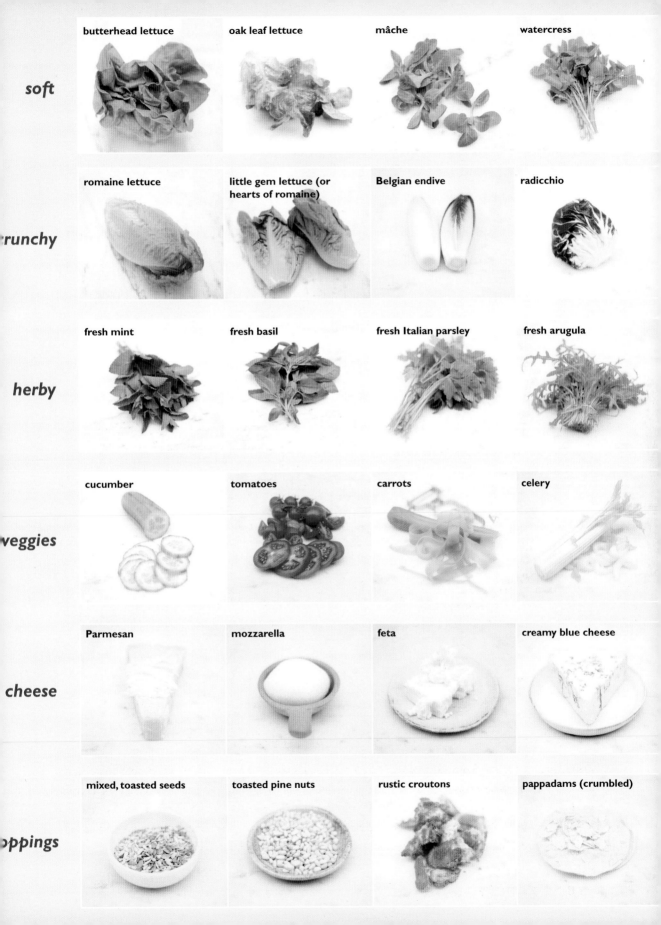

soft
- butterhead lettuce
- oak leaf lettuce
- mâche
- watercress

crunchy
- romaine lettuce
- little gem lettuce (or hearts of romaine)
- Belgian endive
- radicchio

herby
- fresh mint
- fresh basil
- fresh Italian parsley
- fresh arugula

veggies
- cucumber
- tomatoes
- carrots
- celery

cheese
- Parmesan
- mozzarella
- feta
- creamy blue cheese

toppings
- mixed, toasted seeds
- toasted pine nuts
- rustic croutons
- pappadams (crumbled)

THE CHOPPED SALAD FAMILY

Chopped salads are incredibly simple to make – you have to give them a go. If nothing else, they can offer you some chopping practice, so why not make something tasty while you're practicing your knife skills? Anyone can make these salads – just make sure you use a good, sharp chef's knife and your biggest chopping board – and watch your fingers!

What I want to show you here is that the sky's the limit when it comes to the different ingredients you can add to a chopped salad – you can use whatever's available. The only rule I would give you is to always include a couple of handfuls of crunchy lettuce to give your salad a really good texture. Try out different things, and don't feel obliged to use the same old stuff all the time. Bell peppers, tomatoes, herb sprigs, different types of cheese ... you can get any or all of these into a chopped salad.

Everyday green chopped salad

serves 4

4 scallions
½ a cucumber
a handful of fresh basil leaves
2 small, just ripe avocados
1 butterhead lettuce
Large handful sprouted cress or alfalfa

optional: 2 ounces Cheddar cheese
extra virgin olive oil
red wine vinegar
English mustard
sea salt and freshly ground black pepper

Get yourself a big chopping board and a large sharp knife • It's best to start by chopping the harder, crunchier veggies first, so trim and chop your scallions and slice your cucumber • Slice your basil • Bring it all into the center of the board, and continue chopping and mixing together • Halve your avocados around the big pit • Carefully remove the pit and peel the skin off • Add the avocado flesh, lettuce leaves, and cress or alfalfa to the board • Crumble over the cheese, if using, and continue chopping • When everything is well chopped, you'll have a big mound of salad on the board • Make a well in the middle and drizzle in 6 tablespoons of extra virgin olive oil and 2 tablespoons of red wine vinegar • Add a teaspoon of English mustard and a good pinch of salt and pepper • Mix up so everything gets well coated and serve on the board or in a bowl

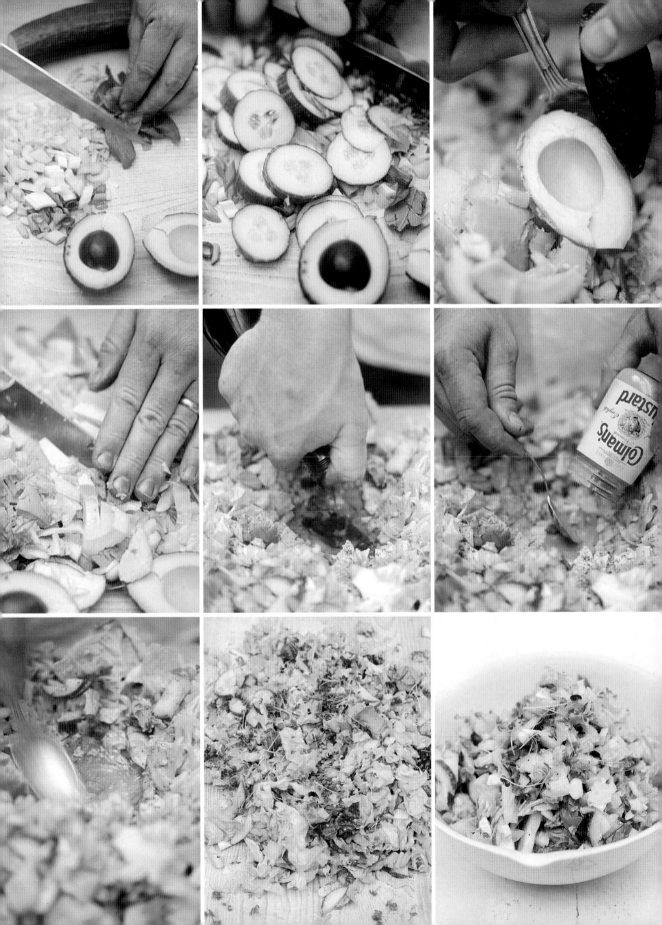

Posh chopped salad

serves 4

1 carrot

1 bulb of fennel

a small handful of radishes

1 Romaine lettuce

2 white Belgian endives

8 ounces smoked salmon

extra virgin olive oil

1 lemon

sea salt and freshly ground black pepper

a small bunch of fresh dill

Get yourself a large chopping board and a large sharp knife • Start chopping the harder, crunchier veggies first • Peel, trim, and chop your carrot, fennel (plus its herby tops) and radishes • Bring it all into the center of the board and continue chopping and mixing together • Add the lettuce and endive leaves and chop them up too • When everything is well chopped, you'll have a big mound of salad on the board • Slice the salmon up into small pieces and mix in • Make a well in the middle and drizzle in 6 tablespoons of olive oil, 2 tablespoons of lemon juice, and a good pinch of salt and pepper • Mix up so everything gets dressed, sprinkle with some chopped dill, and serve straight from the board or in a bowl

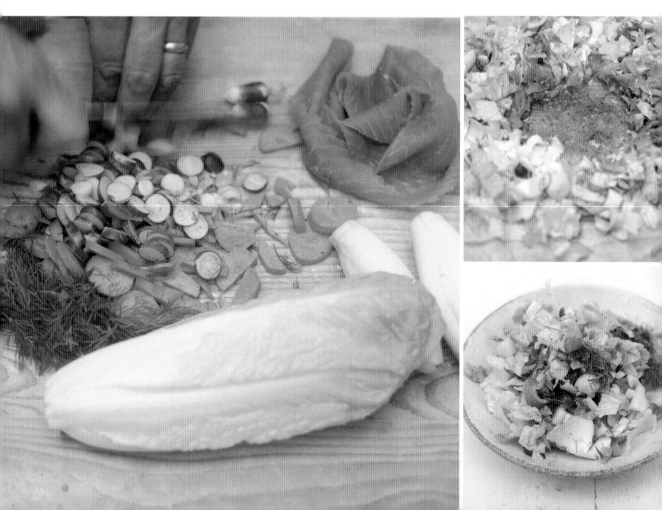

Mediterranean chopped salad

serves 4

a small handful of black olives

½ a red onion

1 red or green chile

3 firm ripe tomatoes

1 Romaine lettuce

a bunch of fresh basil

extra virgin olive oil

balsamic vinegar

sea salt and freshly ground black pepper

Get yourself a large chopping board and a large sharp knife • Press down on the olives with the palm of your hand to squeeze the pits out, then discard the pits • Start chopping the harder, crunchier veggies first • Peel and slice your onion, halve, seed, and finely chop your chile • Chop the olives and the tomatoes • Bring it all into the center of the board and continue chopping and mixing together • Add the lettuce leaves and basil and chop them up too • When everything is well chopped, you'll have a big mound of salad on the board • Make a well in the middle and drizzle in 6 tablespoons of olive oil, 2 tablespoons of balsamic vinegar, and a good pinch of salt and pepper • Mix up so everything gets dressed and serve straight from the board or in a bowl

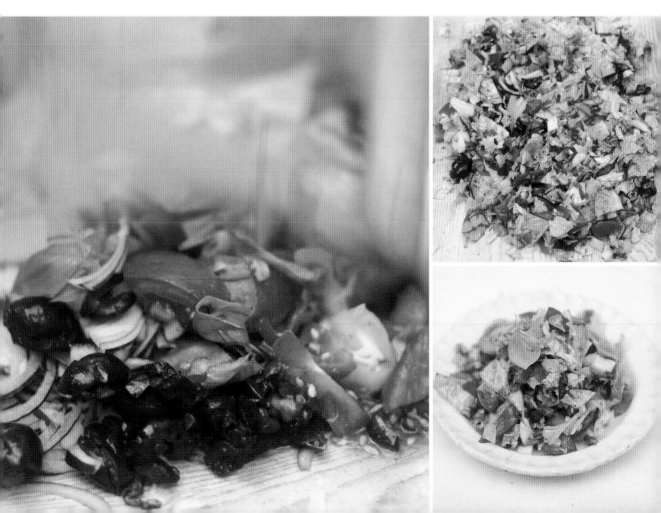

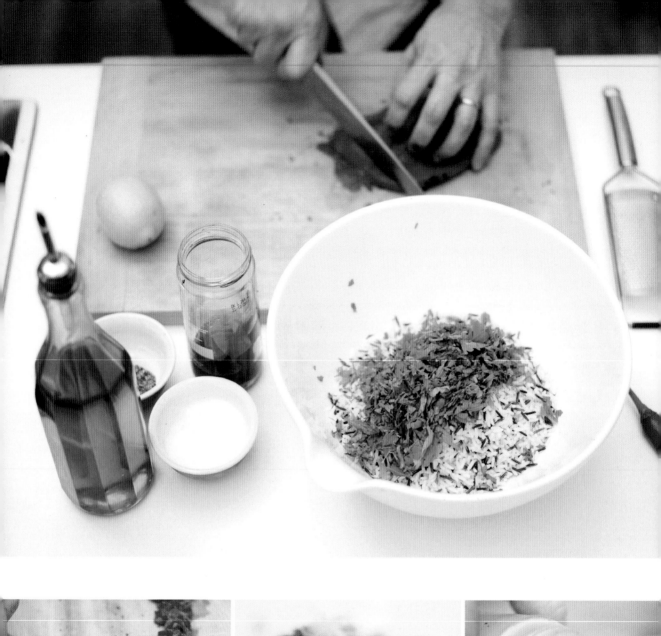

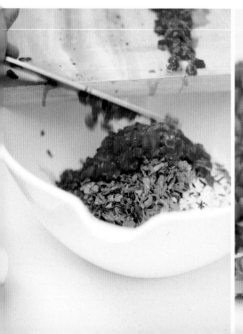

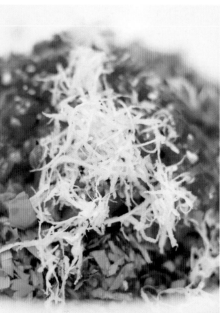

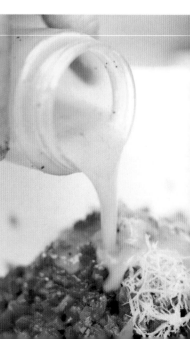

RICE SALAD

Ready-prepared rice salad, like potato salad and coleslaw, is really popular but largely miserable and bland. Have a go at this recipe and you won't go back to buying containers from the grocery store. First, feel free to play with different rice grains – they have a variety of tastes, colors, and textures, which can be a bonus in a rice salad, so have a look around when you're shopping. The big thing to remember, though, is to use good olive oil, a touch of lemon juice, and to get some spice and sweetness into the salad with chiles and roasted red bell peppers (you can use sun-dried tomatoes if you don't have any peppers). You'll have a salad that looks and tastes great. Best eaten at room temperature rather than straight from the refrigerator.

serves 4

sea salt and freshly ground black pepper
1 ¼ cups mixed long grain and wild rice
a few sprigs of fresh basil
a few sprigs of fresh mint
a few sprigs of fresh Italian parsley

8 ounces roasted red bell peppers from a jar or deli counter
½ a fresh red or green chile
¼ cup lemon dressing (see page 107)
1 lemon

Bring a large pan of salted water to a boil • Add the rice and cook it according to the package instructions • Once cooked, drain the rice in a strainer and spread it out on a tray to help it cool down quickly • Meanwhile, pick all the herb leaves off the stalks • Finely chop the bell peppers • Halve, seed, and finely chop your chile • Make your lemon dressing • Put your cooled rice into a big serving bowl • Finely chop your herb leaves and add them to the bowl, together with the bell peppers and chile • Zest over your lemon, add the dressing, and mix well • Taste, add salt and pepper if you think it needs it, and serve

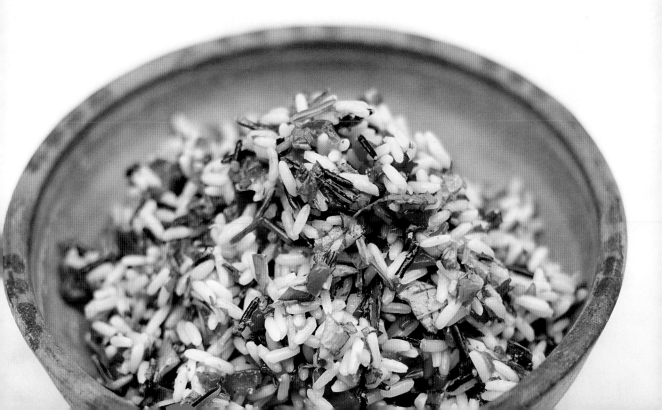

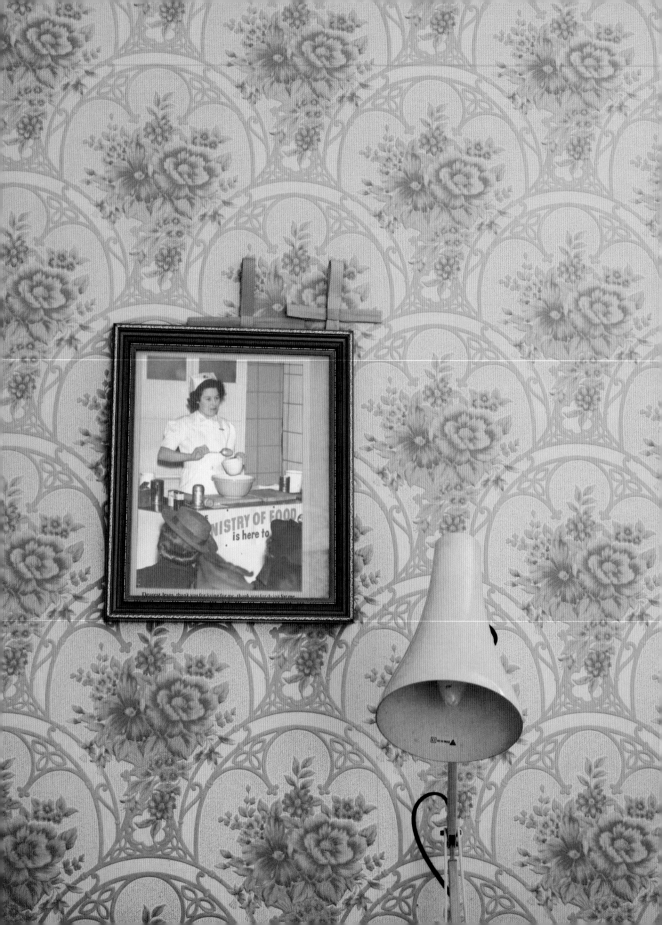

Simple soups

I think it's really important that everyone, from beginners to more advanced cooks, knows how to make a good, simple soup. Ready-made soups, from those in cans to those in Tetrapak cartons, can be found on the shelves and in the refrigerated sections at grocery stores, convenience stores, even gas stations and train station booths – soup is big business! Quite a lot of these ready-made ones are of reasonable quality and taste quite good. However, nothing is better than the real thing, so in this chapter I want to show you how easy it is to turn a bunch of cheap vegetables into a delicious homemade soup.

I think the key to a good soup is cooking the vegetables for the shortest amount of time that they need in order to be soft enough to be liquidized or eaten. This will give you not only better flavor but lots more nutritional value, as the goodness doesn't all cook away. This important short cooking time is much harder for commercial soup operators to achieve because they're cooking in massive containers, but it's easy for us to do at home. Great news, as we all love quick cooking!

So, the idea behind this chapter is simple – one base soup recipe taken in lots of different ways. Once you've got your head around it and made a few, I'm sure you'll be making up your own flavor combinations. And look at page 141, where I give you ideas to "pimp up your soup" with some lovely toppings and flavors.

SPRING VEGETABLE AND BEAN SOUP

This is a lovely soup – very simple and traditional. If you want to give it an Italian vibe, simply add a can of diced tomatoes, the torn leaves from a few sprigs of fresh basil, and some broken spaghetti – delicious.

serves 6–8

2 carrots / 2 celery stalks / 2 medium onions / 2 cloves of garlic / 1¾ quarts chicken or vegetable broth, preferably organic / olive oil / 1 x 15-ounce can of cannellini beans / 2 cups cauliflower / 2 cups broccoli / 7 cups (7 ounces) spinach leaves / 2 large ripe tomatoes / sea salt and freshly ground black pepper / extra virgin olive oil

To make your soup

Peel and roughly slice the carrots • Slice the celery • Peel and roughly chop the onions • Peel and slice the garlic • Put the broth in a saucepan and heat until boiling • Put a large saucepan on a medium heat and add 2 tablespoons of olive oil • Add all your chopped and sliced ingredients and mix together with a wooden spoon • Cook for around 10 to 15 minutes with the lid askew, until the carrots have softened but are still holding their shape, and the onion is lightly golden • Meanwhile, drain your beans • Break up the cauliflower and broccoli into small florets • Roughly chop the spinach • Quarter the tomatoes, removing any stalks • Add the boiling broth to the vegetables in the pan • Add your cannellini beans, cauliflower, broccoli, and quartered tomatoes • Give the soup a good stir and bring to a boil • Reduce the heat and simmer for 10 minutes with the lid on

To serve your soup

Add the spinach to the pan and cook for a further 30 seconds, then remove the pan from the heat • If you like your soup a little less chunky, you can take out half of it, blend it using an immersion blender or liquidizer, then stir it back into the pan • Season carefully with salt and pepper • Ladle the soup into serving bowls and finish with a drizzle of extra virgin olive oil • See page 141 for some great soup topping ideas

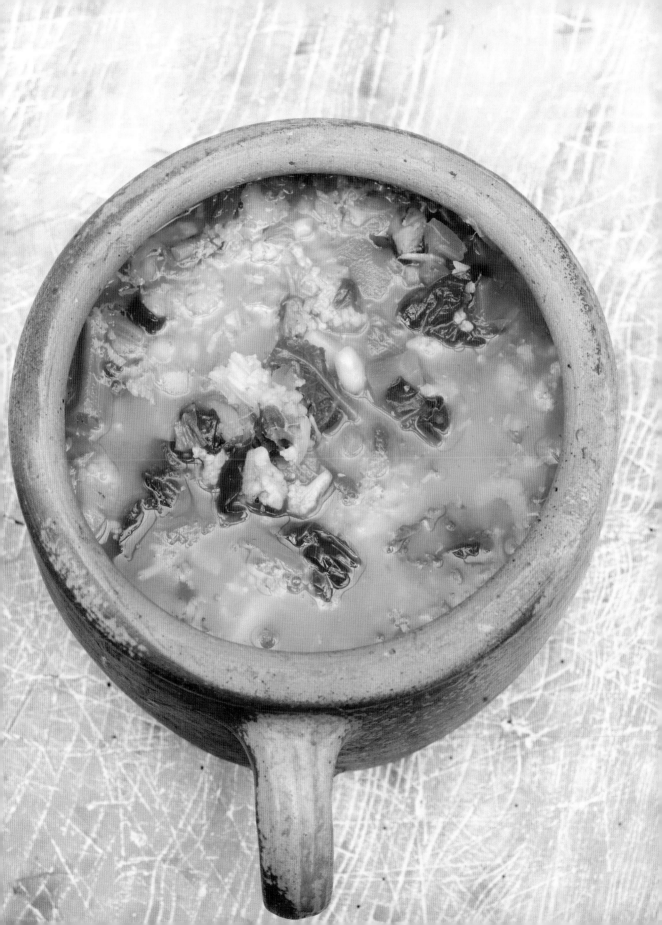

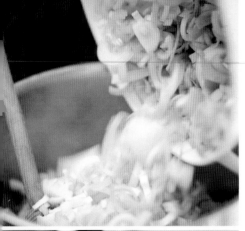
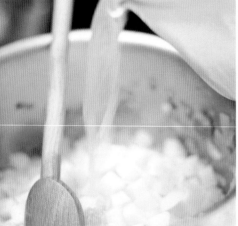

LEEK AND POTATO SOUP

What a classic soup! Usually eaten hot, it's also surprisingly delicious eaten refrigerator-cold on a summer's day with a squeeze of lemon juice and a dollop of natural yogurt.

serves 6–8
2 carrots / 2 celery stalks / 2 medium onions / 1 pound leeks / 2 cloves of garlic / 1¾ quarts chicken or vegetable broth, preferably organic / 1 pound potatoes / olive oil / sea salt and freshly ground black pepper

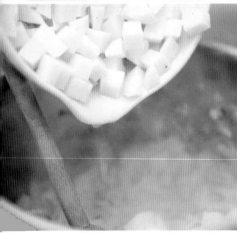

To make your soup
Peel and roughly slice the carrots • Slice the celery • Peel and roughly chop the onions • Cut the ends off the leeks, quarter them lengthways, wash them under running water, and cut them into ¼-inch slices • Peel and slice the garlic • Put the broth in a saucepan and heat until boiling • Place a large saucepan on a high heat and add 2 tablespoons of olive oil • Add all your chopped and sliced ingredients and mix together with a wooden spoon • Cook for around 10 to 15 minutes with the lid askew, until the carrots have softened, but are still holding their shape, and the onion and leeks are lightly golden • Peel the potatoes and cut them into ¼-inch dice • Add the boiling broth to the vegetables • Add your potatoes • Give the soup a good stir and bring to a boil • Reduce the heat and simmer for 10 minutes with the lid on

To serve your soup
Remove the pan from the heat • Season with salt and pepper • Serve like this or pulse until smooth using an immersion blender or liquidizer • Divide between your serving bowls • See page 141 for some great soup topping ideas

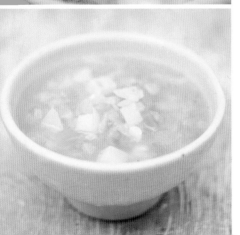

SWEET POTATO AND CHORIZO SOUP

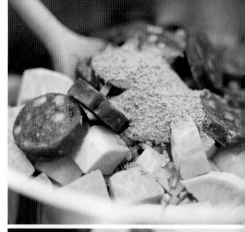

Sweet potatoes or yams have a great flavor. If you can't get hold of any, you can use butternut squash instead. Top with as much chile as you can take, because it's a great flavor to use with squash. If you need to lessen the heat a bit, add a dollop of yogurt to balance it out.

serves 6–8
2 carrots / 2 celery stalks / 2 medium onions / 2 cloves of garlic / 1 ¾ pounds sweet potatoes / 7 ounces chorizo sausage / a small bunch of fresh parsley / 1 ¾ quarts chicken or vegetable broth, preferably organic / olive oil / 1 heaped teaspoon curry powder / sea salt and freshly ground black pepper / 1 fresh red chile

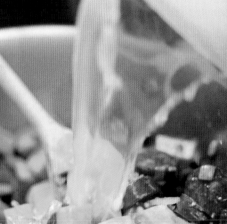

To make your soup
Peel and roughly slice the carrots • Slice the celery • Peel and roughly chop the onions • Peel and slice the garlic • Peel and chop the sweet potatoes • Slice the chorizo • Finely chop the parsley leaves and stalks • Put the broth in a saucepan and heat until boiling • Put a large pan on a high heat and add 2 tablespoons of olive oil • Add all your chopped and sliced ingredients with the curry powder and mix together with a wooden spoon • Cook for around 10 to 15 minutes with the lid askew, until the carrots have softened but are still holding their shape, and the onion is lightly golden • Add the boiling broth to the vegetables • Give the soup a good stir and bring to a boil • Reduce the heat and simmer for 10 minutes, until the sweet potato is cooked through

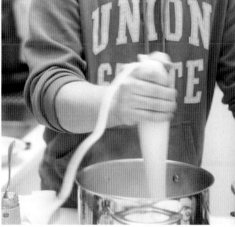

To serve your soup
Season with salt and pepper • Using an immersion blender or liquidizer, pulse the soup until smooth and scatter over a little finely chopped chile • Divide between your serving bowls and tuck in

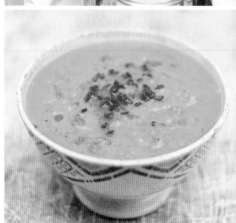

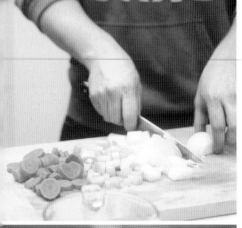

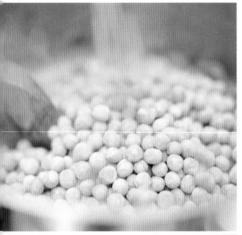

PEA AND MINT SOUP

A delicious soup which is lovely hot, or cold with a squeeze of lemon juice in the summer. My wife likes hers with a portion of fries on the side, to dip into the soup – naughty but nice!

serves 6–8

2 carrots / 2 celery stalks / 2 medium onions / 2 cloves of garlic / 1 ¾ quarts chicken or vegetable broth, preferably organic / olive oil / 5½ cups frozen peas / a small bunch of fresh mint / sea salt and freshly ground black pepper / optional: ¾ pound cooked ham, preferably free-range or organic

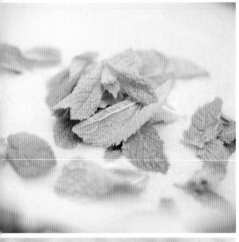

To make your soup

Peel and roughly slice the carrots • Slice the celery • Peel and roughly chop the onions • Peel and slice the garlic • Put the broth in a saucepan and heat until boiling • Put a large saucepan on a medium heat and add 2 tablespoons of olive oil • Add all your chopped and sliced ingredients to the pan and mix together with a wooden spoon • Cook for around 10 to 15 minutes with the lid askew, until the carrots have softened but are still holding their shape, and the onion is lightly golden • Add the boiling broth to the vegetables • Add your peas • Give the soup a good stir and bring to a boil • Once boiling, allow to simmer for 10 minutes • Meanwhile, pick your mint leaves

To serve your soup

When the peas have softened, remove the pan from the heat • Season with salt and pepper and add the mint leaves • Using an immersion blender or liquidizer, pulse the soup until smooth • If using ham, chop it up and stir in • Heat through before dividing between your serving bowls • Really nice served with a toasted slice of ciabatta, drizzled with extra virgin olive oil

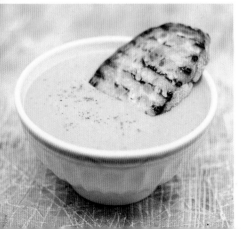

TOMATO SOUP

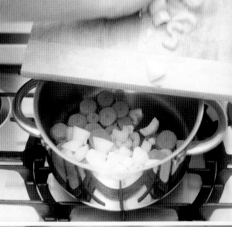

A wonderful classic soup – if you get the seasoning right, you'll be surprised at the difference between your homemade version and the canned stuff. It's also great to use as a quick base sauce for dishes such as cannelloni or lasagne.

serves 6–8

2 carrots / 2 celery stalks / 2 medium onions / 2 cloves of garlic / 1¾ quarts chicken or vegetable broth, preferably organic / olive oil / 2 x 14-ounce cans of plum tomatoes / 6 large ripe tomatoes / a small bunch of fresh basil / sea salt and freshly ground black pepper

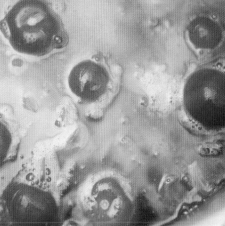

To make your soup

Peel and roughly slice the carrots • Slice the celery • Peel and roughly chop the onions • Peel and slice the garlic • Put the broth in a saucepan and heat until boiling • Put a large saucepan on a medium heat and add 2 tablespoons of olive oil • Add all your chopped and sliced ingredients and mix together with a wooden spoon • Cook for around 10 to 15 minutes with the lid askew, until the carrots have softened but are still holding their shape, and the onion is lightly golden • Add the boiling broth to the pan with your canned and fresh whole tomatoes, including the green stalks that may still be attached to some of them (these give an amazing flavor – trust me!) • Give it a good stir and bring to a boil • Reduce the heat and simmer for 10 minutes with the lid on • Meanwhile, pick your basil leaves

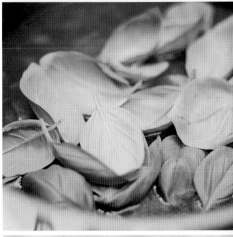

To serve your soup

Remove the pan from the heat • Season with salt and pepper and add the basil leaves • Using an immersion blender or liquidizer, pulse the soup until smooth • Season again before dividing between your serving bowls • See page 141 for some great soup topping ideas

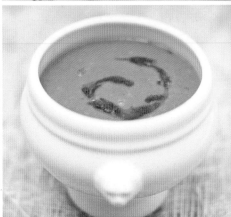

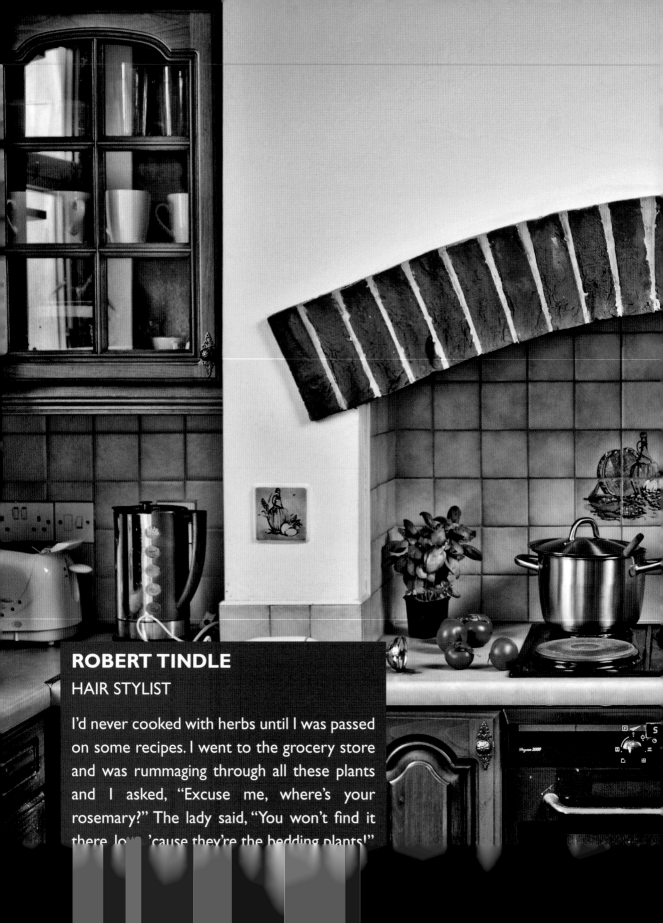

ROBERT TINDLE
HAIR STYLIST

I'd never cooked with herbs until I was passed on some recipes. I went to the grocery store and was rummaging through all these plants and I asked, "Excuse me, where's your rosemary?" The lady said, "You won't find it there lo... 'cause they're the bedding plants!"

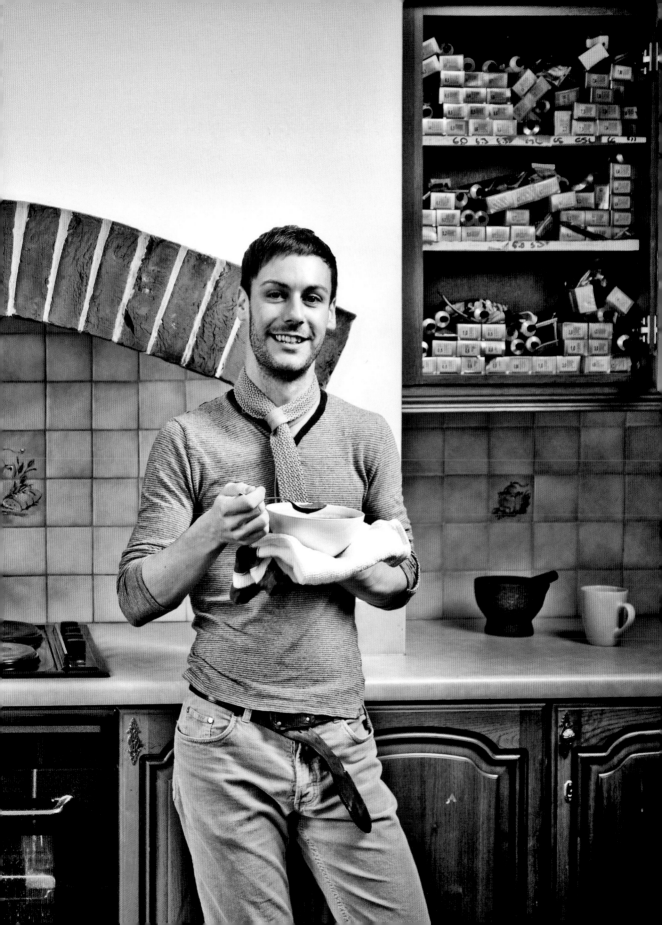

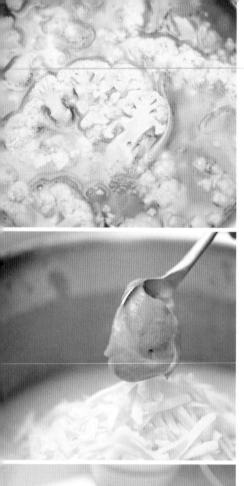
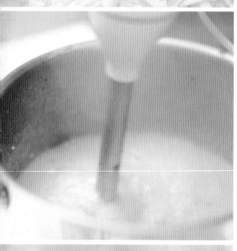
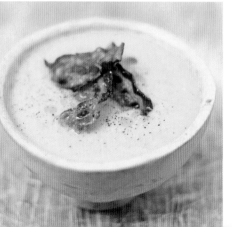

CAULIFLOWER CHEESE SOUP

What a vegetable dish, and what a soup! Try this once and you'll be hooked. The better the quality of the cheese, the better the soup will be. Try an artisan-produced Cheddar, available in farmers' markets and some grocery stores.

serves 6–8

2 carrots / 2 celery stalks / 2 medium onions / 2 cloves of garlic / 8 cups cauliflower florets / olive oil / 1¾ quarts chicken or vegetable broth, preferably organic / sea salt and freshly ground black pepper / 8 ounces Cheddar cheese / 1 teaspoon English mustard / optional: nutmeg

To make your soup

Peel and roughly slice the carrots • Slice the celery • Peel and roughly chop the onions • Peel and slice the garlic • Cut your cauliflower into ½ inch slices • Put the broth in a saucepan and heat until boiling • Put a large saucepan on a medium heat and add 2 tablespoons of olive oil • Add all your chopped and sliced ingredients and mix together with a wooden spoon • Cook for around 10 to 15 minutes with the lid askew, until the carrots have softened but are still holding their shape, and the onion is lightly golden • Grate the Cheddar into a bowl and put to one side for later • Add the boiling broth to the vegetables • Give the soup a good stir and bring to a boil • Reduce the heat and simmer for 10 minutes with the lid on

To serve your soup

Remove the pan from the heat • Season with salt and pepper and add the cheese and mustard • Using an immersion blender or liquidizer, pulse the soup until silky smooth • Divide between your serving bowls and grate over some nutmeg, if you like • Lovely topped with some lightly fried crispy bacon, or see page 141 for some other great soup topping ideas

LENTIL AND SPINACH SOUP

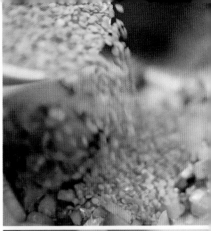

This soup works really well if you make it with yellow split peas or dried green peas, as well as with greens like spinach, cabbage, and Swiss chard.

serves 6–8

2 carrots / 2 celery stalks / 2 medium onions / 2 cloves of garlic / 1 ¾ quarts chicken or vegetable broth, preferably organic / olive oil / a thumb-sized piece of fresh root ginger / ½–1 fresh red chile, to your taste / 10 grape or cherry tomatoes / 2 cups red lentils / 7 cups (7 ounces) spinach / sea salt and freshly ground black pepper / 1 cup natural yogurt

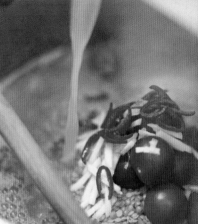

To make your soup

Peel and roughly slice the carrots • Slice the celery • Peel and roughly chop the onions • Peel and slice the garlic • Put the broth in a saucepan and heat until boiling • Put a large saucepan on a medium heat and add 2 tablespoons of olive oil • Add all your chopped and sliced ingredients and mix together with a wooden spoon • Cook for around 10 to 15 minutes with the lid askew, until the carrots have softened but are still holding their shape, and the onion is lightly golden • Meanwhile, peel and finely slice the ginger • Seed and slice the chile • Remove the stalks from the grape or cherry tomatoes and slice the tomatoes in half • Add the boiling broth to the pan with the lentils, ginger, chile, and tomatoes • Give the soup a good stir and bring to a boil • Reduce the heat and simmer for 10 minutes with the lid on, or until the lentils are cooked • Add the spinach and continue to cook for 30 seconds

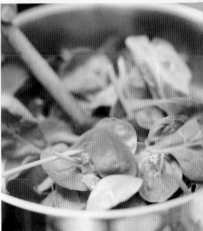

To serve your soup

Season well with salt and pepper • You can now serve the soup just as it is, or, using an immersion blender or liquidizer, pulse until smooth • Divide between your serving bowls • Delicious topped with a dollop of natural yogurt, or see page 141 for some other great soup topping ideas

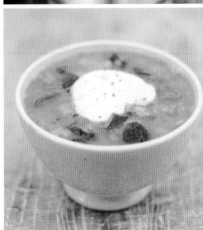

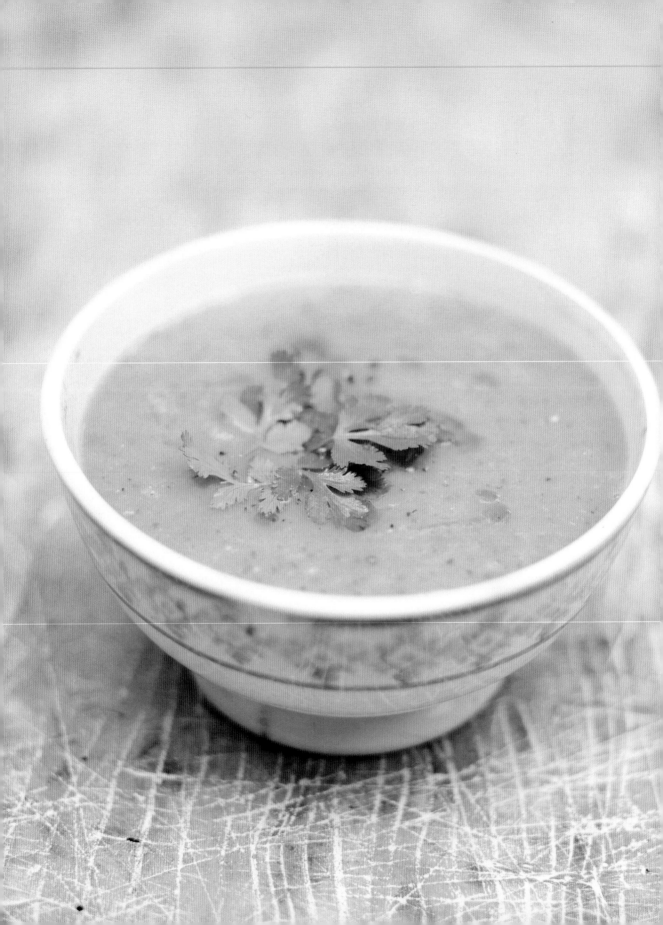

PARSNIP AND GINGER SOUP

This is a great soup with an unusual combination of flavors. The parsnips work fantastically well with the fragrance of the ginger. My own favorite way to serve this is with some crunchy croutons, fried with smoked bacon, scattered over the top.

serves 6–8

2 carrots / 2 celery stalks / 2 medium onions / 1¾ pounds parsnips / a thumb-sized piece of fresh root ginger / 2 cloves of garlic / 1¾ quarts chicken or vegetable broth, preferably organic / olive oil / 4 sprigs of fresh cilantro / sea salt and freshly ground black pepper

To make your soup

Peel and roughly slice the carrots • Slice the celery • Peel and roughly chop the onions, parsnips, and ginger • Peel and slice the garlic • Put the broth in a saucepan and heat until boiling • Put a large saucepan on a medium heat and add 2 tablespoons of olive oil • Add all your chopped and sliced ingredients and mix together with a wooden spoon • Cook for around 10 to 15 minutes with the lid askew, until the carrots have softened but are still holding their shape, and the onion is lightly golden • Add the boiling broth to the vegetables • Give the soup a good stir and bring to a boil • Reduce the heat and simmer for 10 minutes with the lid on • Pick the cilantro leaves and discard the stalks

To serve your soup

Season with salt and pepper • Using an immersion blender or liquidizer, pulse the soup until smooth • Divide between your serving bowls and sprinkle over the cilantro leaves, or see page 141 for some great topping ideas

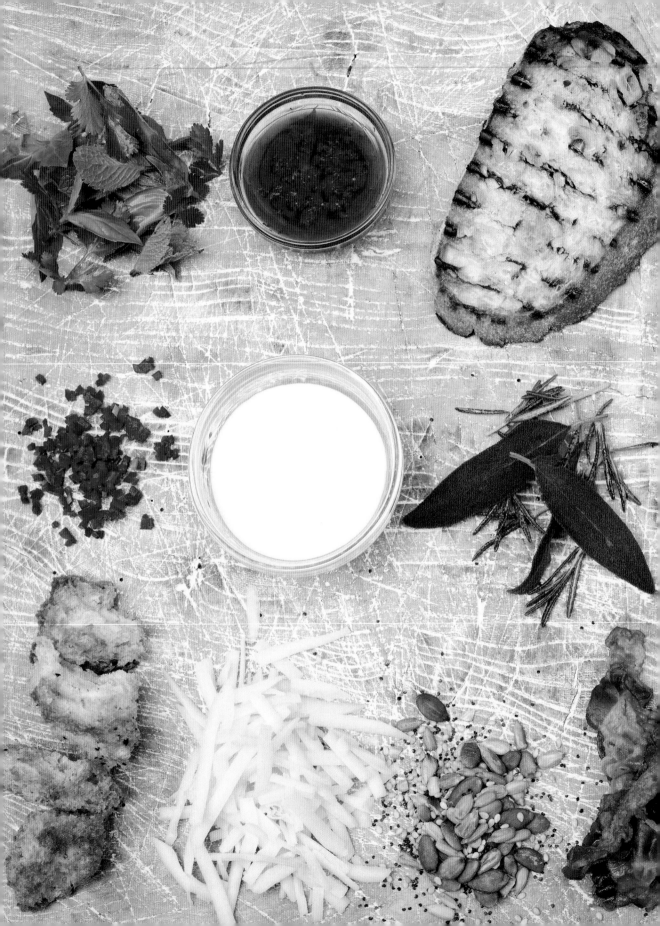

PIMP UP YOUR SOUP

Soup doesn't have to be boring or predictable, so once you've mastered making these easy soups, pimp them up a bit! I'm not going to give you recipes, just a few ideas …

- Try grilling, toasting, or baking chunky croutons or slices of ciabatta bread

- Tear in soft fresh herbs like basil, parsley, and mint

- Try bashing up soft fresh herbs like basil and parsley, and mixing them with some olive oil and lemon juice

- Fry woody herbs like sage, thyme, and rosemary in a little butter and olive oil, until crisp and delicious

- Crunchy bacon (preferably free-range or organic), crumbled over, is always a winner

- Toasted seeds and nuts can be interesting on creamy soups

- Things like chopped fresh chile can add a little heat

- All sorts of different cheeses can be crumbled and grated over, or stirred in

- Try a nice dollop of mascarpone, crème fraîche, or sour cream

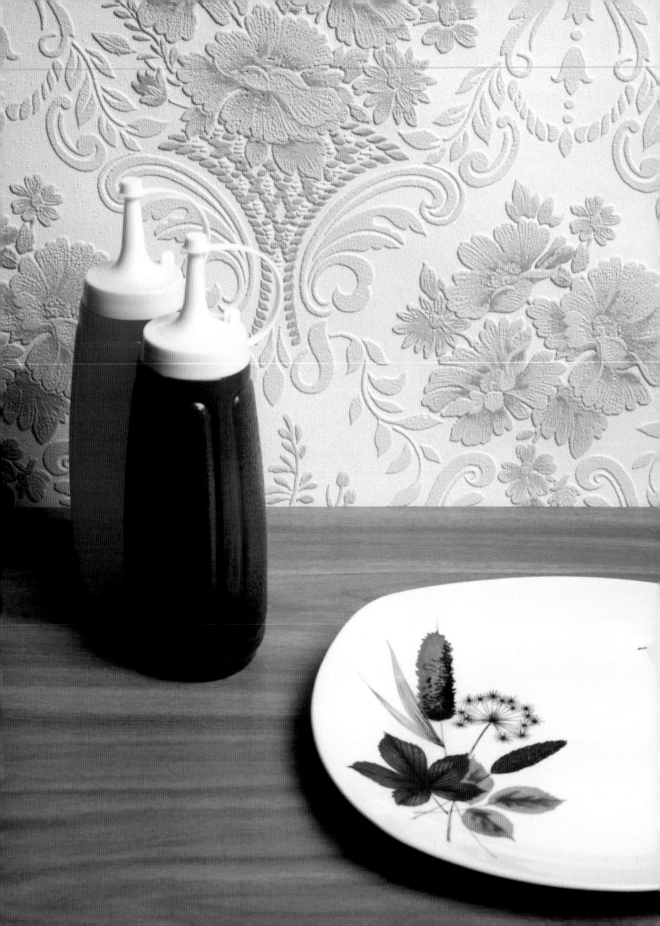

Homely ground beef

Ground meat might not be the most glamorous aspect of the meat world, but it absolutely deserves its own place in this book because it's the biggest-selling area of the meat section in the grocery stores. You buy more of this stuff than anything else. With this in mind, I want to help you understand it a bit more by showing you a whole handful of quick recipes so that you can really make the most of it. A good ground meat dish can put a smile on even the toughest foodie's face!

There are two types of ground meat recipe – you can either mold a drier mixture into burgers or meatballs, or you can stew the meat in liquid, which takes it into the realms of pie fillings and things like Bolognese sauce and chili con carne. Both ways of treating ground meat have had an impact on just about every country I can think of, from the moussaka of Greece to the Bolognese of Italy, to the ground beef and onion pie of England.

Ground meat is cheap – always has been and always will be. Therefore it allows you to get meat into your diet cheaply and regularly and it also means you can look to buy organic, as this is relatively affordable when it comes to ground meat. Most grocery stores actually do have very high standards for ground meat these days. Some of them, and also some butchers, now sell lean ground beef, which means low in fat. If you buy this, you can make some pretty healthy ground meat dishes.

I totally endorse buying and cooking larger batches of ground meat, because there's relatively little difference in the time it takes to cook for 4 or for 16 people. And it's great to be able to bag up stewed beef, or meatballs and burgers, in portioned sandwich bags for freezing. They can be defrosted very quickly and cooked the same day. Real loyal staples to have in your freezer to help you out when ambushed by hungry kids or friends!

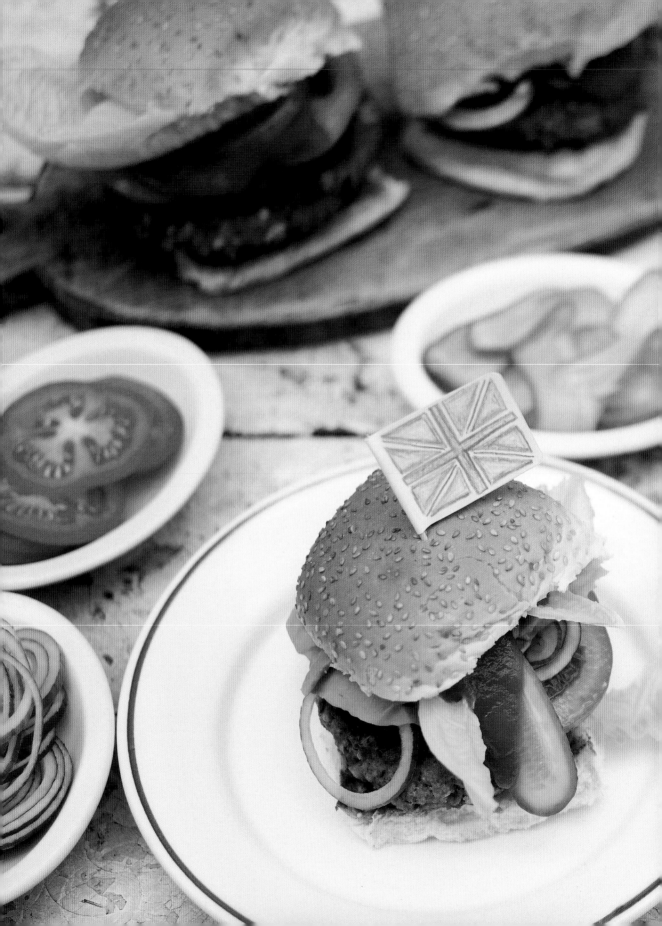

A CRACKING BURGER

There's nothing better than a homemade burger. Everyone loves them, they're easy to make and, if made with quality, fresh ingredients (and not overladen with greasy stuff), they certainly don't have to be unhealthy, especially if served with a salad. Once you've mastered this tasty basic recipe, you can make it your own with different herbs, spices and toppings. The sky's the limit – that's why cooking is so exciting.

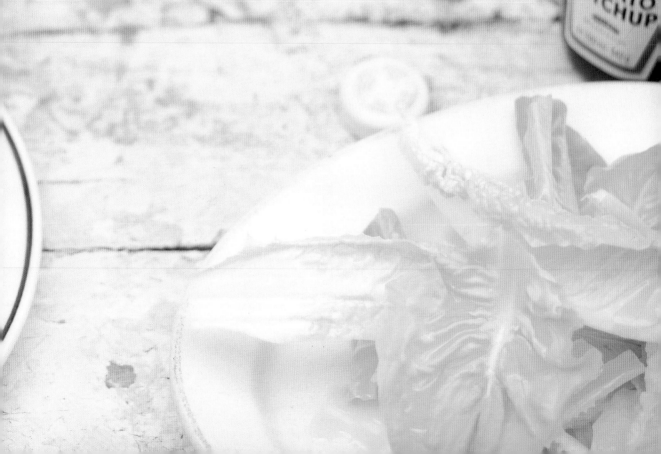

A CRACKING BURGER

serves 6

36 unsalted saltine crackers
8 sprigs of fresh Italian parsley
2 heaped teaspoons Dijon mustard
1 pound good-quality ground beef
1 large egg, preferably free-range or organic
sea salt and freshly ground black pepper
olive oil

1 romaine or butterhead lettuce
3 tomatoes
1 red onion
3 or 4 pickles
6 burger buns
optional: 6 slices of Cheddar cheese

To make your burger

Wrap the crackers in a kitchen towel and smash up until fine, breaking up any big bits with your hands, and put them into a large bowl • Finely chop the parsley, including the stalks • Add the parsley, mustard, and ground beef to the bowl • Crack in the egg and add a good pinch of salt and pepper • With clean hands, scrunch and mix everything up well • Divide into 6 and pat and mold each piece into a roundish shape about ¾ inch thick • Drizzle the burgers with oil, put on a plate, cover and place in the refrigerator until needed (this helps them to firm up)

To cook your burger

Preheat a large grill pan or frying pan for about 4 minutes on a high heat • Turn the heat down to medium • Place the burgers on the grill pan or in the frying pan and use a turner to lightly press down on them, making sure the burger is in full contact • Cook them to your liking for 3 or 4 minutes on each side – you may need to cook them in two batches

To serve your burger

Wash and dry a few small lettuce leaves, tearing up the larger ones • Slice the tomatoes • Peel and finely slice the red onion • Slice the pickles lengthways as thinly as you can • Place all this on a platter and put in the middle of the table with plates, cutlery, ketchup, and drinks • Remove your burgers to another plate and carefully wipe your frying pan or grill pan clean with paper towels • Halve your burger buns and lightly toast them on the grill pan or in the frying pan • Also great with a chopped salad (see pages 120–23)

PS I'd still make this quantity even if it was just for 4 people. I'd wrap the extra 2 burgers in plastic wrap and put them into the freezer.

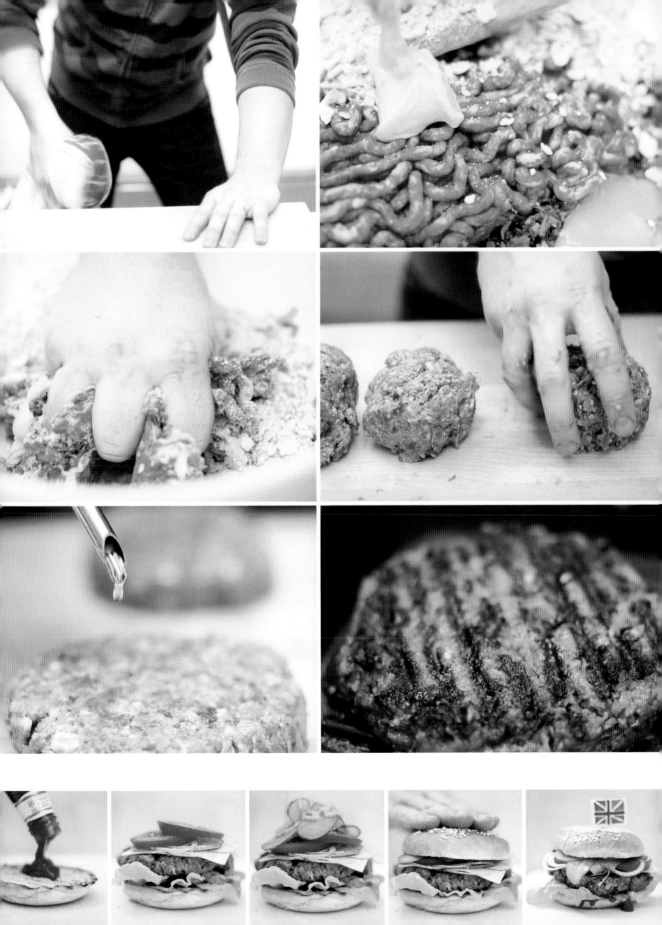

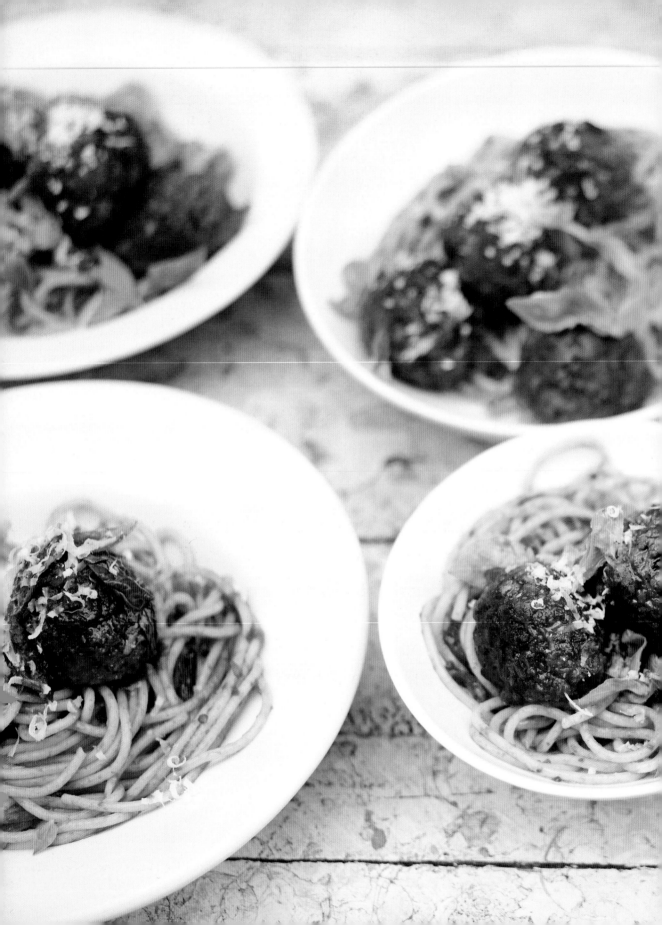

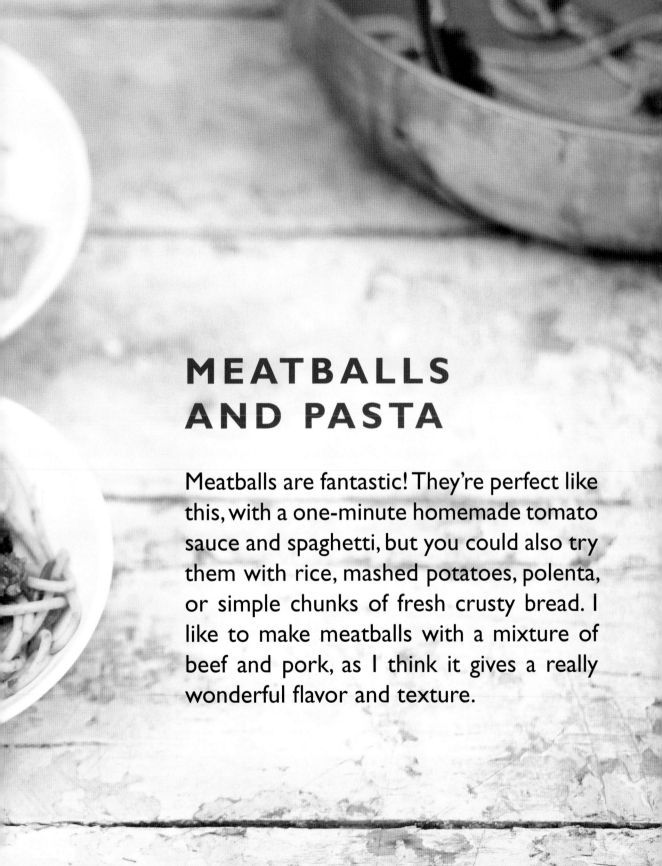

MEATBALLS
AND PASTA

Meatballs are fantastic! They're perfect like this, with a one-minute homemade tomato sauce and spaghetti, but you could also try them with rice, mashed potatoes, polenta, or simple chunks of fresh crusty bread. I like to make meatballs with a mixture of beef and pork, as I think it gives a really wonderful flavor and texture.

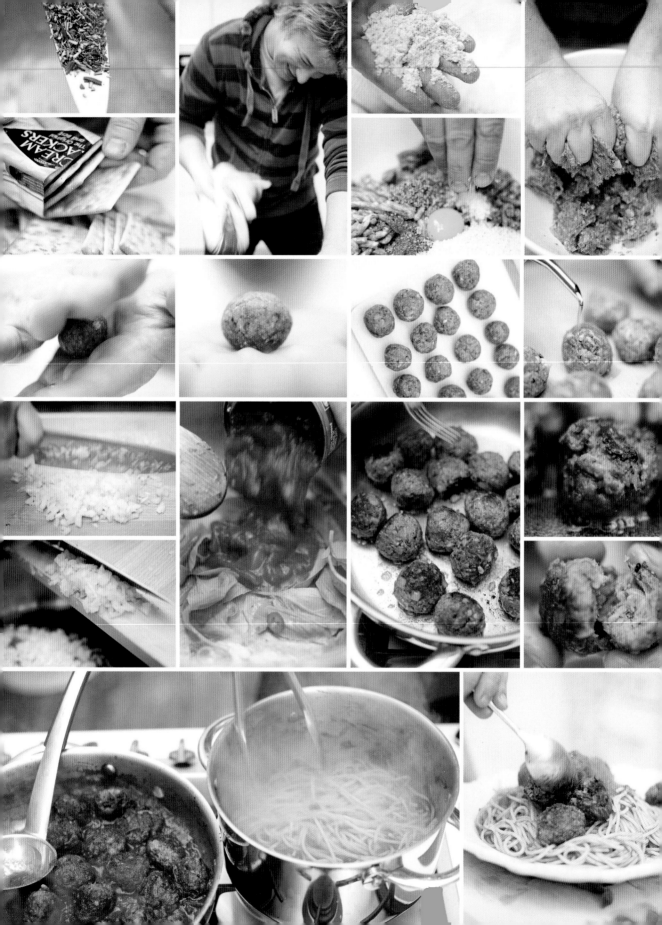

MEATBALLS AND PASTA

serves 4–6

4 sprigs of fresh rosemary

36 unsalted saltine crackers

2 heaped teaspoons Dijon mustard

1 pound good-quality ground beef, pork, or a mixture
  of the two

1 heaped tablespoon dried oregano

1 large egg, preferably free-range or organic

sea salt and freshly ground black pepper

olive oil

a small bunch of fresh basil

1 medium onion

2 cloves of garlic

½ a fresh or dried red chile

2 x 14-ounce cans of diced tomatoes

2 tablespoons balsamic vinegar

1 pound dried spaghetti or penne

Parmesan cheese, for grating

To make your meatballs

Pick the rosemary leaves off the woody stalks and finely chop them • Wrap the crackers in a kitchen towel and smash up until fine, breaking up any big bits with your hands • Add to the bowl with the mustard, ground meat, chopped rosemary, and oregano • Crack in the egg and add a good pinch of salt and pepper • With clean hands, scrunch and mix up well • Divide into 4 large balls • With wet hands, divide each ball into 6 and roll into little meatballs – you should end up with 24 • Drizzle them with olive oil and jiggle them about so they all get coated • Put them on a plate, cover, and place in the refrigerator until needed

To cook your pasta, meatballs, and sauce

Pick the basil leaves, keeping any smaller ones to one side for later • Peel and finely chop the onion and the garlic • Finely slice the chile • Put a large pan of salted water on to boil • Next, heat a large frying pan on a medium heat and add 2 lugs of olive oil • Add your onion to the frying pan and stir for around 7 minutes or until softened and lightly golden • Then add your garlic and chile, and as soon as they start to get some color add the large basil leaves • Add the tomatoes and the balsamic vinegar • Bring to the boil and season to taste • Meanwhile, heat another large frying pan and add a lug of olive oil and your meatballs • Stir them around and cook for 8–10 minutes until golden (check they're cooked by opening one up – there should be no sign of pink) • Add the meatballs to the sauce and simmer until the pasta is ready, then remove from the heat • Add the pasta to the boiling water and cook according to the package instructions

To serve your meatballs

Saving some of the cooking water, drain the pasta in a colander • Return the pasta to the pan • Spoon half the tomato sauce into the pasta, adding a little splash of your reserved water to loosen • Serve on a large platter, or in separate bowls, with the rest of the sauce and meatballs on top • Sprinkle over the small basil leaves and some grated Parmesan

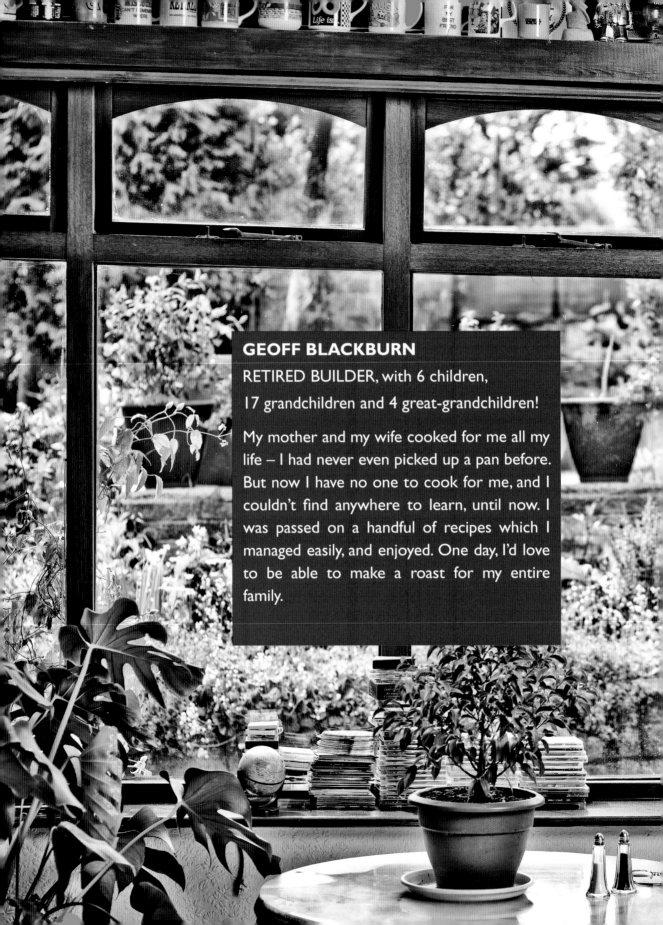

GEOFF BLACKBURN

RETIRED BUILDER, with 6 children,
17 grandchildren and 4 great-grandchildren!

My mother and my wife cooked for me all my life – I had never even picked up a pan before. But now I have no one to cook for me, and I couldn't find anywhere to learn, until now. I was passed on a handful of recipes which I managed easily, and enjoyed. One day, I'd love to be able to make a roast for my entire family.

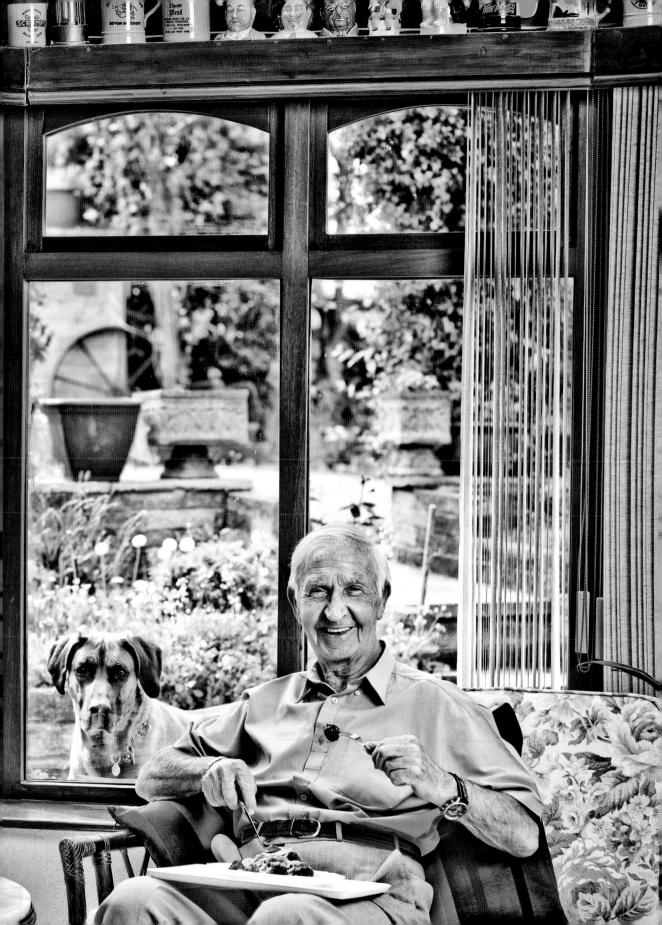

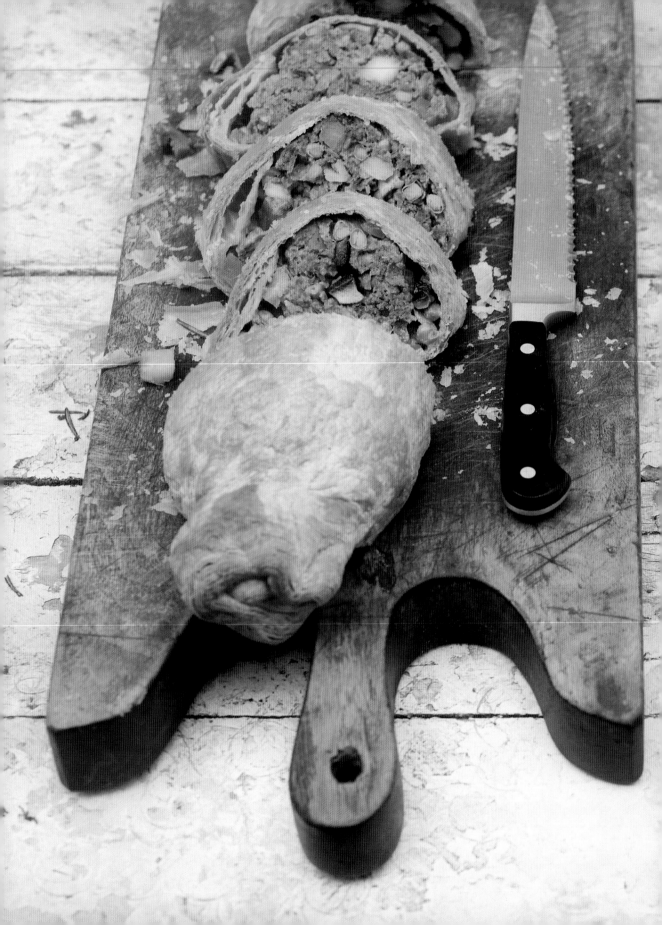

GROUND BEEF WELLINGTON

This is a great alternative to a traditional roast dinner, especially if you don't have enough time to roast a large piece of meat. It's also a cheap dish to make and, since puff pastry is so easily available in grocery stores, you can make something that's absolutely delicious in a relatively short space of time. You can make one large one, as I'm doing here, or smaller individual ones.

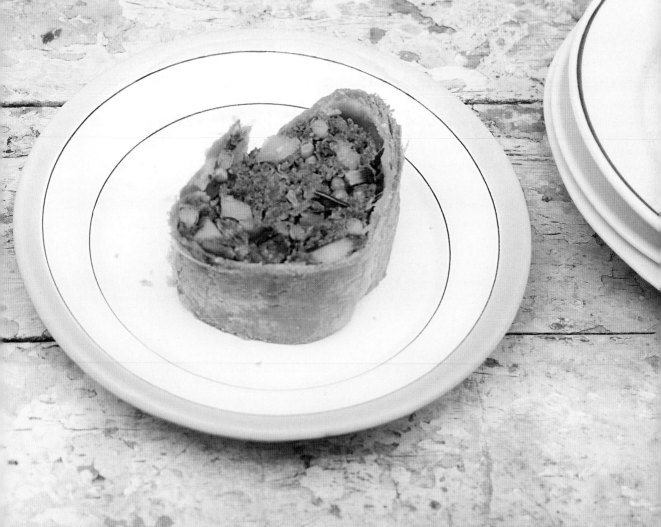

GROUND BEEF WELLINGTON

serves 4–6

1 medium onion	4 sprigs of fresh rosemary
1 carrot	a big handful of frozen peas
1 celery stalk	1 large egg, preferably free-range or organic
1 potato	1 pound good-quality ground beef
2 cloves of garlic	sea salt and freshly ground black pepper
2 portobello mushrooms	all-purpose flour, for dusting
olive oil	2 sheets puff pastry, defrosted if frozen

To prepare your ground beef

Preheat the oven to 350°F • Peel and chop the onion, carrot, celery, and potato into ¼-inch-sized-dice • Finely grate the garlic • Clean and roughly chop the mushrooms so they're about the same size as your other veggies • Place all the vegetables into a large frying pan on a medium low heat with 2 lugs of olive oil • Pick the rosemary leaves off the woody stalks, finely chop them, and add to the pan • Fry and stir for around 8 minutes or until the vegetables soften and color lightly • Add the frozen peas and cook for another minute • Put the vegetable mixture into a large bowl to cool completely • Crack the egg into a cup and beat it up • Add the ground beef to the bowl with a good pinch of salt and pepper and half the beaten egg • With clean hands, scrunch and mix up well

To roll and fill your pastry

Lightly dust your clean work surface and rolling pin with flour and lay the puff pastry sheets one on top of the other. Roll out the puff pastry so it is roughly a rectangle 12 x 16 inches • Dust with flour as you go • Turn your pastry so you have a long edge in front of you and place the ground beef mixture along this edge • Mold it into an even, long sausage shape • Brush the edges of the pastry with a little of the beaten egg • Roll the ground beef up in the pastry until it's covered completely • Squeeze the ends together – it will look like a big Christmas cracker! • Dust a large cookie pan with flour and place your Wellington on top • Brush all over with the rest of the beaten egg • Bake in the preheated oven for an hour until golden

To serve your Wellington

Slice the Wellington up into portions at the table • Lovely served with some lightly boiled or steamed greens, cabbage tossed in a little butter, or mashed potatoes

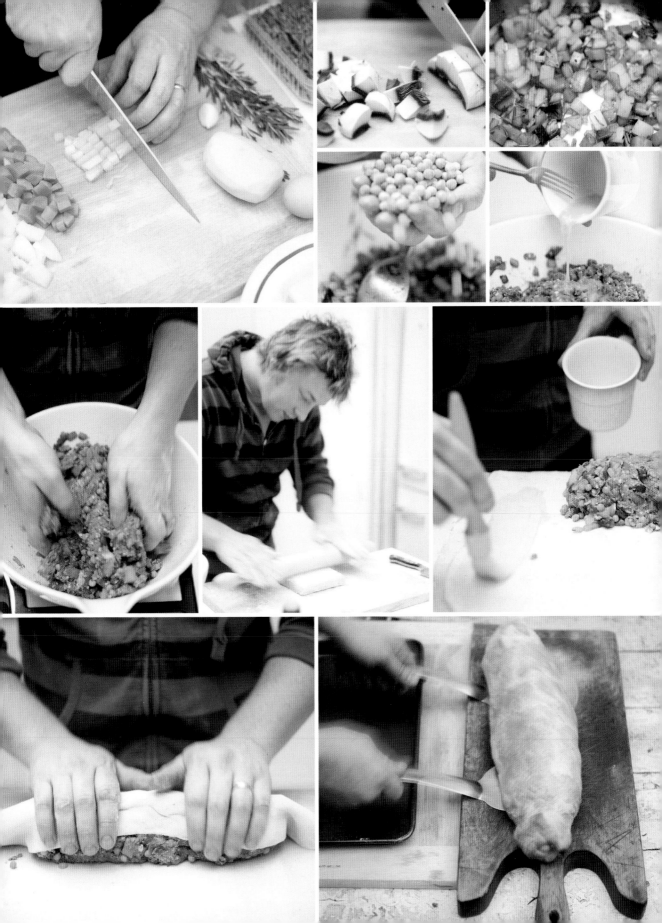

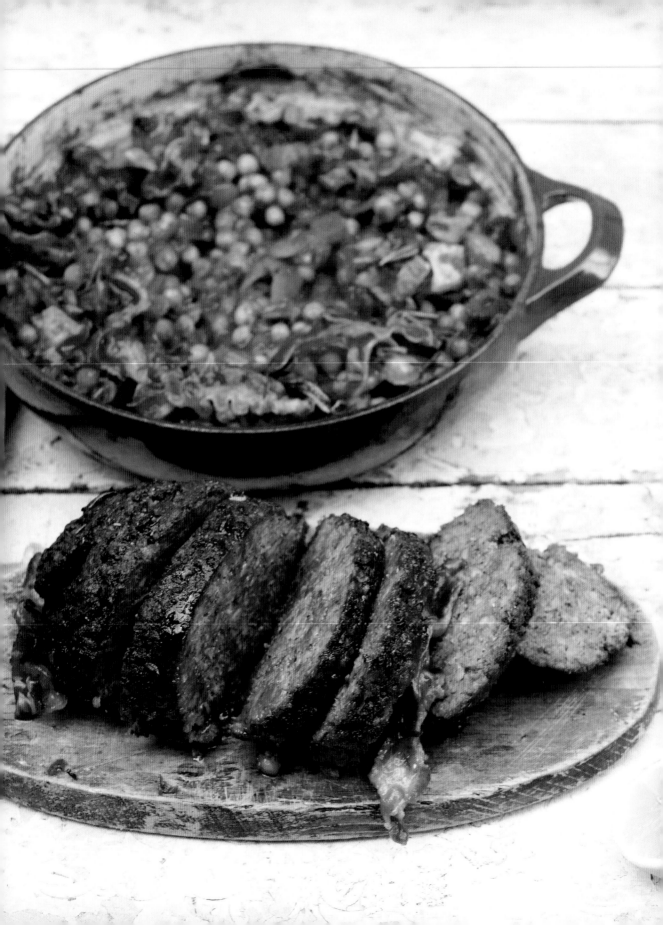

POT-ROAST MEATLOAF

A good meatloaf with freshly made tomato sauce is great comfort food. I think this also makes a tasty change from the traditional British Sunday lunch and I flavor it and treat it as if I'm roasting a big joint of meat. I used to make this a lot for staff dinners at the restaurant. It's made along similar lines to meatballs and burgers, and trust me – people love this just as much.

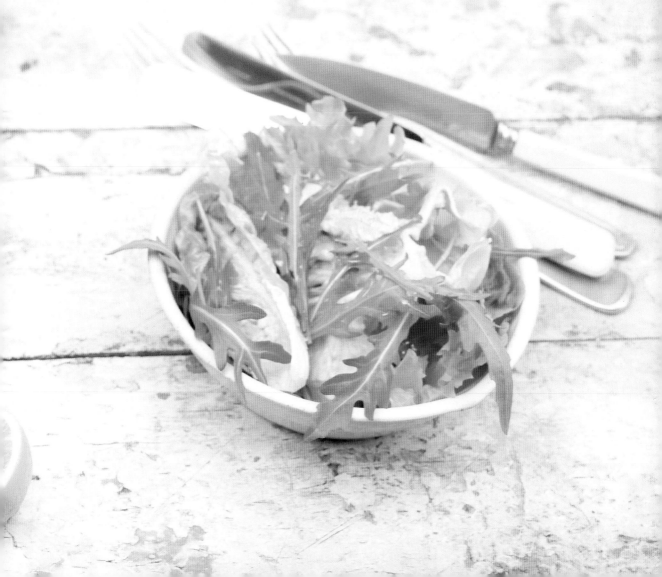

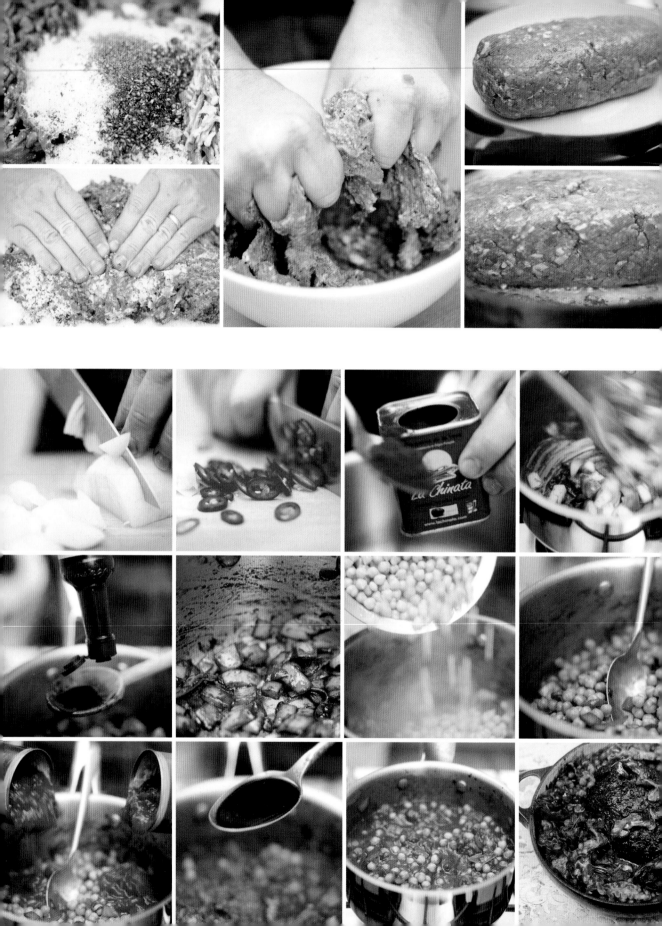

POT-ROAST MEATLOAF

serves 4–6

2 medium onions

olive oil

sea salt and freshly ground black pepper

1 level teaspoon ground cumin

1 heaped teaspoon ground coriander

36 unsalted saltine crackers

2 teaspoons dried oregano

2 heaped teaspoons Dijon mustard

1 pound good-quality ground beef

1 large egg, preferably free-range or organic

2 cloves of garlic

½–1 fresh red or green chile, to your taste

1 teaspoon smoked paprika

2 tablespoons Worcestershire sauce, such as Lea & Perrins

1 x 15-ounce can of garbanzo beans, drained

2 x 14-ounce cans of diced tomatoes

2 tablespoons balsamic vinegar

2 sprigs of fresh rosemary

12 slices of smoked bacon, preferably free-range or organic

1 lemon

To make your meatloaf

Preheat the oven to full whack (475°) • Peel and finely chop one of the onions – don't worry about technique, just chop away until fine • Place in a large frying pan on a medium high heat with 2 lugs of olive oil and a pinch of salt and pepper • Add the ground cumin and coriander • Fry and stir every 30 seconds for around 7 minutes or until softened and lightly golden, then put into a large bowl to cool • Wrap the crackers in a kitchen towel and smash up until fine, breaking up any big bits with your hands • Add to the bowl of cooled onions with the oregano, mustard, and ground beef • Crack in the egg and add another good pinch of salt and pepper • With clean hands, scrunch and mix up well • Move the meat mixture to a board, then pat and mold it into a large football shape • Rub it with a little oil • You can either cook it straight away or put it on a plate, cover, and place in the refrigerator until needed • Place the meatloaf in a Dutch oven–type pan or baking dish, put it into the preheated oven, and turn down the temperature immediately to 400°F • Bake for half an hour

To make your meatloaf sauce

Peel the other onion and chop into ¼-inch pieces • Peel and slice the garlic • Finely slice the red chile • Place the onion, garlic, and chile in a large pan on a medium high heat with 2 lugs of olive oil, the paprika, and a pinch of salt and pepper • Cook for around 7 minutes, stirring every 30 seconds until softened and lightly golden • Add the Worcestershire sauce, garbanzo beans, tomatoes, and balsamic vinegar • Bring to a boil, then turn the heat down and let it slowly simmer for 10 minutes • Taste the sauce and season with salt and pepper if needed

To finish off and serve your meatloaf

Pick the rosemary leaves off the woody stalks and put them into a little bowl • Remove the meatloaf from the oven and pour all the fat from the pan over the rosemary leaves and mix up well • Spoon your sauce around the meatloaf • Lay the slices of bacon over the top of the meatloaf and sauce • Scatter over the rosemary leaves • Put the pan back into the oven for 10 to 15 minutes, until the bacon turns golden and the sauce is bubbling and delicious • Serve with a mixed leaf salad and some wedges of lemon for squeezing over – this will add a nice sharp twang

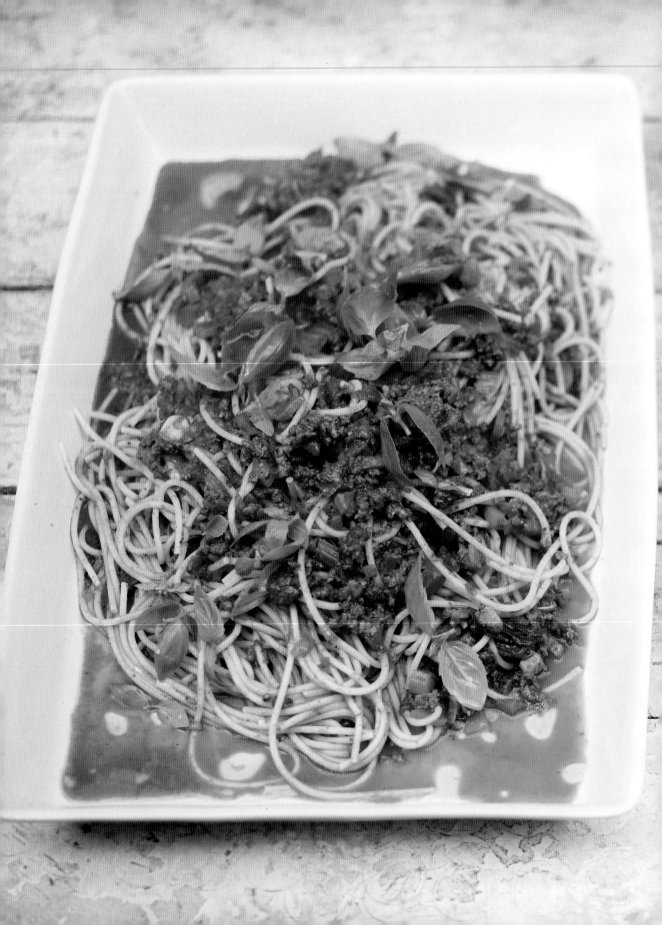

BOLOGNESE SAUCE

A good Bolognese sauce is an Italian classic. In Italy it is made in many different ways, using all sorts of wines and herbs, but I like this way because it's really reliable, tasty, and simple. The classic pastas to serve this with are spaghetti, tagliatelle, and penne, but this sauce can also be used for many other things, like filling cannelloni or layering up a lasagne. With so many options, it's well worth bagging up any leftover sauce and freezing it for another day.

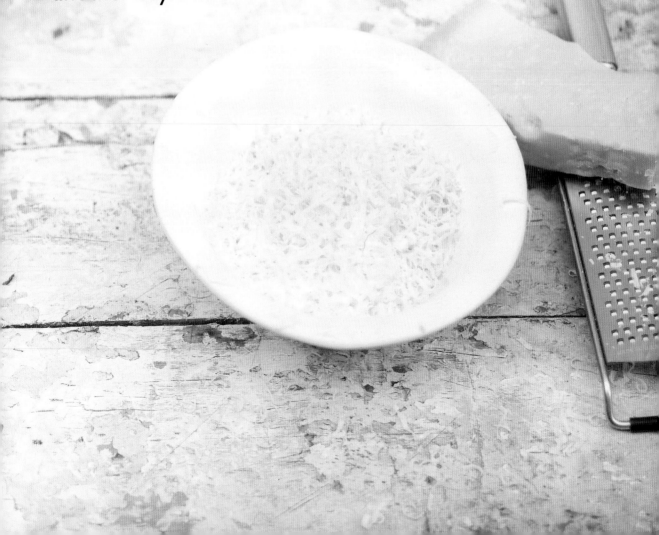

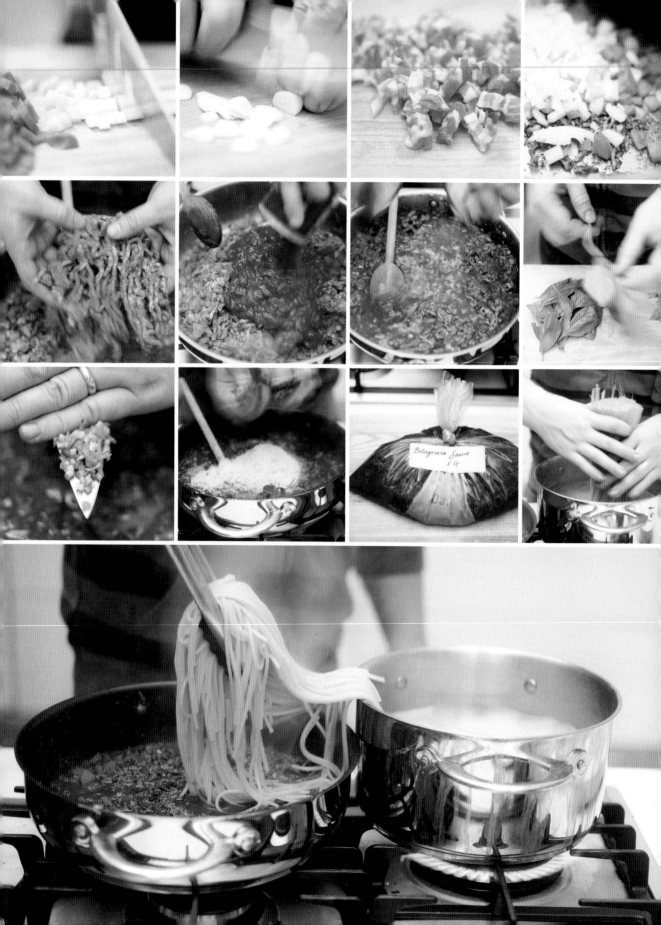

BOLOGNESE SAUCE

serves 4–6

2 slices of smoked bacon, preferably free-range or
  organic

2 medium onions

2 cloves of garlic

2 carrots

2 celery stalks

olive oil

2 heaped teaspoons dried oregano

1 pound good-quality ground beef, pork, or (even
  better!) a mixture of the two

2 x 14-ounce cans of diced tomatoes

sea salt and freshly ground black pepper

a small bunch of fresh basil

4 ounces Parmesan cheese

1 pound dried spaghetti or penne

To make your sauce

Finely slice the bacon • Peel and finely chop the onions, garlic, carrots, and celery – don't worry about
technique, just chop away until fine • Place a large casserole-type pan on a medium to high heat • Add 2
lugs of olive oil, your sliced bacon, and the oregano and cook and stir until the bacon is lightly golden • Add
the vegetables to the pan and stir every 30 seconds for around 7 minutes or until softened and lightly
colored • Stir in the ground meat and the canned tomatoes • Fill one of the empty cans with water and
add to the pan • Stir in a good pinch of salt and pepper • Pick the basil leaves and place in the refrigerator
for later • Finely chop the basil stalks and stir into the pan • Bring to a boil • Turn the heat down and
simmer with the lid slightly askew for 1 hour, stirring every now and again • Take the lid off and cook for
another 30 minutes, stirring occasionally • Keep an eye on the sauce as it cooks, and if you think it's
starting to dry out, add a splash of water • Remove the Bolognese sauce from the heat • Finely grate the
Parmesan and stir half into the sauce • Tear and stir in any larger basil leaves, keeping the smaller ones
for sprinkling over before serving • Mix up, have a taste, and season with a little more salt and pepper if
needed – congratulations! You now have a beautiful Bolognese sauce • At this stage you can allow it to
cool, bag it up and freeze it, or eat it straightaway with the pasta below

To cook your pasta and serve

Bring a large pan of salted water to a boil • Add your pasta and stir, following the package cooking times
– don't let it cook any longer or it will become too soft – you want it to have a bit of bite • Saving a little
of the cooking water, drain the pasta in a colander • Put the drained pasta back into the pan • Add half
the Bolognese sauce to the cooked pasta and mix well, adding a little of the reserved cooking water to
loosen • Divide between your plates and spoon the remaining sauce over the top • Drizzle with olive oil,
sprinkle over the rest of the Parmesan, and scatter with the small basil leaves – bellissima!

LASAGNE

I couldn't do a ground beef chapter without including lasagne. The ground beef used here is basically the same recipe as for the Bolognese sauce on page 165, with added instructions for how to build up a lasagne and make a quick white sauce.

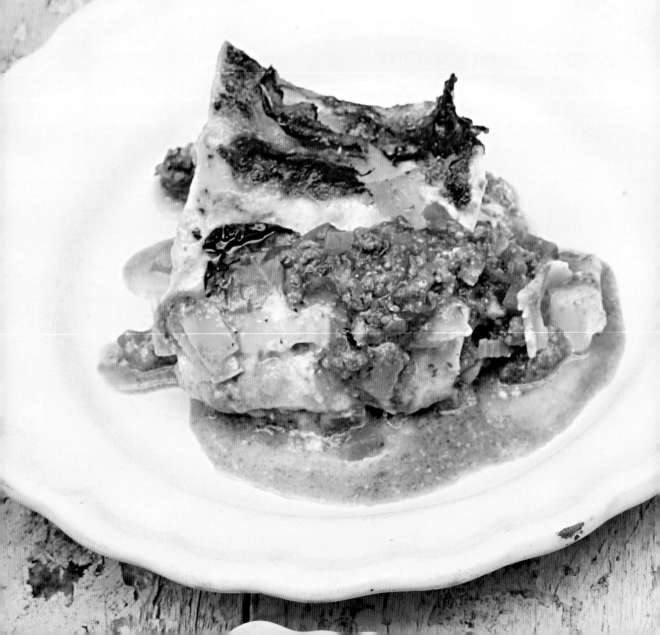

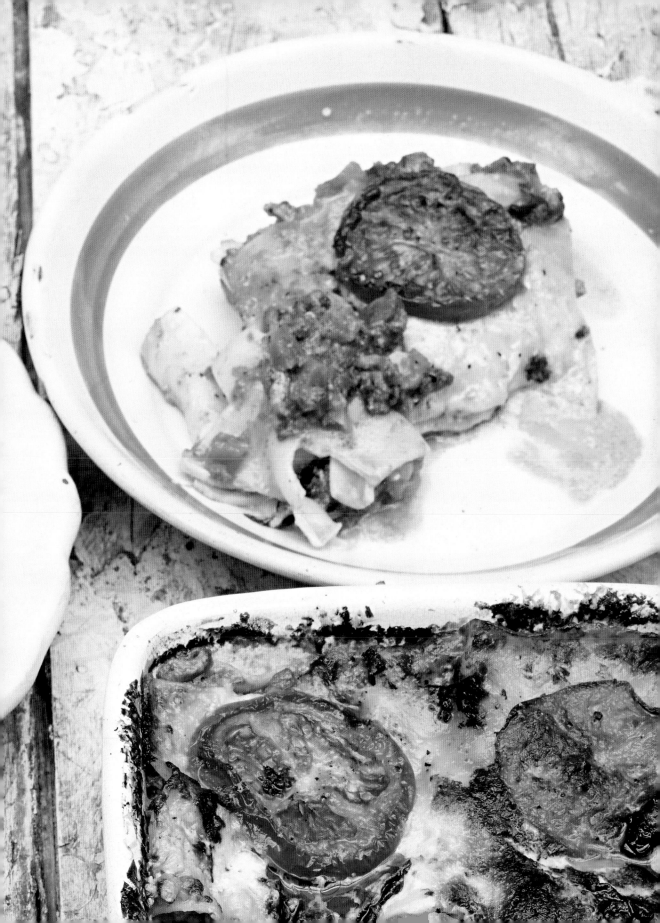

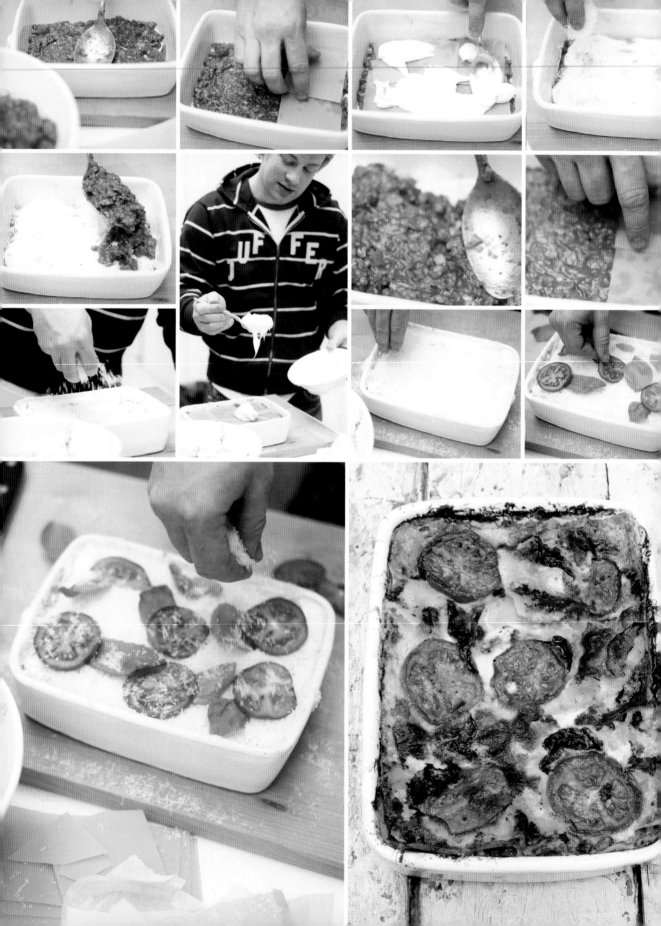

LASAGNE

serves 6–8

For the Bolognese sauce

2 slices of smoked bacon, preferably free-range or
   organic

2 medium onions

2 cloves of garlic

2 carrots

2 celery stalks

olive oil

2 heaped teaspoons dried oregano

1 pound good-quality ground beef, pork, or (even
better!) a mixture of the two

2 x 14-ounce cans of diced tomatoes

sea salt and freshly ground black pepper

a small bunch of fresh basil

For the lasagne

8 ounces dried egg lasagne sheets

4 ounces Parmesan cheese

2½ cups of crème fraîche or 2½ cups thick sour
   cream

1 large ripe tomato, sliced

To make your Bolognese sauce

Finely slice the bacon • Peel and finely chop the onions, garlic, carrots, and celery – don't worry about technique; just chop away • Place a large casserole-type pan on a medium to high heat • Add 2 lugs of olive oil, your sliced bacon, and the oregano and cook and stir until the bacon is lightly golden • Add the vegetables to the pan and stir every 30 seconds for around 7 minutes or until softened and lightly colored • Stir in the ground meat and the canned tomatoes • Fill one of the empty cans with water and add to the pan • Stir in a good pinch of salt and pepper • Pick the basil leaves and place in the refrigerator for later • Finely chop the basil stalks and stir into the pan • Bring to a boil • Turn the heat down and simmer with the lid askew for 1 hour, stirring every now and again • Take the lid off and cook for another 30 minutes, stirring occasionally • Keep an eye on the sauce as it cooks, and if you think it's starting to dry out, add a splash of water

To finish the sauce

Preheat the oven to 375°F • Remove the Bolognese sauce from the heat • Tear and stir in any larger basil leaves, keeping the smaller ones aside for later • Have a taste of the sauce, and season with a little more salt and pepper if you think it needs it • Boil some water in a kettle and pour it into a large pan, then add your lasagne sheets with a drizzle of oil and blanch (slightly soften) for 3 to 4 minutes • Drain the sheets in a colander and carefully pat them dry with some paper towels to absorb any excess water • Finely grate the Parmesan and stir most of it through the crème fraîche

To make your lasagne

Spoon a third of your Bolognese sauce into the bottom of an earthenware ovenproof dish (approximately 9 x 13 inches) • Follow with a layer of lasagne sheets and another third of your Bolognese sauce, then dollop over a third of your crème fraîche • Sprinkle with a good pinch of salt and pepper and top with another layer of lasagne sheets • Spoon over the rest of the Bolognese sauce and another third of the crème fraîche • Finish with a final layer of lasagne sheets and top with the rest of the crème fraîche • Scatter over the remaining Parmesan • Top with some slices of tomato, scatter over the small basil leaves and drizzle with olive oil • Cover with aluminum foil, place in the preheated oven and bake for 30 minutes • After that, remove the foil and cook for a further 20 minutes until the lasagne is bubbling and golden • Serve on the table with a fresh green salad and let everyone help themselves

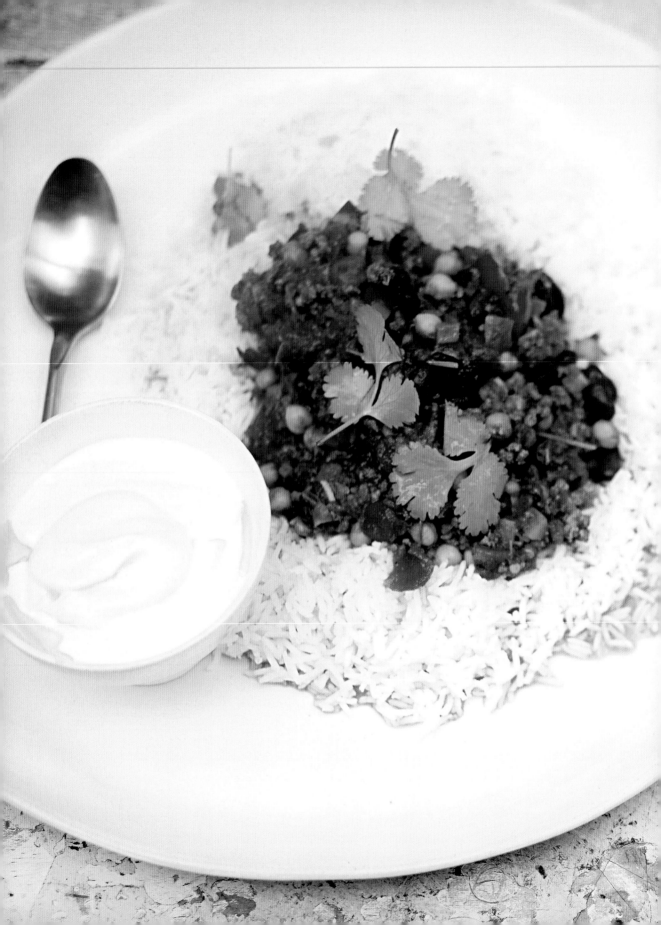

GOOD OLD CHILI CON CARNE

What a classic this dish is. Most of my mates love the garbanzo beans, but butter beans or even cubed potatoes will work well in their place. Feel free to pep up this dish with more chili powder depending on your taste. This will make enough for six portions, so simply freeze the extra if you're only cooking for four — it's so damn good the next day, even on a baked potato!

GOOD OLD CHILI CON CARNE

serves 6

2 medium onions	1 x 15-ounce can garbanzo beans
2 cloves of garlic	1 x 15-ounce can of red kidney beans
2 medium carrots	2 x 14-ounce cans of diced tomatoes
2 celery stalks	1 pound good-quality ground beef
2 red bell peppers	1 small bunch of fresh cilantro
olive oil	2 tablespoons balsamic vinegar
1 heaped teaspoon chili powder	2 cups basmati rice
1 heaped teaspoon ground cumin	2 cups natural yogurt
1 heaped teaspoon ground cinnamon	1 cup guacamole
sea salt and freshly ground black pepper	1 lime

To make your chili

Peel and finely chop the onions, garlic, carrots, and celery – don't worry about the technique, just chop away until fine • Halve the bell peppers, remove the stalks and seeds, and roughly chop • Place your largest casserole-type pan on a medium high heat • Add 2 lugs of olive oil and all your chopped vegetables • Add the chili powder, cumin, and cinnamon with a good pinch of salt and pepper • Stir every 30 seconds for around 7 minutes until softened and lightly colored • Add the drained garbanzo beans, drained kidney beans, and the canned tomatoes • Add the ground beef, breaking any larger chunks up with a wooden spoon • Fill one of the empty tomato cans with water and pour this into the pan • Pick the cilantro leaves and place them in the refrigerator • Finely chop the washed stalks and stir in • Add the balsamic vinegar and season with a good pinch of salt and pepper • Bring to a boil and turn the heat down to a simmer with the lid slightly askew for 1 hour and 15 minutes, stirring every now and then • Take the lid off and cook for another 15 minutes, stirring occasionally • Keep an eye on it as it cooks, and if you think it's starting to dry out, add a splash of water

To serve your chili

This is fantastic served with fluffy rice (see pages 95–96) • Just divide the rice and chili into big bowls or serve in the middle of the table and let everyone help themselves • If you don't fancy rice it's equally good with a nice hunk of fresh crusty bread, over a baked potato, or with couscous • Put a small bowl of natural yogurt, some guacamole, and a few wedges of lime on the table, and sprinkle the chili with the cilantro leaves • I love to add a nice green salad to round it off

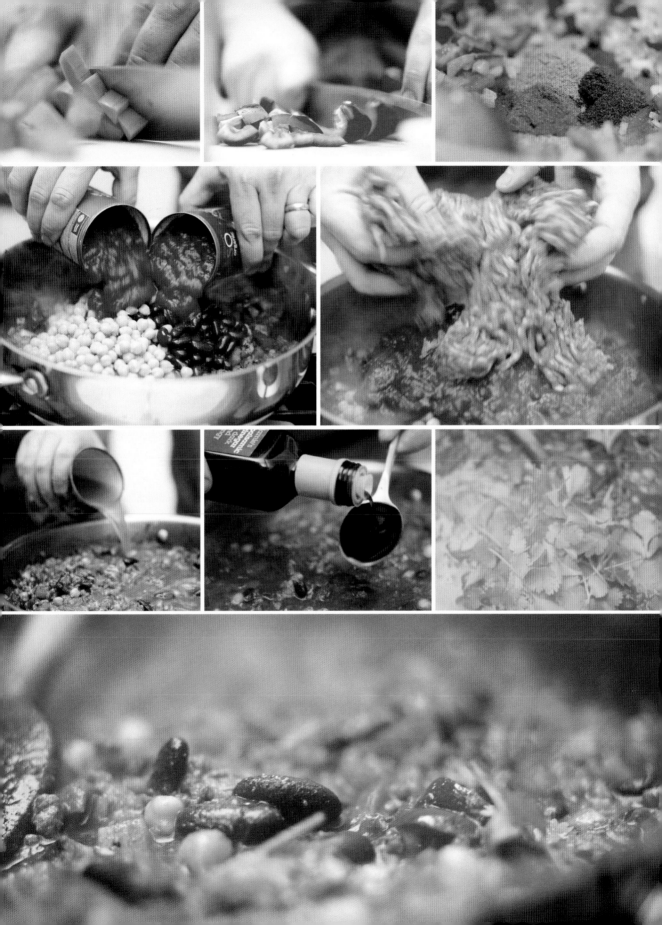

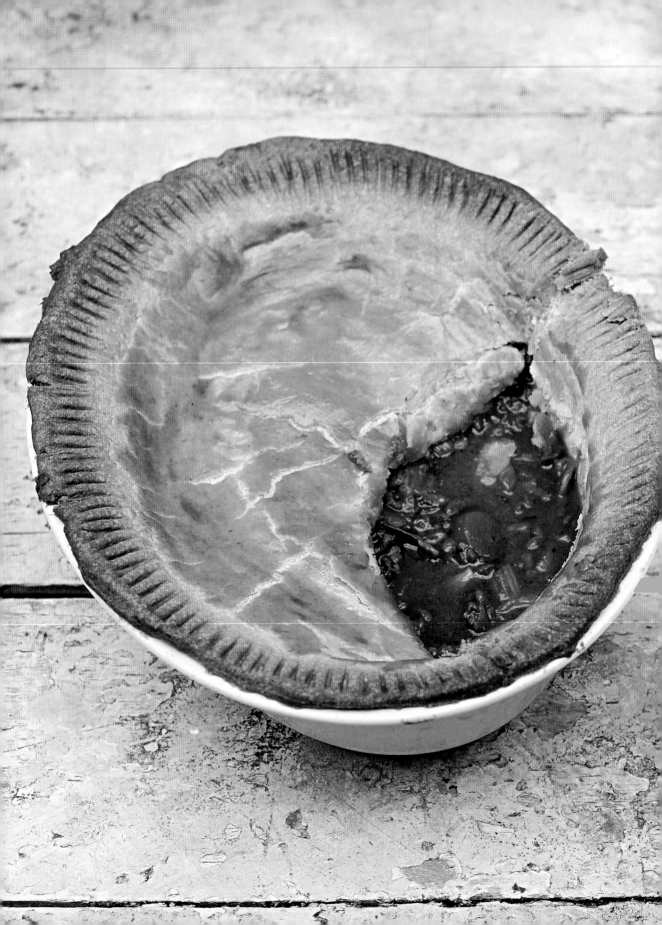

BRITISH BEEF AND ONION PIE

I think a nice slice of pie is such a treat and this one is a great British classic. It's comforting, damn tasty, and also cheap to make. There's great satisfaction in making a lovely meat pie, and I can promise you that everyone at your table will be coming back for more.

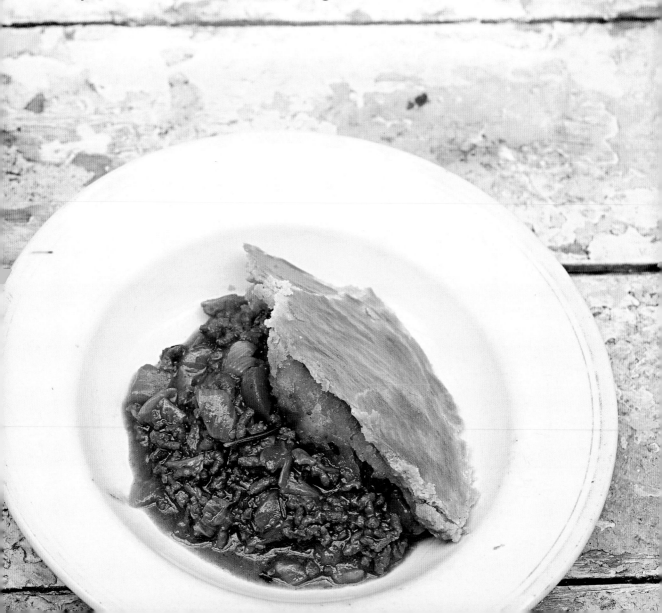

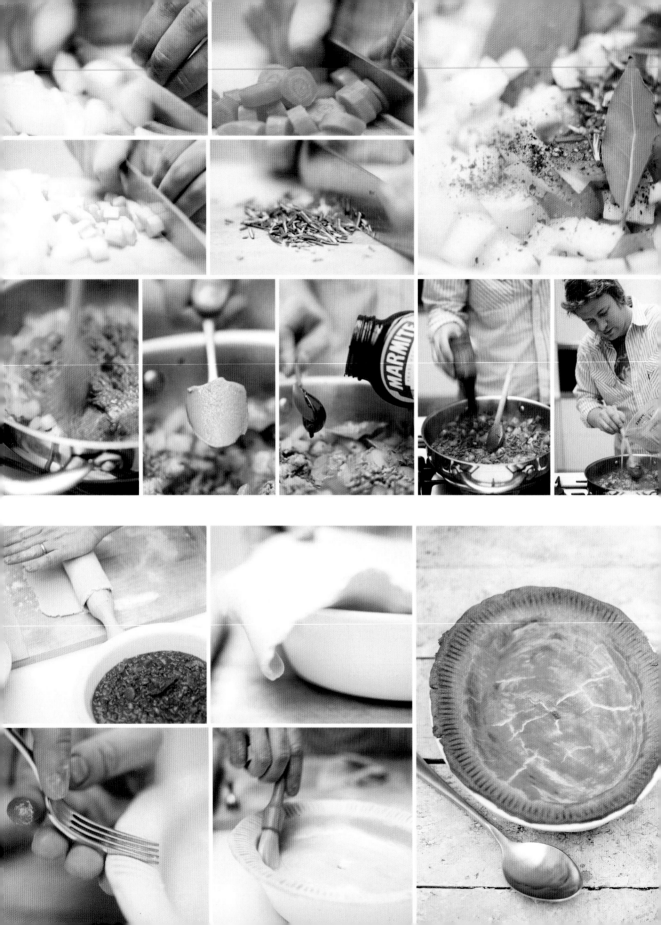

BRITISH BEEF AND ONION PIE

serves 4

3 medium onions

2 carrots

2 stalks celery

2 sprigs of fresh rosemary

olive oil

2 bay leaves

I pound good-quality ground beef

I teaspoon English mustard

optional: I teaspoon Marmite

I tablespoon Worcestershire sauce, such as Lea & Perrins

2 teaspoons all-purpose flour, plus extra for dusting

I quart beef broth, preferably organic

2 x 9 inch pie crusts

I large egg, preferably free-range or organic, or a splash of milk

To make your beef filling

Peel and roughly chop your onions, carrots, and celery – don't worry about technique, just chop away until fine • Remove the rosemary leaves from the woody stalks and chop finely • Place a large casserole-type pan on a high heat • Add 2 lugs of olive oil, all the vegetables, the rosemary, and the bay leaves • Stir every minute for around 10 minutes or until the veggies have softened and lightly, colored • Stir in the ground beef, breaking up any large chunks with a wooden spoon • Add the mustard, Marmite, Worcestershire sauce, and 2 teaspoons of flour • Add the beef broth and bring to a boil • Turn the heat down and simmer with the lid slightly askew for about an hour, stirring every now and again to stop it catching

To make your pie

Fill a large baking dish with the beef filling and allow it to cool down • Remove the pastry from the refrigerator 10 minutes before you need to roll it out • Preheat the oven to 350°F • Dust a clean work surface and your rolling pin with some flour and lay the pie crusts one on top of the other, then fold in half and roll out the pastry to ⅛ inch thick • Once it's large enough to cover your serving dish easily, wind the pastry around the rolling pin and unroll it over the dish (don't worry if it breaks or tears, just patch it up – you'll get the hang of it!) • Run a knife around the edge of the dish to trim off any excess pastry • Using a fork, press down around the edge of the pastry to "crimp" it • Make a hole in the middle of the pastry using the tip of a knife • Brush the top of the pastry with beaten egg or a little milk • Bake on the bottom shelf of the preheated oven for 40 minutes, or until the pastry is golden and crisp

To serve your pie

Place the pie in the middle of the table for everyone to help themselves • As it's so scrummy and rich, it's best served with some simply steamed greens like broccoli or peas tossed in a little butter

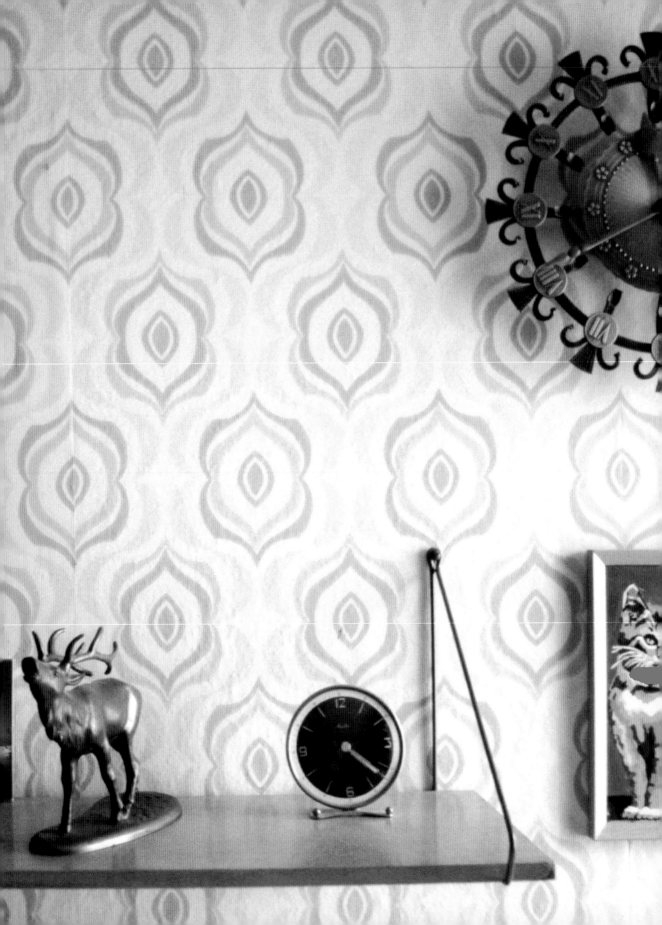

Comforting stews

A good stew is delicious, comforting, nutritious, homely, nostalgic, cheap to make, and can be eaten and enjoyed in so many different ways.

Some people think stewing meat cuts are bad or low grade, because they don't cost much compared to prime cuts like tenderloin, top loin, or sirloin. This is not the case at all. Yes, the cuts are cheaper, but in simple layman's terms that meat just comes from a part of the animal that has done lots of work – parts like the legs (lots of walking) and the neck area (holding the head while it constantly dips down to the ground to eat!). The outcome is that this meat contains more connective tissue, which is pretty much impossible to make tender if quickly cooked like a steak. Instead, if you cook these cuts slowly the tough tissues will eventually melt away, making the meat incredibly tender and even more tasty. So this makes them perfect for stews.

This chapter is not full of different kinds of stew recipes. I'm actually going to concentrate on teaching you how to make just one basic stew that works every single time. The way I've written it as a principal recipe allows you to chop and change it easily, using different meats, herbs, and liquids, and very quickly I think you will gain confidence and be comfortable enough to start making up some of your own variations on the story. Stews are great to serve up for family dinners and dinner parties, because once they're cooking away in the oven you're free to do other things.

A good stew with crusty bread and some greens is a delicious dinner, but I've also given you four different ways of topping your stew so you can take it in different directions: pastry, mashed potatoes, sliced potatoes, and dumplings. All great ways of finishing off a stew. And all very simple as well.

BASIC STEW RECIPE

You are going to love this slow-cooked stew recipe, because it's so simple and gives consistently good results. Try each of the different options below. It's a good idea to stick to the meat and booze combinations I've given you, but if you want to pick and mix the herbage feel free! For each of the four options below the meat should be cut into approximately ¾-inch cubes. Packages from most grocery stores are often about that size.

In stew recipes you're often told to brown off the meat first. But I've done loads of tests and found the meat is just as delicious and tender without browning it first, so I've removed this usual stage from these recipes.

For each stew you will need:

serves 4–6

2 stalks celery
2 medium onions
2 carrots
olive oil

1 heaped tablespoon all-purpose flour
1 x 14-ounce can of diced tomatoes
sea salt and freshly ground black pepper

Then choose one of the following:

Beef and ale (3 hours)

3 fresh or dried bay leaves
1 pound diced stewing beef
2 cups brown ale, Guinness or stout

Chicken and white wine (1½ hours)

3 sprigs of fresh thyme
1 pound diced, boneless, skinless chicken thighs
2 cups white wine

Pork and cider (2½ hours)

3 sprigs of fresh sage
1 pound diced stewing pork, preferably free-range or organic
2 cups medium-dry hard cider

Lamb and red wine (2½ hours)

3 sprigs of fresh rosemary
1 pound diced stewing lamb
2 cups red wine

If using the oven to cook your stew, preheat it to 350°F • Trim the ends off your celery and roughly chop the stalks • Peel and roughly chop the onions • Peel the carrots, slice lengthways, and roughly chop • Put a Dutch oven on a medium heat • Put all the vegetables and your chosen herb into the pan with 2 lugs of olive oil and fry for 10 minutes • Add your meat and flour • Pour in the booze and canned tomatoes • Give it a good stir, then season with a teaspoon of sea salt (less if using table salt) and a few grinds of pepper • Bring to a boil, put the lid on, and either simmer slowly on your cooktop or cook in an oven for the times shown above • Remove the lid for the final half hour of simmering or cooking and add a splash of water if it looks a bit dry • When done, your meat should be tender and delicious • Remove any bay leaves or herb stalks before serving, and taste it to see if it needs a bit more salt and pepper

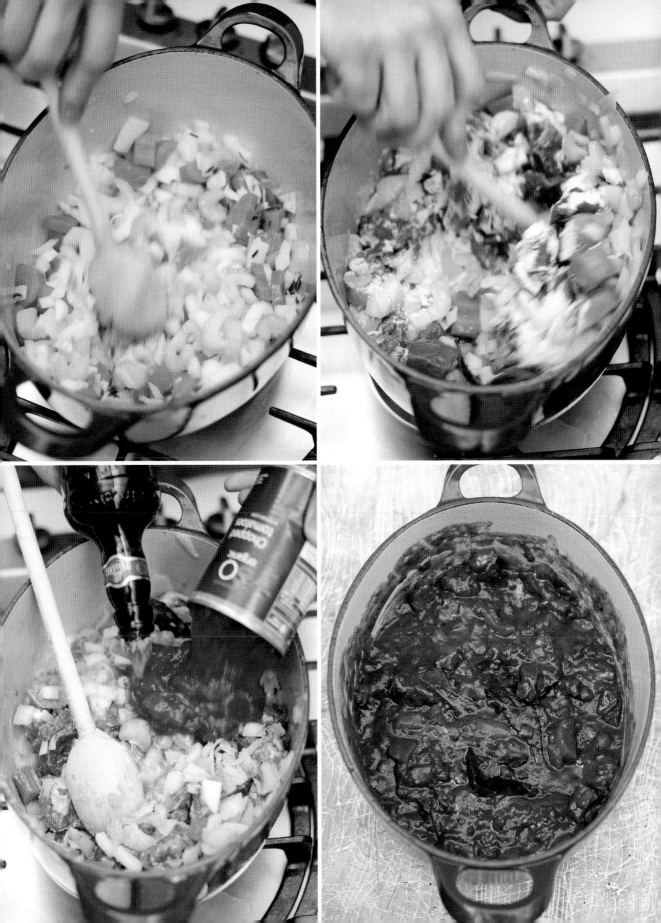

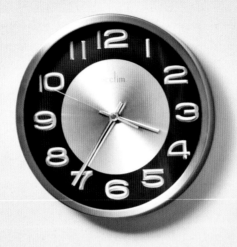

MATTHEW BORRINGTON
BRICKLAYER

I'm single and I've got my own house. My parents aren't here to cook for me any more so I thought it was a good time to learn how. Now that I've been passed on a few recipes, I'm doing stuff I never would have imagined doing. People actually want me to cook for them, and it makes me proud when I see that they've enjoyed something I've made.

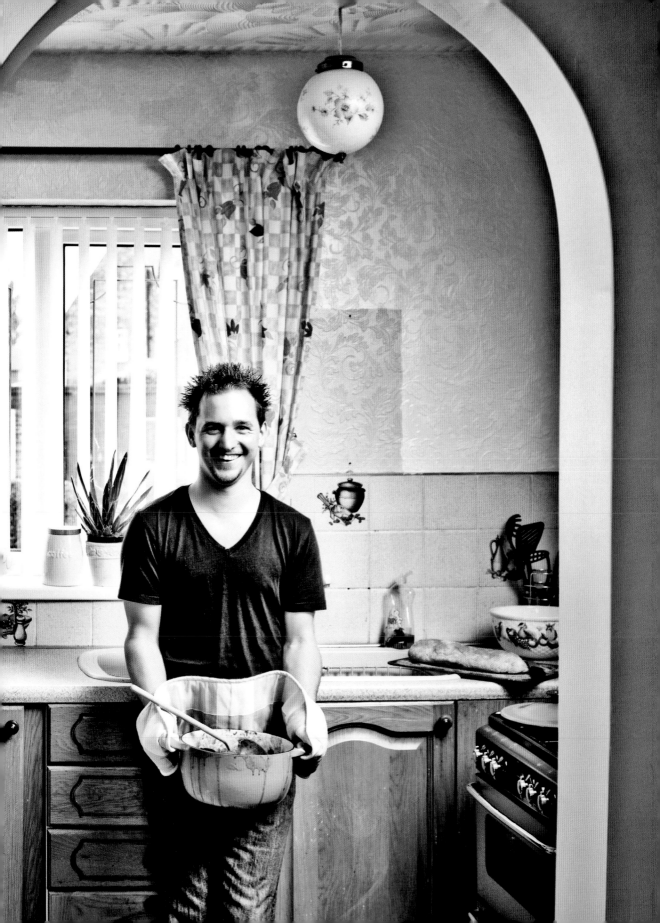

Why not add a puff pastry lid to your stew?

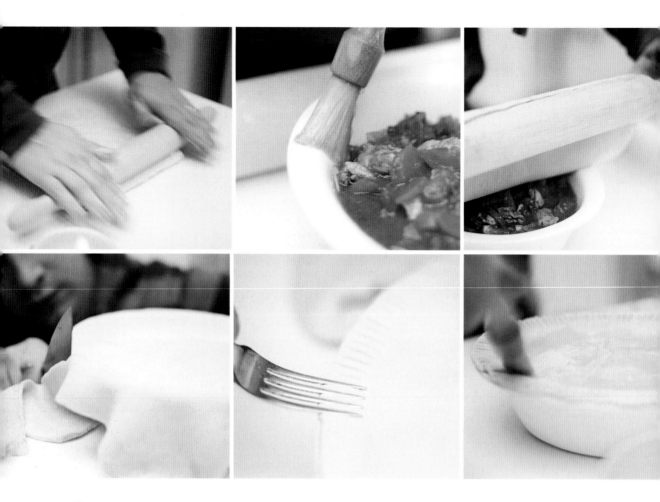

For your pastry lid:

2 sheets puff pastry, defrosted if frozen • all-purpose flour for dusting • 1 large egg, preferably free-range or organic • a splash of milk

Preheat your oven to 350°F • Transfer your fully cooked stew to a large pie dish and let it cool completely • Remove the puff pastry from the refrigerator 10 minutes before you need to roll it out • Dust a clean work surface and your rolling pin with flour and lay one sheet on top of the other, then roll out the pastry until it's ⅛ inch thick and large enough to cover your pie dish easily • Crack the egg into a small bowl, add a splash of milk, and beat with a fork • Brush the edge of the pie dish with a little of the egg mixture – this will help the pastry to stick • Wind the pastry around the rolling pin, then unroll it over the dish (if it tears, don't worry, just patch it up and keep going) • Run a knife around the side of the dish to trim off any excess pastry • Using a fork, lightly press down around the edge of the pastry to "crimp" it • Brush the top of the pie with a little more of the egg mixture • Using the tip of a knife, make a small hole in the middle of the pastry to let the steam escape • Bake in the bottom of the oven for 40 minutes, or until the pastry is golden and crisp

Or serve it with lovely dumplings?

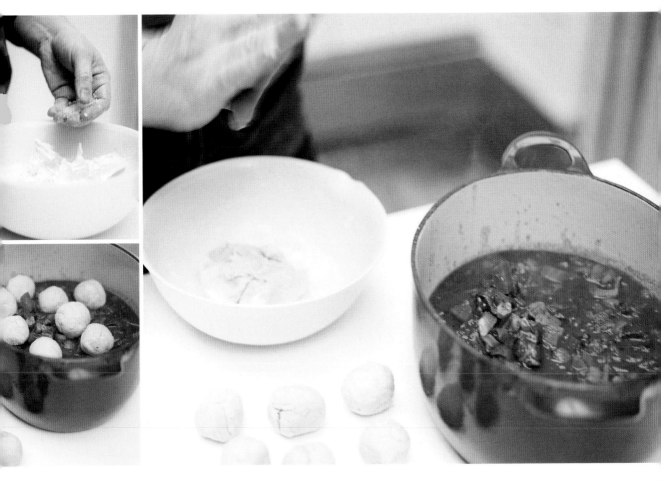

For your dumplings:

2 cups self-rising flour • 9 tablespoons really cold butter • sea salt and freshly ground black pepper

Preheat your oven to 375°F • Put your flour into a mixing bowl • Using a coarse grater, grate your cold butter into the flour • Add a pinch of salt and pepper • Using your fingers, gently rub the butter into the flour until it begins to resemble breadcrumbs • Add a splash of cold water to help bind it into a dough • Divide the dough into 12 pieces and gently roll each into a round dumpling • The dumplings will suck up quite a bit of moisture, so if your stew looks dry, add a cup of boiling water and give it a good stir • Place the dumplings on top of your fully cooked stew and press down lightly so that they're half submerged • Cook in the oven or on the stovetop over a medium heat with the lid on for 30 minutes

Or make it into a kinda hot-pot?

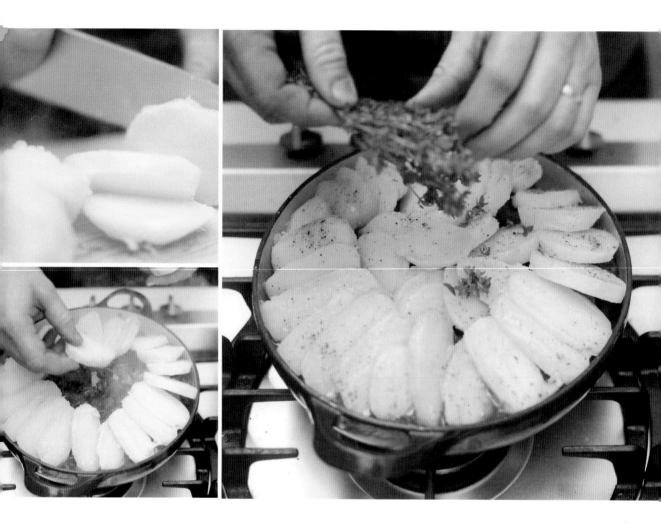

For your hot-pot topping:

1 ¼ pounds medium potatoes • sea salt and freshly ground black pepper • olive oil or a pat of butter • a few sprigs of fresh thyme

Preheat your oven to 375°F • Fill a large baking dish with the fully cooked stew • Peel the potatoes and put them into a pan of boiling, salted water • Boil for 10 minutes • Drain them in a colander and put to one side for 5 minutes to cool slightly • Slice the potatoes lengthways into ¼-inch-thick slices and lay these over the top of your stew • Drizzle with a little olive oil or melt the butter and brush this over the potatoes • Pick the thyme leaves off the stalks and sprinkle them over the potatoes with a pinch of salt and pepper • Cook in the oven for 40 minutes

Or a sort of cottage pie?

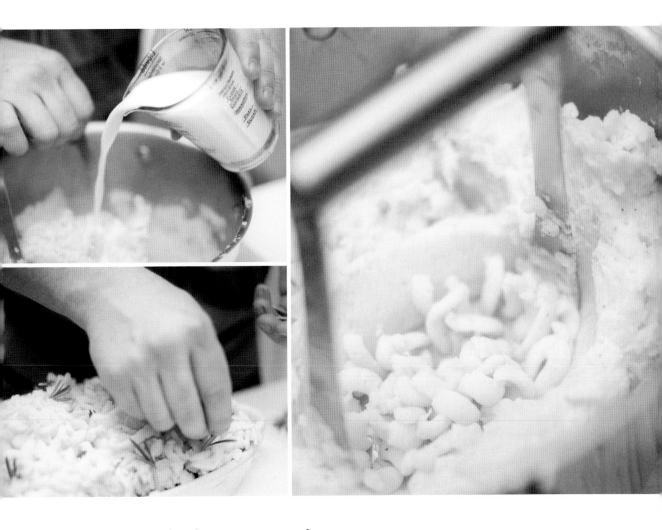

For your mashed potato topping:

2¼ pounds potatoes • a splash of milk • a tablespoon of butter • sea salt and freshly ground black pepper • a sprig of fresh rosemary • olive oil

Preheat the oven to 375°F • Fill a large baking dish with the fully cooked stew • Peel the potatoes, cut them in half, and put them into a pan of salted, boiling water • Boil for about 10 minutes until tender • Stick a knife into them to check they're soft all the way through • Drain in a colander and return them to the pan • Add the milk, butter, and a pinch of salt and pepper • Mash until smooth and creamy, adding another splash of milk if necessary • Roughly top the stew with the mashed potatoes – don't worry about it being smooth and even • Pick a few rosemary leaves off the woody stalk and lightly push them into the potato • Drizzle your pie with some olive oil, lightly coating the rosemary leaves • Cook in the oven for 25 minutes

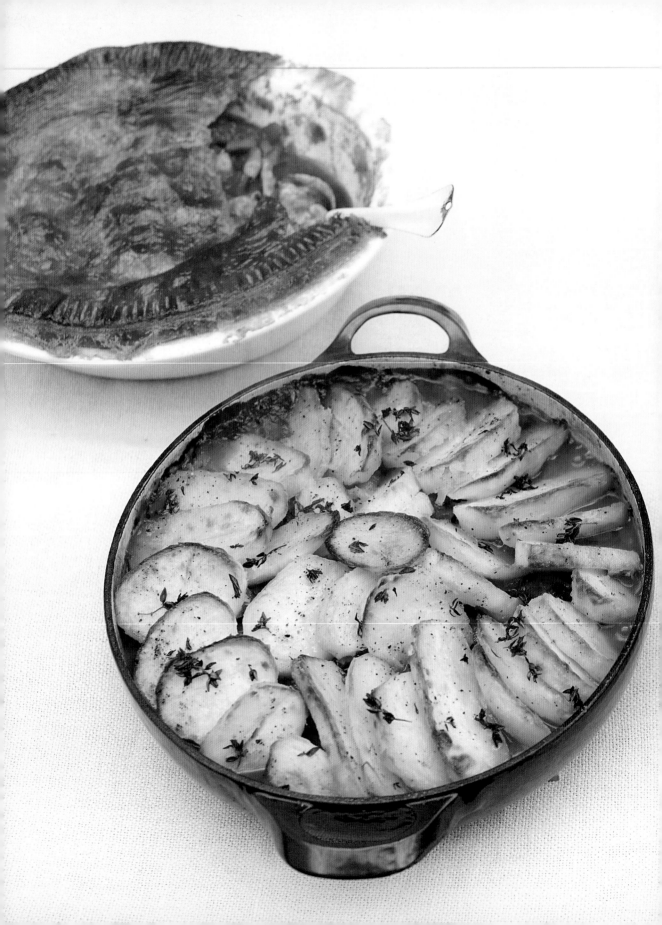

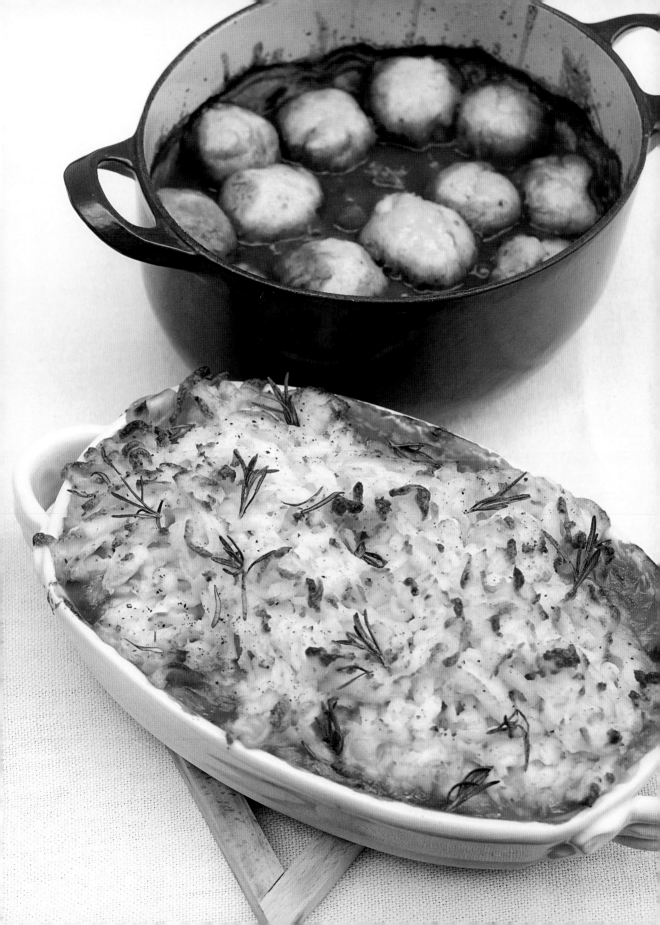

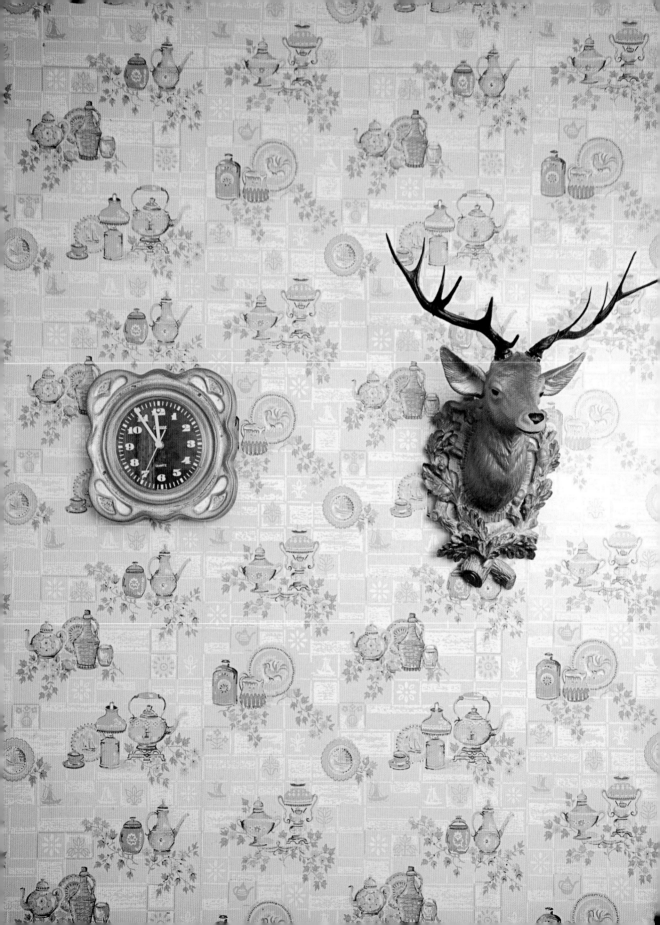

Family roast dinners

If you've never had a go at roasting a straightforward chicken, leg of lamb, or cut of beef with all the trimmings, you're missing out on what's probably one of the most satisfying and nostalgic social meals, because roast dinners are loved by everyone, including some of the most awkward kids, teenagers, and fussy friends. Traditionally in Britain a roast dinner has always been cooked on the weekend, and historically, up until about twenty or thirty years ago, your roast bird or cut of meat was something that was planned, saved up for, and looked forward to as a treat.

Even though food has become cheaper, buying a good roasting cut will still cost you a few dollars, especially if you're buying quality meat (you'll probably have to visit the meat counter at the grocery store for your pork and beef, or pay a visit to your local butcher). So the fear of ruining it or getting it wrong will definitely add extra pressure, more than with any other meal. However, a proper roast is a million times better than a rôtisserie chicken from the grocery store, or pre-roasted frozen potatoes, or a microwaveable roast dinner. So I'm going to hold your hand through the recipes and try to get you making some of the best, most memorable roast dinners, which will serve you, your family, and your friends well for many happy years! Oh, and don't forget, guys, you can roast a mega free-range chicken, with all the trimmings, for less than it costs to buy one of those greasy buckets of fried chicken.

I think the reason a roast dinner is one of the most important things you can learn to make is because it's usually cooked for a whole group of friends or family. To be able to absolutely nail it, with crispy roasted potatoes and a hint of rosemary, with a juicy bit of meat that isn't dry and overcooked, and with ass-kicking gravy — I mean, really, if you can do all these things, the rest is history. I've also given you a page of delicious but quick sauces — apple, bread, horseradish, and mint — that will leave your guests' jaws on the floor.

PERFECT ROAST BEEF

I've used a top round here because it is by far the most widely available roasting cut, but you can also use a rib of beef. The meat has to be rested after cooking for at least half an hour and sliced really thinly for you to enjoy the tenderness. The timings below are just a guide, as they can differ depending on the type of oven you have or the size of the cut.

serves 4–6

3¼ pounds beef top round
2 medium onions
2 carrots
2 celery stalks
1 bulb of garlic

a small bunch of fresh thyme, rosemary, bay, or sage,
 or a mixture
olive oil
sea salt and freshly ground black pepper

To prepare your beef

Take your beef out of the refrigerator 30 minutes before it goes into the oven • Preheat your oven to 475°F • There's no need to peel the vegetables – just give them a wash and roughly chop them • Break the garlic bulb into cloves, leaving them unpeeled • Pile all the vegetables, garlic, and herbs into the middle of a large roasting pan and drizzle with olive oil • Drizzle the beef with olive oil and season well with salt and pepper, rubbing it all over the meat • Place the beef on top of the vegetables

To cook your beef

Place the roasting pan in the preheated oven • Turn the heat down immediately to 400°F and cook for 1 hour for medium beef • If you prefer it medium-rare, take it out 5 to 10 minutes earlier • For well done, leave it in for another 10 to 15 minutes • If you're doing roasted potatoes and veggies, this is the time to crack on with them (see page 202) – get them into the oven for the last 45 minutes of cooking • Baste the beef halfway through cooking and if the vegetables look dry, add a splash of water to the pan to stop them burning • When the beef is cooked to your liking, take the pan out of the oven and transfer the beef to a board to rest for 15 minutes or so • Cover it with a layer of aluminum foil and a kitchen towel and put aside while you make your gravy (see page 205), horseradish sauce (see page 210), and Yorkshire puddings (see page 209)

To carve your beef

Remove the string from the meat • Use a good, long, sharp knife to carve the meat and a fork (preferably a carving fork) to hold it steady • Serve with your piping hot gravy, your horseradish sauce, roasted veggies, and Yorkshire puddings

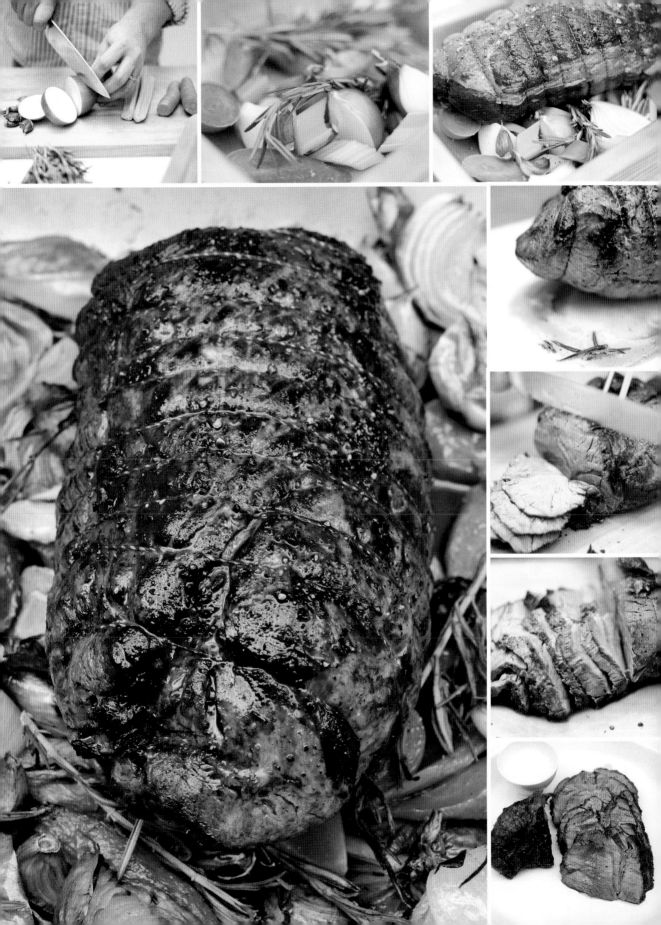

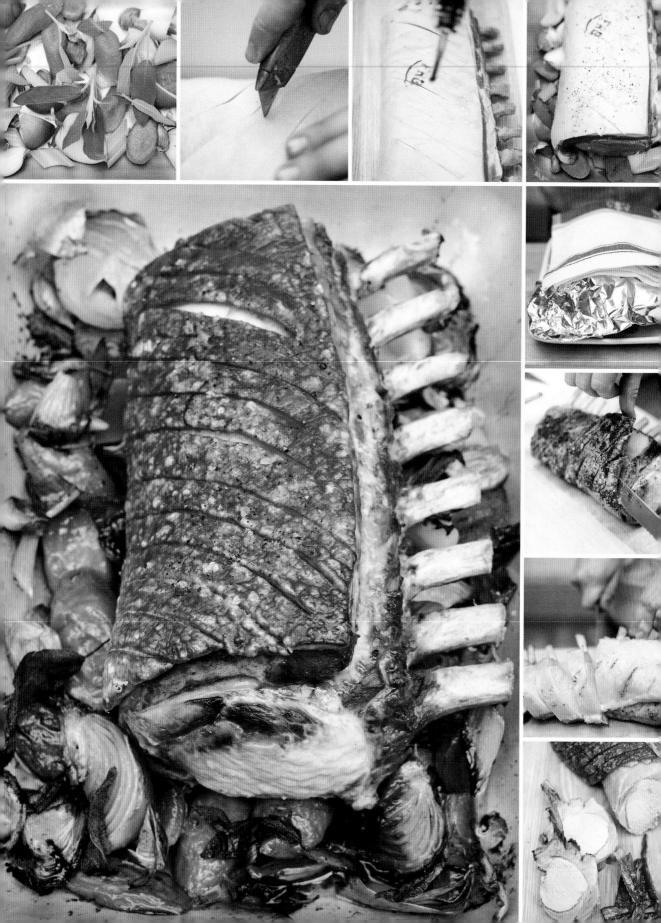

PERFECT ROAST PORK

Your pork loin will come in one of two ways, either on or off the bone. Either way it's fine, but if it's on the bone you'll have to cook it for an extra 20 minutes. You'll need a box cutter knife to score the fat (or ask your butcher to do this for you).

serves 4–6

1 x approximately 4-pound center cut pork loin, with bones (or 3-pound boneless loin), preferably free-range or organic

2 medium onions

2 carrots

2 celery stalks

1 bulb of garlic

a small bunch of fresh thyme, rosemary, bay, or sage, or a mixture

olive oil

sea salt and freshly ground black pepper

To prepare your pork

Take your pork out of the refrigerator 30 minutes before it goes into the oven • Preheat your oven to 475°F • There's no need to peel the vegetables – just give them a wash and roughly chop them • Break the garlic bulb into cloves, leaving them unpeeled • Pile all the vegetables, garlic, and herbs into the middle of a large roasting pan and drizzle with olive oil • Using a box cutter or a very sharp kitchen knife, score the skin all the way along at ¼-inch intervals (unless your butcher has done this for you) – make sure that it's just the skin and fat that you're cutting and not the meat underneath • Drizzle the pork with olive oil and season it well with salt and pepper, pushing the seasoning right into the scored skin and rubbing it all over the meat • Place the pork on top of the vegetables

To cook your pork

Place the roasting pan in the preheated oven • Turn the heat down immediately to 400°F and cook for 1 hour and 20 minutes – if you're roasting a pork loin on the bone add an extra 20 minutes • If you're doing roasted potatoes and veggies, this is the time to crack on with them (see page 202) – get them into the oven for the last 45 minutes of cooking • Baste the pork halfway through cooking and if the vegetables look dry, add a splash of water to the pan to stop them burning • When the pork is cooked to your liking, take the pan out of the oven and transfer the pork to a board to rest • How does the crackling look? If it doesn't look crispy enough for you, use a sharp knife to peel the skin away from the layer of fat and the meat • Pop this crackling into a separate pan on the top shelf of the oven or under the broiler for 5 to 10 minutes until golden and crisp • Cover the meat with a layer of aluminum foil and a kitchen towel and put aside to rest for 15 minutes or so while you make your gravy (see page 205) and applesauce (see page 210)

To carve your pork

If the crackling is still on the meat, use a sharp knife to peel it away from the layer of fat and the meat • If the pork loin is on the bone you can carve the meat into individual chunky chops • If a boneless cut, hold your meat steady with a carving fork and carve into thick or thin slices • Lay all the meat on a big serving platter with plenty of crackling • Serve with your piping hot gravy, your applesauce, and your roasted veggies

PERFECT ROAST CHICKEN

Having learned the things I've learned about chickens over the last few years, of course I'm going to suggest that you buy free-range or organic. A bird that's had a happy life is going to taste miles better than one that's been fattened too fast in a tiny cage or dark, overcrowded barn, so it's worth spending a few extra dollars when you can.

serves 4–6

1 x approximately 3½-pound chicken, preferably
  free-range, organic, or higher welfare
2 medium onions
2 carrots
2 stalks celery
1 bulb of garlic

olive oil
sea salt and freshly ground black pepper
1 lemon
a small bunch of fresh thyme, rosemary, bay, or sage,
  or a mixture

To prepare your chicken

Take your chicken out of the refrigerator 30 minutes before it goes into the oven • Preheat your oven to 475°F • There's no need to peel the vegetables – just give them a wash and roughly chop them • Break the garlic bulb into cloves, leaving them unpeeled • Pile all the vegetables and garlic into the middle of a large roasting pan and drizzle with olive oil • Drizzle the chicken with olive oil and season well with salt and pepper, rubbing it all over the bird • Carefully prick the lemon all over, using the tip of a sharp knife (if you have a microwave, you could pop the lemon in there for 40 seconds at this point as this will really bring out the flavor) • Put the lemon inside the chicken's cavity, with the bunch of herbs

To cook your chicken

Place the chicken on top of the vegetables in the roasting pan and put it into the preheated oven • Turn the heat down immediately to 400°F and cook the chicken for 1 hour and 20 minutes • If you're doing roasted potatoes and veggies, this is the time to crack on with them (see page 202) – get them into the oven for the last 45 minutes of cooking • Baste the chicken halfway through cooking and if the vegetables look dry, add a splash of water to the pan to stop them burning • When cooked, take the pan out of the oven and transfer the chicken to a board to rest for 15 minutes or so • Cover it with a layer of aluminum foil and a kitchen towel and put aside while you make your gravy (see page 205) and bread sauce (see page 210)

To carve your chicken

Remove any string from the chicken and take off the wings (break them up and add to your gravy for mega flavor) • Carefully cut down between the leg and the breast • Cut through the joint and pull the leg off • Repeat on the other side, then cut each leg between the thigh and the drumstick so you end up with four portions of dark meat • Place these on a serving platter • You should now have a clear space to carve the rest of your chicken • Angle the knife along the breastbone and carve one side off, then the other • When you get down to the fussy bits, just use your fingers to pull all the meat off, and turn the chicken over to get all the tasty, juicy bits from underneath • You should be left with a stripped carcass, and a platter full of lovely meat that you can serve with your piping hot gravy, roasted veggies, and bread sauce

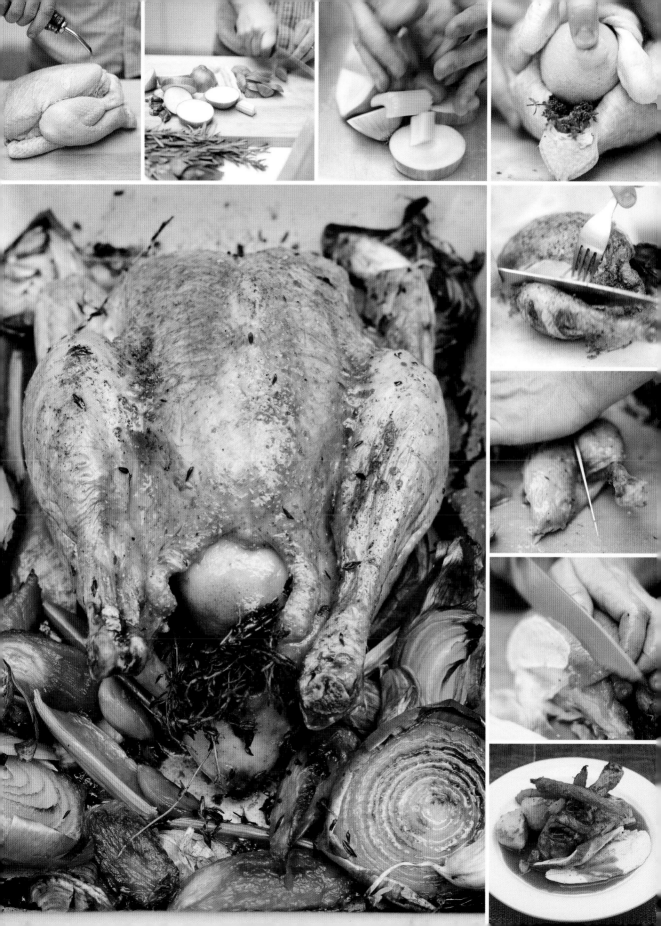

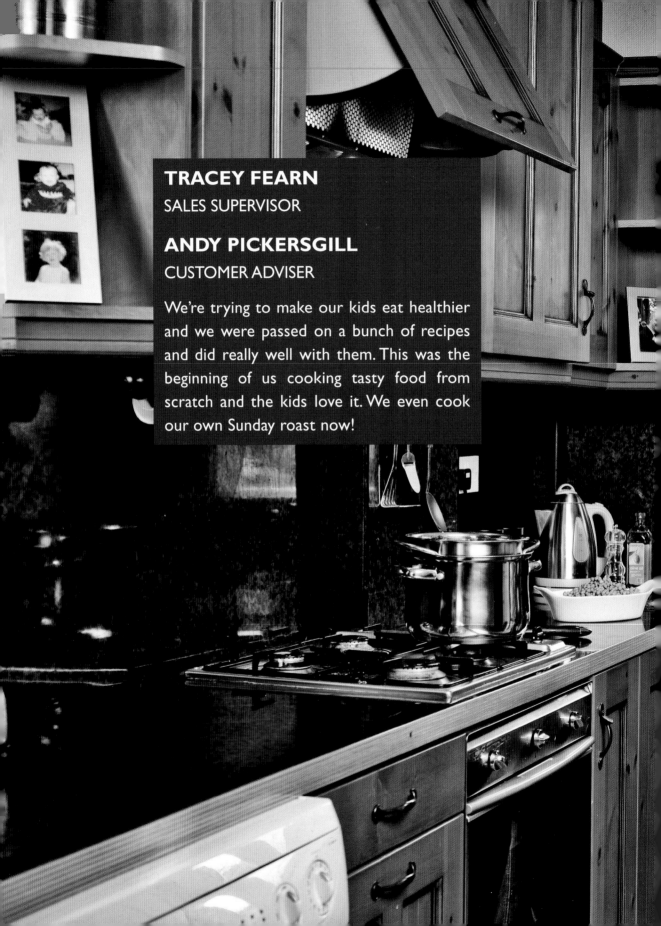

TRACEY FEARN
SALES SUPERVISOR

ANDY PICKERSGILL
CUSTOMER ADVISER

We're trying to make our kids eat healthier and we were passed on a bunch of recipes and did really well with them. This was the beginning of us cooking tasty food from scratch and the kids love it. We even cook our own Sunday roast now!

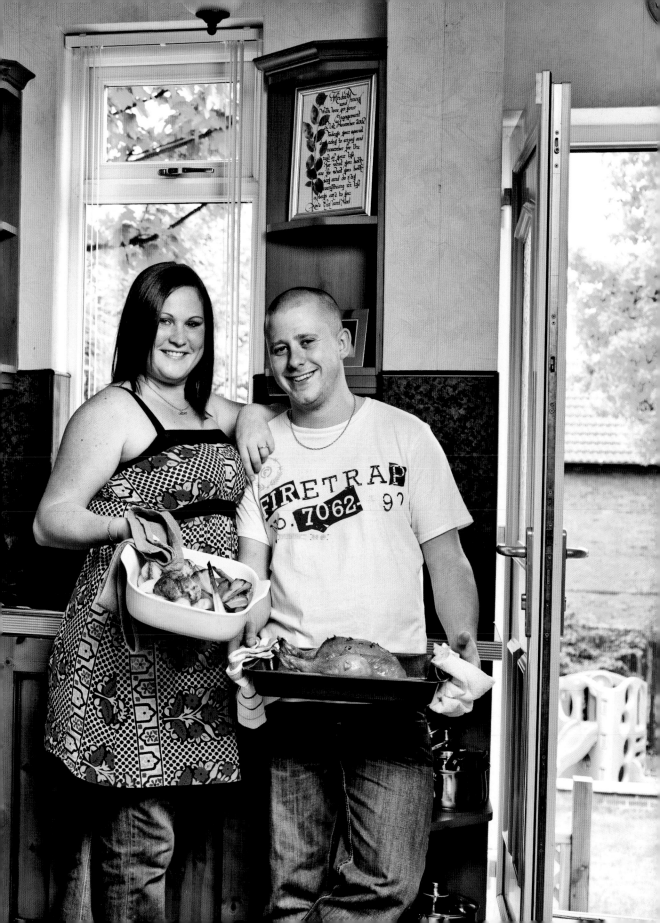

PERFECT ROAST LAMB

Roasting a leg of lamb is a dream. There will be different sizes of leg available throughout the year, so you're going to have to tell your butcher how many you're cooking for and ask his advice. You're going to want about 10 ounces per person on the bone.

serves 4–6

1 x approximately 4½-pound leg of lamb

2 medium onions

2 carrots

2 stalks celery

1 bulb of garlic

olive oil

sea salt and freshly ground black pepper

a small bunch of fresh thyme, rosemary, bay, or sage,
* or a mixture*

To prepare your lamb

Take your lamb out of the refrigerator 30 minutes before it goes into the oven • Preheat the oven to 475°F • There's no need to peel the vegetables – just give them a wash and roughly chop them • Break the garlic bulb into cloves, leaving them unpeeled • Pile all the vegetables, garlic, and herbs into the middle of a large roasting pan and drizzle with olive oil • Drizzle the lamb with olive oil and season well with salt and pepper, rubbing it all over the meat • Place the lamb on top of the vegetables

To cook your lamb

Place the roasting pan in the preheated oven • Turn the heat down immediately to 400°F and cook for 1 hour and 30 minutes for blushing pink meat • If you're doing roasted potatoes and veggies, this is the time to crack on with them (see page 202) – get them into the oven for the last 45 minutes of cooking • Baste the lamb halfway through cooking, and if the vegetables look dry, add a splash of water to the pan to stop them burning • When cooked to your liking, take the tray out of the oven and transfer the lamb to a board to rest for 15 minutes or so • Cover it with a layer of aluminum foil and a kitchen towel and put aside while you make your gravy (see page 205) and mint sauce (see page 210)

To carve your lamb

With lamb I don't think there's a right way or a wrong way when it comes to carving • Wrap a clean kitchen towel around the end of the bone and hold it firmly • Use a sharp knife to carve the lamb – away from you – in nice slices so you get a good cross-section of meat • When you get down to bones, just rotate the leg and start carving again • Lay all the carved meat on a serving platter and serve with your piping hot gravy, your mint sauce, and your roasted veggies

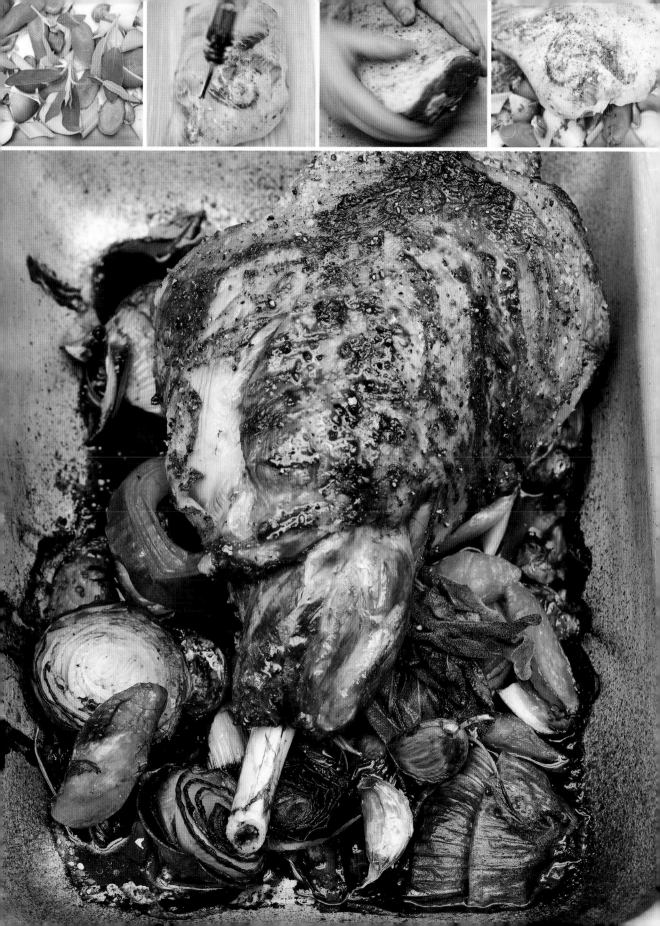

ROASTED POTATOES, PARSNIPS, AND CARROTS

In my eyes, a good roasted potato is one of the most important things in cooking. How is it that such a humble little vegetable can make people so happy? Have a go at this recipe – it will give you potatoes that are perfectly crispy on the outside and fluffy in the middle. The principle of parcooking in boiling water, then tossing in flavored oil, and roasting until deliciously golden and crisp, is just about the same for any other root vegetables, particularly parsnips and carrots, so I've included these in this recipe too.

You want your veggies to cook for about an hour in total, so the best time to put them into the oven is about 45 minutes before the meat is ready to come out. Once you've taken your meat out to rest for 15 minutes there'll be more space in the oven and you'll be able to move the veggies up to the top shelf and finish them off to perfection.

serves 4–6
2½ pounds potatoes
6 parsnips
6 carrots

1 bulb of garlic
3 sprigs of fresh rosemary
sea salt and freshly ground black pepper
olive oil

To prepare your vegetables
If you're cooking these separately and not as part of one of the roast meats in this chapter, preheat your oven to 400°F • Peel the vegetables and halve any larger ones lengthways • Break the garlic bulb into cloves, leaving them unpeeled, and bash them slightly with the palm of your hand • Pick the rosemary leaves from the woody stalks

To cook your vegetables
Put the potatoes and carrots into a large saucepan — you may need to use two — of salted, boiling water on a high heat and bring back to a boil • Allow to boil for 5 minutes, then add the parsnips and cook for another 4 minutes • Drain in a colander and allow to steam dry • Take out the carrots and parsnips and put to one side • Fluff up the potatoes in the colander by shaking it around a little – it's important to "chuff them up" like this if you want them to have all those lovely crispy bits when they're cooked • Put a large roasting pan over a medium heat and either add a few generous lugs of olive oil or carefully spoon a little of the fat from the meat you're cooking • Add the garlic and rosemary leaves • Put the vegetables into the pan with a good pinch of salt and pepper and stir them around to coat them in the flavors • Spread them out evenly into one layer – this is important, as you want them to roast, not steam as they will if you have them all on top of each other • Put them into the preheated oven for about 1 hour, or until golden, crisp, and lovely • Serve immediately, with your roast meat and your gravy (see page 205)

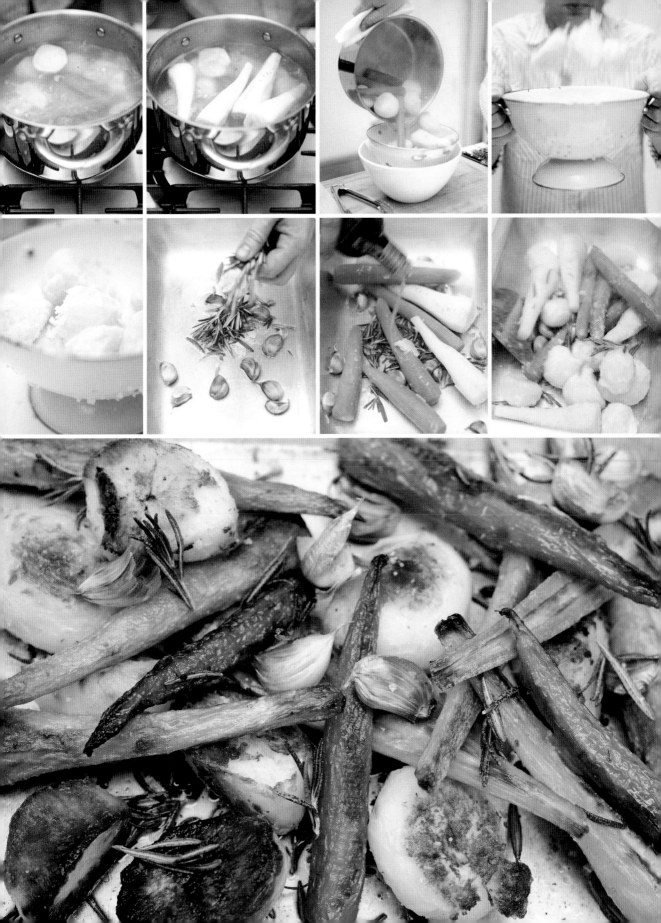

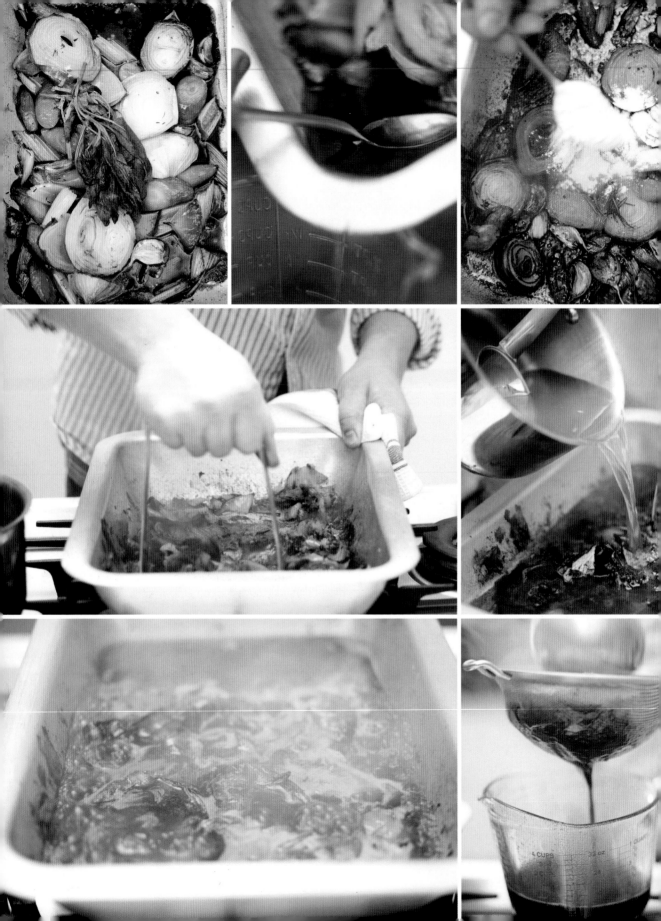

A CONSISTENTLY GOOD GRAVY

There are two things that make a good gravy: a vegetable trivet, which is the layer of vegetables in the bottom of your roasting tray that your meat sits on; and the juices from a roasted piece of good-quality meat.

As long as you always use a vegetable trivet and buy good-quality meat, your gravy will taste like heaven whether you use water or stock. Follow my method for making gravy and you'll never look back.

serves 4–6

As well as your roasted vegetables (listed in each meat recipe), you'll need:

1 heaped dessertspoon all-purpose flour

a wineglass of red wine, white wine, or cider, or a good splash of port or sherry

1 quart vegetable, chicken, or beef broth, preferably organic

To make your gravy

By the time you need to turn to this page your meat will be covered and resting and you'll have your pan of meat juices and vegetable trivet in front of you • Using a spoon, carefully remove 90 per cent of the hot fat from the tray by angling it away from yourself and scooping off the fatty layer that settles on top • Put the pan back on the cooktop over a high heat • Add the flour, stir it around, and, holding the pan steady with a kitchen towel in one hand, use a potato masher to mash all the veg to a pulp – don't worry if it's lumpy • If you're making chicken gravy, you can rip the wings off the chicken and break them up into the tray to add more flavor at this point • When everything is mixed and mashed up, add the alcohol to give a little fragrance before you add your stock (the alcohol will cook away) • Keep it over the heat and let it boil for a few minutes • Pour the stock into the pan, or add 1 quart of hot water • Bring everything in the pan to a boil, scraping all the goodness from the bottom of the pan as you go • Reduce the heat and simmer for 10 minutes, or until you've achieved the gravy consistency you're looking for

To serve your gravy

Get yourself a large jug, bowl, or saucepan and put a coarse strainer over it • Pour your gravy through the strainer, using a ladle to really push all the goodness through • Discard any vegetables or meat left behind • At this point you've got a really cracking gravy, and you can either serve it straightaway or put it back on the heat to simmer and thicken up • Depending on which meat I'm serving it with, I'll add a teaspoonful of horseradish, mustard, red-currant jelly, cranberry, mint, or apple sauce – you certainly don't have to, but I think the little edge of complementary flavor you get from doing this is brilliant

DELICIOUS SAGE AND ONION STUFFING

This is a classic recipe, and I like to cook it in an earthenware pot so it gets nice and crispy on the sides and the top. Obviously, the better the sausage meat and the bread, the better the stuffing will be. Little extras like chestnuts and dried fruits add lovely textures and flavors. It goes well with any type of roasted meat, and leftover stuffing is great in cold meat sandwiches.

Start making this as soon as your meat goes into the oven, so the mixture has time to cool completely before you add the sausage meat. Then simply put it into the oven 50 minutes before you're ready to eat.

serves 4–6

3 medium onions
a small bunch of fresh sage
½ a large loaf of stale unsliced bread
olive oil
1 tablespoon butter

optional: a handful of roasted, peeled chestnuts (from a vacuum pack or a jar), or a handful of dried fruit such as sour cherries or apricots
1¾ pounds good-quality sausage meat, preferably free-range or organic
sea salt and freshly ground black pepper

To prepare your stuffing
Preheat your oven to 400°F • Peel, halve, and roughly chop your onions • Pick the sage leaves from the stalks and roughly slice • Cut the crusts off the bread and discard • Tear the bread into large chunks • Fill a bowl with cold water

To cook your stuffing
Put a large frying pan on a medium heat and add a good lug of olive oil and the butter • Add your onions and cook gently for 7 to 10 minutes, until soft and golden • Stir in the sage leaves • Take handfuls of the bread and dip them into the bowl of water • Squeeze the water out well, then add the wet bread to the pan, stirring and breaking up any big chunks with a wooden spoon • Let it cook for a few minutes • At this point you can add any lovely extras, like roasted, peeled, and roughly chopped chestnuts or chopped dried fruit • Remove the pan from the heat, spoon the contents into a large bowl, and put aside to cool down completely • Once it's cooled, mix the sausage meat into the onion mixture and season well with salt and pepper • If you want to freeze the stuffing, now's the time to bag it up • To cook it straight away, put the stuffing into an oil-rubbed dish and bake it at the bottom of the preheated oven for 50 minutes, until really golden and crispy on top • Serve with your roast meat, veggies (see page 202), and gravy (see page 205)

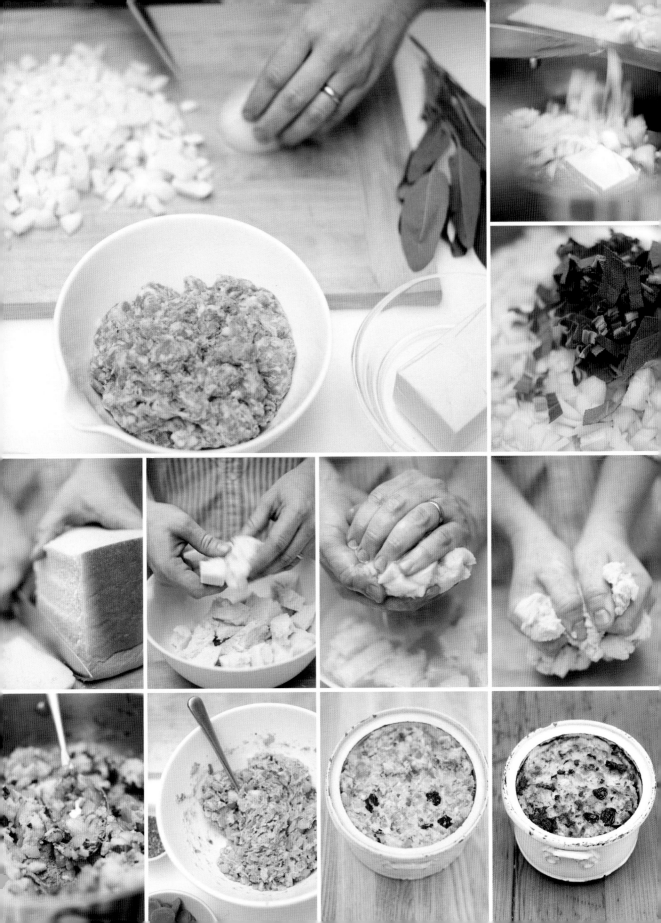

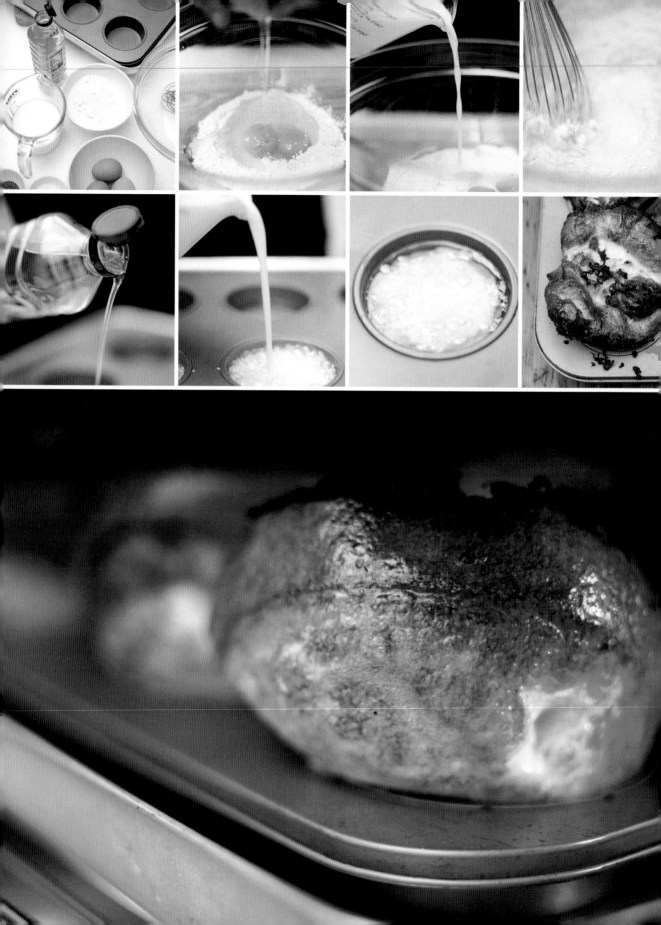

YORKSHIRE PUDDINGS

Traditionally we Brits eat our Yorkshire puddings with a roast beef dinner, but they're so tasty you can eat them in loads of different ways. Try them with onions and gravy, or cook one large one with sausages to make "toad-in-the-hole." Believe it or not, they're even good eaten with fruit as a sweet treat. The key to making great Yorkshires is to cook them in a really, really hot oven and to keep the door shut. If you do this, the rest should be no trouble.

makes 12

3 eggs, preferably free-range or organic
1 cup all-purpose flour
a pinch of sea salt

scant 1¼ cups milk
vegetable oil

To prepare your Yorkshires

Whisk the eggs, flour, salt, and milk together really well in a bowl to make your batter • Pour the batter into a jug and put to one side to rest for 30 minutes before you use it – this will help to make it smoother, giving you wonderfully light and crispy puddings

To cook your Yorkshires

Turn the oven up to the highest temperature (475°) and let it preheat fully • As it's warming up, put a muffin pan on to a cookie sheet and place on the top shelf of the oven • When the oven is up to temperature, carefully remove the pan and sheet, close the oven door, and add a tablespoon of vegetable oil to each muffin hole in the muffin pan • Pop the pan and sheet back into the oven for 5 minutes, until the oil is smoking hot • Open the oven door and slide the shelf with the pan and sheet on it halfway out • Quickly fill each muffin hole with batter, then slide the shelf carefully back into the oven • Leave the oven door shut for at least 15 minutes, and don't open it even once to check on how the Yorkshires are doing, otherwise they'll end up all sunken • After 15 minutes, the Yorkshires will be crisp and golden with a soft, fluffy center, which is how I like them • If you prefer them to be crispy all the way through, turn the oven down to 300°F and cook them for another 10 minutes • Remove the pan from the oven once the puddings are crisp, golden, and puffed up • Serve as soon as possible with your roast beef and gravy . . . or anything else you fancy

PS Don't wash your muffin pan out, just wipe it clean – if you keep it just for making Yorkshire puddings, the non-stick surface will improve every time you make them, as will the ability of the puddings to rise

ROAST DINNER SAUCES

Applesauce serves 4–6

3 good eating apples such as Macintosh / ½ an orange / a pat of butter / ¼ cup sugar / ¼ teaspoon ground cinnamon / ¼ of a nutmeg / ¼ teaspoon ground cloves

Peel and core your apples and chop them into roughly 1-inch pieces • Zest your orange half over a small saucepan and squeeze in the juice • Add the butter, sugar, and ground cinnamon • Grate over the nutmeg and add the ground cloves • Put the pan over a low heat and let the butter gently melt • Stir until the butter looks all foamy, then stir in all your apple pieces • Place a lid on the pan and cook for 20 to 25 minutes on a medium to low heat, stirring occasionally until you have a soft, chunky sauce • At this point, taste and add a bit more sugar if you think it needs it • Serve the applesauce warm or cold – it's delicious either way!

Bread sauce serves 4–6

½ a medium onion / 2 cups milk / 2 bay leaves / 2 cloves / 6 slices of good, stale bread / ½ teaspoon English mustard / sea salt and freshly ground black pepper

Peel and finely chop the onion half • Put in a small saucepan over a low heat with the milk, bay leaves, and cloves • Simmer for 10 minutes, then remove and discard the bay leaves and cloves • Slice the crusts off the bread and discard • Place the bread in the pan and simmer it for 5 minutes, until the bread has absorbed all the milk and softened • Stir now and again • Stir in the mustard and season well to taste with salt and pepper • The finished sauce should have a loose, oatmeal-like consistency • You can simmer it for a little while longer to thicken it up, or loosen it by adding a splash of water

Horseradish sauce serves 4–6

¼ cup grated fresh horseradish or 1 tablespoon fiery jarred horseradish / 1 lemon / 5 tablespoons crème fraîche or sour cream / extra virgin olive oil / sea salt and freshly ground black pepper

Put your horseradish into a small bowl • Finely zest over your lemon, then cut it in half and squeeze the juice into the bowl • Add the crème fraîche (or sour cream) and a good drizzle of extra virgin olive oil, and season with a pinch of salt and pepper • Mix together well • Taste and add more horseradish and seasoning if you think it needs it

Mint sauce serves 4–6

1 big handful of fresh mint leaves / 1 heaped tablespoon sugar / 2 tablespoons red wine vinegar / sea salt and freshly ground black pepper

Finely chop the mint leaves and place in a small bowl • Dissolve the sugar in scant ½ cup of boiling water and pour straight over the mint • Add the vinegar – this will give the sauce a nice twang and make it a bit looser in consistency • Add a pinch of salt and pepper to taste and balance the flavor by adding a touch more sugar or vinegar

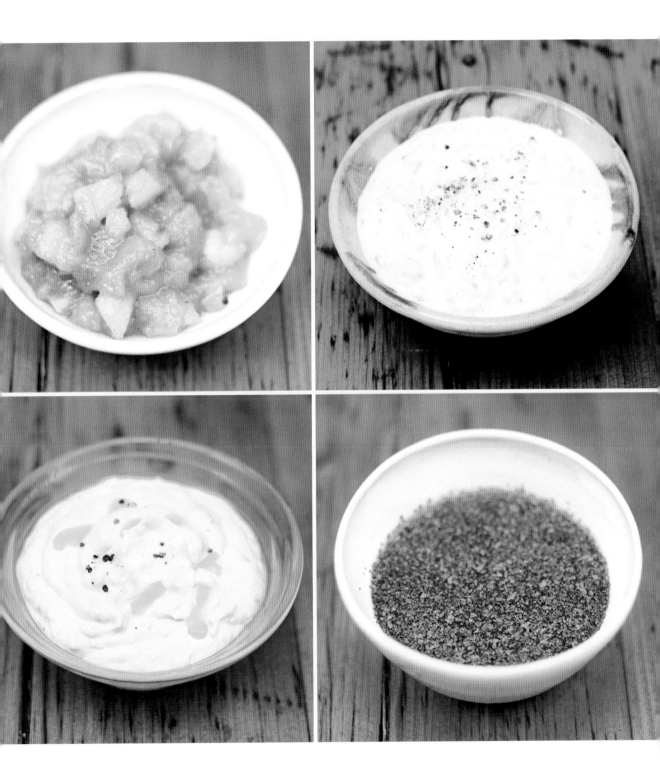

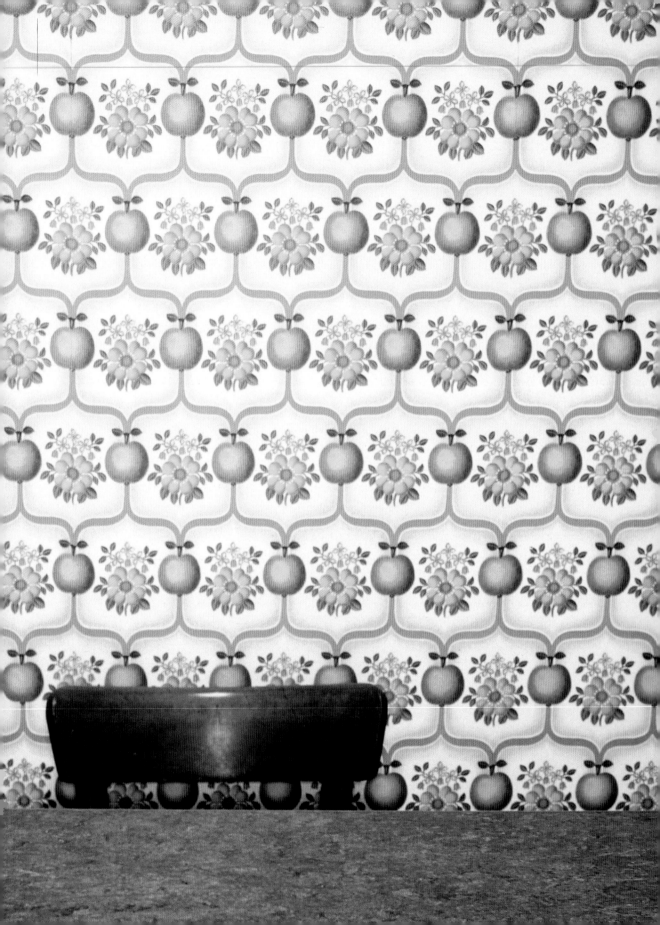

Delish veggies

This chapter is all about making vegetables taste delicious. And it's especially for those of you who think you hate veggies – I promise that you will love these recipes. Over the past few years, I've had so many conversations with people who tell me they can't stand eating vegetables. It only takes me about 10 seconds to work out why, and I'm not surprised. More often than not, they will boil their vegetables until they're completely overcooked and soggy, and then serve them without any dressing or flavoring. And this is missing out on the key thing – vegetables, like any good salad, need to be dressed with fantastic flavors.

So this chapter is made up of twelve recipes. Each recipe is very close to my heart, because these are the ones I love to cook all the time when I'm at home.

There are lots of messages being given to us these days about five-a-day and what we should have or what we shouldn't have, but I think that when it comes to salads and vegetables you should *want* to eat them, not *have* to eat them. And if you're one of the many people out there who boil the hell out of vegetables until all their texture, color, and taste have gone, give these recipes a go.

BAKED CARROTS IN A BAG

serves 4–6

Preheat your oven to 400°F • Peel 1¾ pounds of **carrots** • Leave them whole if small, chopping any larger ones up • Get yourself a sheet of aluminum foil about 2 feet long, fold it in half to make a crease, and then open it out again • Pile your carrots in the middle of the aluminum foil on one side of the crease • Finely slice 1 rasher of **smoked bacon, preferably free-range or organic** • Pick the leaves off 2 sprigs of **fresh rosemary** and finely chop • Peel 1 clove of **garlic** and finely slice • Scatter the bacon, rosemary, and garlic over the carrots • Grate over the zest of ½ an **orange**, and add 1 teaspoon of **marmalade**, 2 pats of **butter**, and a pinch of **salt and pepper** • Fold the other half of the aluminum foil over the carrots and scrunch and seal the two sides of the aluminum foil bag together, leaving one end open • Halve the orange and squeeze all the juice into the bag • Seal up the final side • Place your aluminum foil bag on a baking tray in the preheated oven for around 50 minutes • To serve, carefully pour the carrots and all their juices into a nice big serving dish

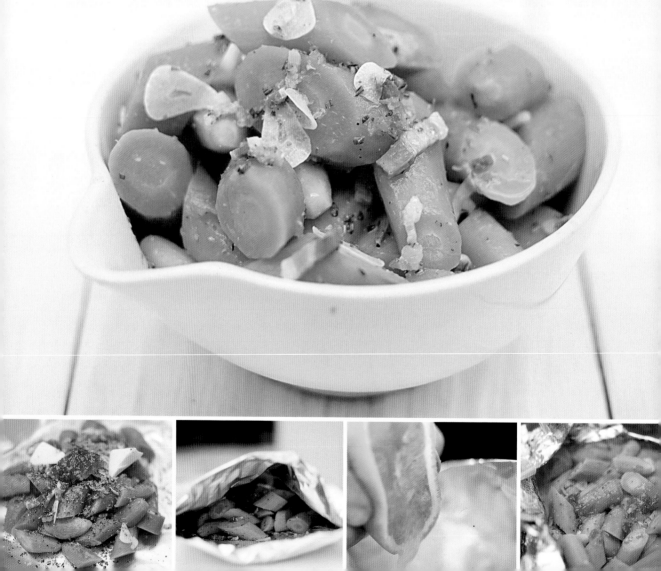

DRESSED ASPARAGUS

serves 4–6

Put a saucepan of water on to boil • Get I pound of **asparagus** and bend the base of each stalk to click the woody ends off, leaving you with the tender tips • Add a teaspoon of **salt** to the saucepan, and all the asparagus • Place a lid on, bring back to a boil, and cook for I to 2½ minutes, depending on how thick your asparagus spears are • Put 3 tablespoons of **extra virgin olive oil**, I teaspoon of **Dijon mustard**, I tablespoon of **red wine vinegar,** and a pinch of chopped **parsley** into a bowl and whisk together with a pinch of salt and **pepper** • Drain the asparagus, place on a serving dish, and drizzle over the vinaigrette, making sure that all the spears are coated

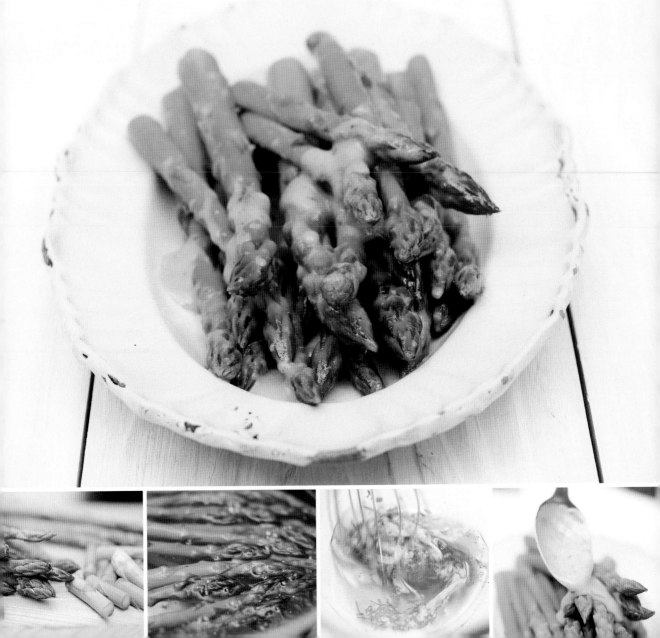

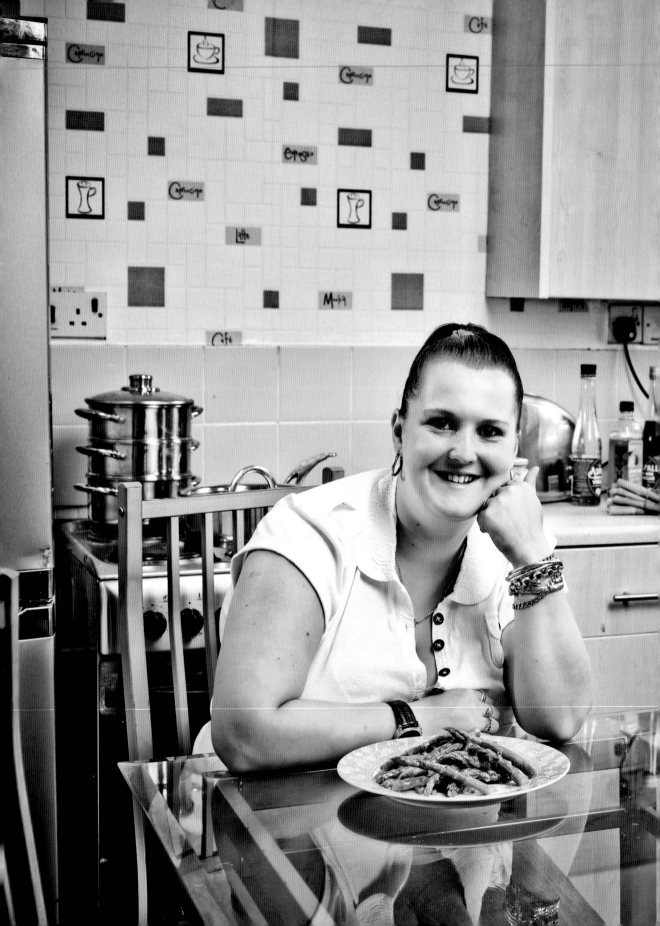

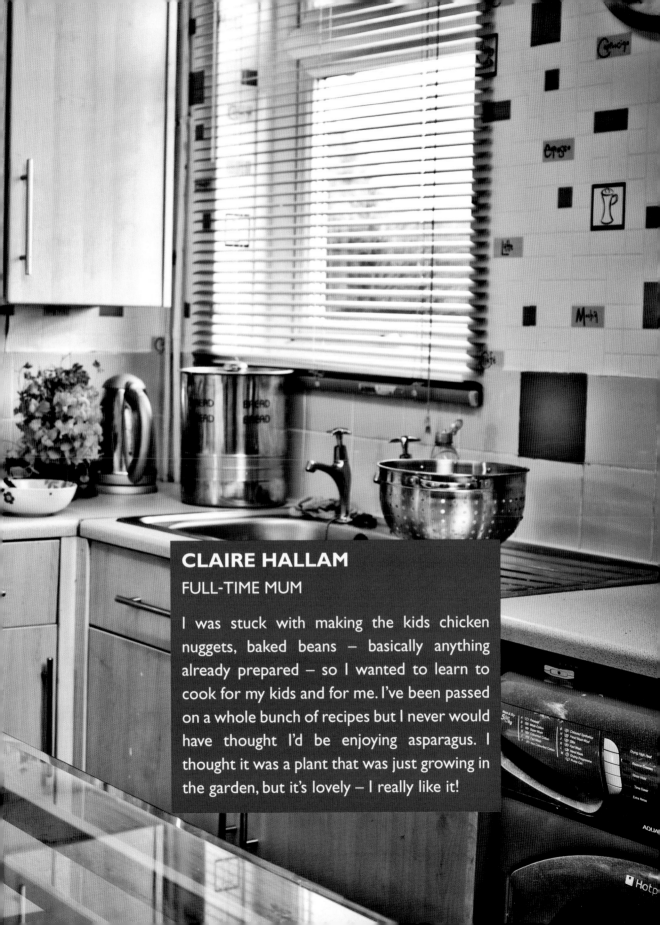

CLAIRE HALLAM

FULL-TIME MUM

I was stuck with making the kids chicken nuggets, baked beans — basically anything already prepared — so I wanted to learn to cook for my kids and for me. I've been passed on a whole bunch of recipes but I never would have thought I'd be enjoying asparagus. I thought it was a plant that was just growing in the garden, but it's lovely — I really like it!

BEST BABY POTATOES

serves 4–6

Get yourself 1¾ of **baby potatoes** • You can either leave the skins on, as they're full of vitamin C and very good for you, or you can rub or scrape them off • Half fill a large saucepan with boiling water from your kettle and add a pinch of **salt** • Add the potatoes and boil fast for 10 to 15 minutes • Stick a knife into them to test if they're done • Drain them in a colander, put them into a large bowl with 3 pats of **butter,** and season nicely with salt and **pepper** • Pick the leaves from 4 or 5 sprigs of **fresh mint** and finely chop • Add to the bowl, squeeze over the juice of 1 **lemon,** and toss well before serving • Use any leftovers cold as a salad, or even roast them in a really hot oven until crisp and golden

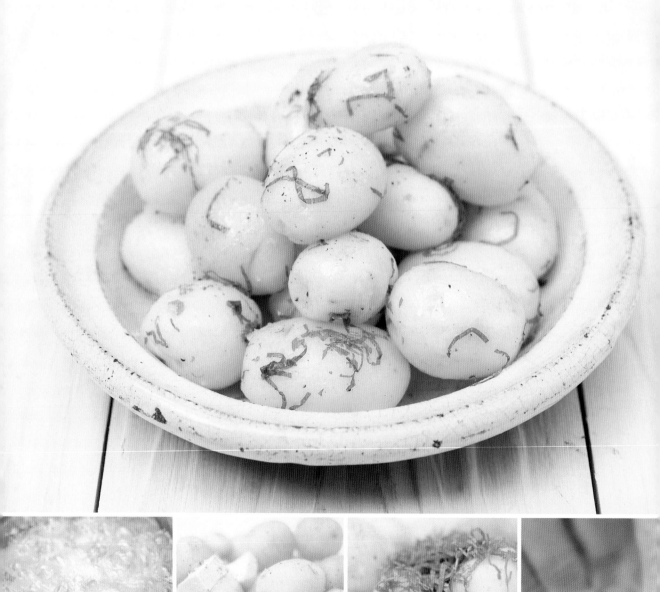

BUTTERED SPINACH

serves 4–6

Preheat your largest frying pan or wok until hot • Wash and drain 1 pound of **spinach or baby spinach** • Peel and finely slice 2 cloves of **garlic** • Tilt the pan and add a lug of olive oil, immediately followed by the garlic • Shake the pan around so the garlic cooks evenly • When the garlic goes slightly golden, tip in your spinach and mix it around quickly, using a pair of tongs • Season with a pinch of **salt and pepper** • In just 1 minute the spinach will cook down – you'll be amazed how quickly it happens! • Put it into a colander and let any excess water drain away • Put the pan back on the heat and add 2 pats of **butter** • As soon as the butter starts to bubble, put the spinach back into the pan and squeeze over the juice of 1 **lemon** • Stir it around, taste, and add more salt and pepper if you think it needs it • Serve immediately

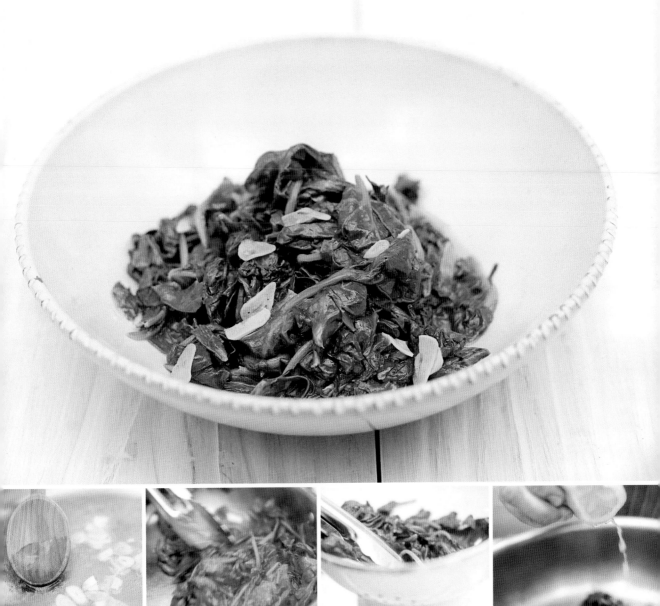

BROCCOLI WITH ASIAN DRESSING

serves 4–6

Get yourself around 1¼ pounds of **broccoli or broccolini or broccoli rabe** • Heat your steamer pan or put a large pan of water on to boil • Break the broccoli up into little pieces and slice up the stalks • Place the broccoli in your steamer or in a colander placed over the pan of boiling water and cover with a tight-fitting lid or some aluminum foil • Steam for around 6 minutes, until the stalks are tender • Meanwhile, make your dressing • Peel a thumb-sized piece of **fresh ginger** and a clove of **garlic** and grate into a bowl • Halve, seed, and finely chop a **fresh red or green chile** and add to the bowl • Stir in 1 tablespoon of **sesame oil**, 3 tablespoons of **extra virgin olive oil**, 1 tablespoon of **soy sauce,** and the juice from 1 **lime** • Drizzle in a teaspoon of **balsamic vinegar** • Whisk the dressing together and have a taste • What you're looking for is a flavor balance between saltiness from the soy sauce, sweetness from the balsamic vinegar, acid from the lime, and heat from the chile • When the broccoli is cooked, place it on a big serving platter • Mix up the dressing one last time before pouring it over • Absolute heaven!

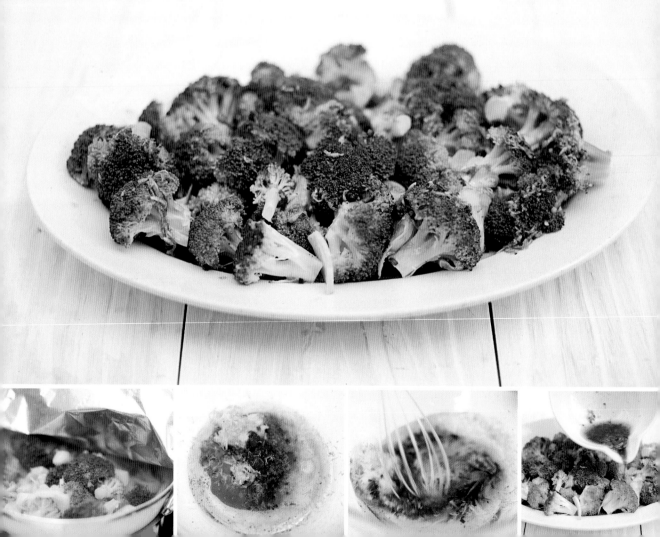

MINTED PEAS

serves 4–6

Trim and finely slice 2 **scallions** • Wash and finely slice 1 **butterhead lettuce** or 1 **romaine heart** • Put the scallions into a saucepan with 2 good pats of **butter** • Fry for a minute or so, then stir in 2 heaped teaspoons of **all-purpose flour** • Add 4 cups of **frozen or fresh peas** and the lettuce • Pour in ½ cup of water • Crumble in 1 **vegetable or chicken bouillion cube**, stir it in, and simmer for 5 minutes • Season to taste with a good pinch of **salt and pepper** • Pick the leaves from 4 sprigs of **fresh mint**, finely chop, and stir in

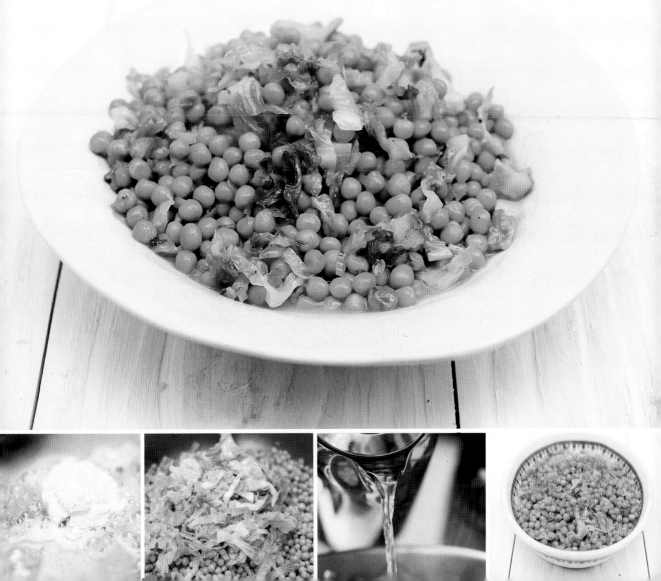

BEST EVER FRENCH BEANS

serves 4–6

Line up 1¼ pounds of **French or other green beans** on a chopping board • Cut off the stalks, leaving the wispy ends as they are – they look nice! • Put the beans into a large saucepan of boiling water with a pinch of **salt** and cook for about 6 minutes • Try one – if it's soft and not squeaky when you eat it, they're done • Drain them in a colander, reserving some of the cooking water, and set them aside to steam dry • Peel and slice 3 cloves of **garlic** • Finely grate 1½ cups of **Parmesan cheese** • Put the pan back on the heat, add a good lug of **extra virgin olive oil** and the sliced garlic, and give it a stir • When the garlic starts to turn golden, add the beans and jiggle the pan around to coat them in the garlicky oil • Add a ladleful of the reserved cooking water, the Parmesan, and the juice of ½ a **lemon** • Stir and simmer until the water and cheese start to form an oozy, sticky sauce, then remove from the heat and serve immediately

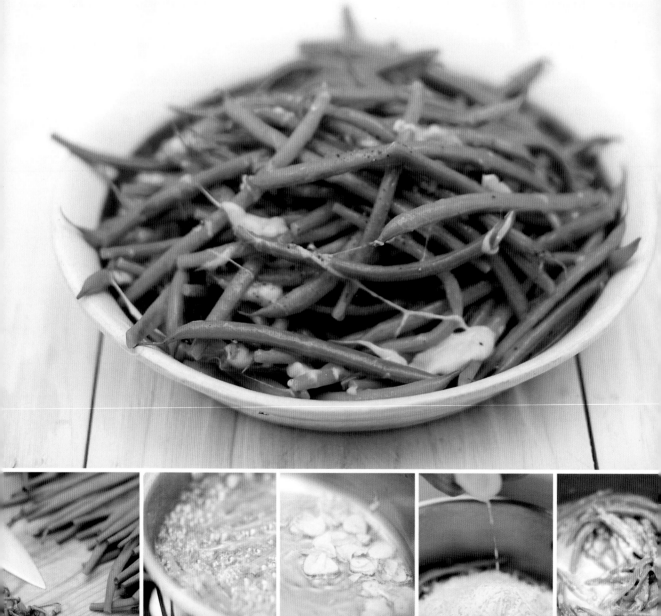

BAKED CREAMY LEEKS

serves 4–6

Preheat your oven to 400°F • Get yourself 1¾ pounds of **leeks**, peel back the scruffy outer leaves, trim the ends and discard, then quarter the leeks lengthways and roughly chop them • Put them into a colander, give them a really good wash to get rid of any dirt, and drain • Peel and finely slice 2 cloves of **garlic** • Put a large pan on a medium heat and add 2 pats of **butter**, a lug of **olive oil**, and the garlic • Pick the leaves off 6 sprigs of **fresh thyme**, discarding the stalks • Just as the garlic begins to take on the smallest amount of color, add all the leeks and thyme leaves and give them a stir • Turn the heat up and cook for about 10 minutes, until the leeks have softened • Meanwhile, grate 1 cup of **Cheddar cheese** • Remove the pan of leeks from the heat and season with a couple of good pinches of **salt and pepper** • Add just under 1 cup of **heavy cream** and half the grated cheese • Mix everything up and transfer into an earthenware dish that will give you a layer of leeks about 1 inch thick • Sprinkle over the rest of the cheese and bake in the preheated oven for about 20 minutes, until golden and bubbling

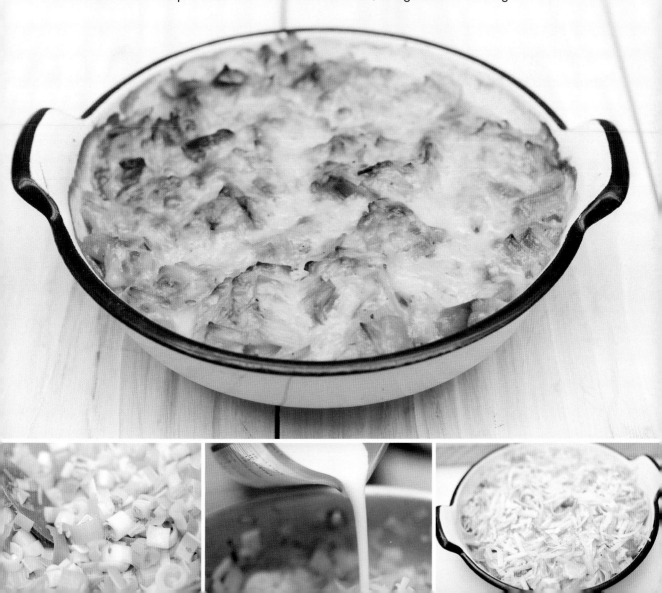

BAKED FRENCH POTATOES

serves 4–6

Preheat your oven to 400°F • Put 3½ cups chicken or vegetable broth in a saucepan and bring to a boil • Peel and finely slice 1¾ poundsof **potatoes** • Peel, halve, and finely slice 1 pound of **medium onions** and 3 cloves of **garlic** • Pick the leaves from a small handful of **fresh Italian parsley** and finely chop • Pour a couple of lugs of **olive oil** into a large, hot pan with the onions, garlic, and parsley • Slowly fry for 10 minutes, until the onions are soft and lightly golden • Add a good pinch of **salt and pepper** • In a large baking dish place a layer of potatoes, a sprinkling of salt and pepper, and a layer of onions • Continue, repeating until you've used everything up, but try to finish with a layer of potatoes on top • Pour in the hot broth to just cover the top of the potatoes • Break up 2 pats of **butter** and dot over the top • Rub some aluminum foil with olive oil, place it, oil-side down, over the dish, and seal tight • Place in the preheated oven for 45 minutes, then remove the aluminum foil, push the potatoes down, and return to the oven for 20 to 40 minutes until golden and crisp

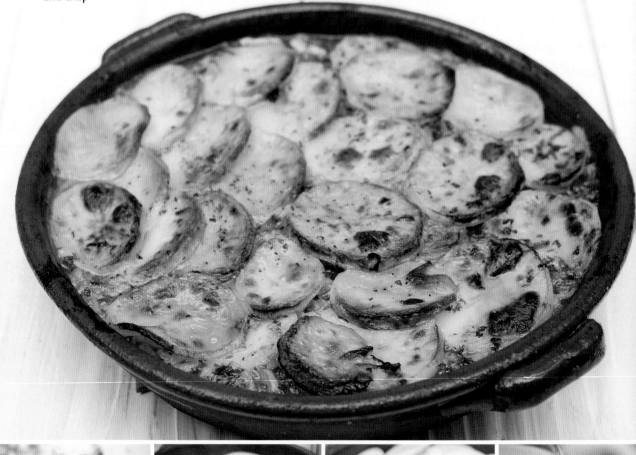

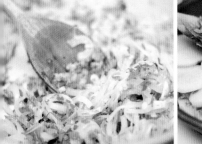
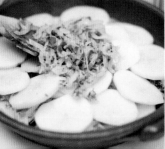
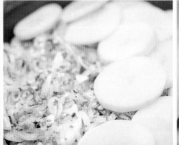
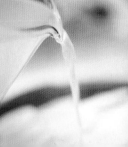

CAULIFLOWER CHEESE

serves 4–6

Preheat your oven to 350°F • Put a large saucepan of water on to boil • Remove the outer green leaves from 1 **large cauliflower** and discard • Break the cauliflower into small pieces and slice up the stalk • Pick the leaves off 2 sprigs of **fresh rosemary** • Add all the cauliflower to the pan of boiling water with a pinch of **sea salt** and boil for 5 minutes • Chop up 4 **anchovy fillets** and put them into a bowl with 1 ⅔ cups of **crème fraîche or heavy cream** • Stir in 1 cup of grated **Cheddar cheese** and season with **salt and pepper** • Pour a lug of **extra virgin olive oil** into a food processor and add 4 slices of **bread** with the crusts left on, a slice of **smoked bacon, preferably free-range or organic,** and the rosemary leaves • Whiz everything up until you have breadcrumbs • By now your cauliflower should be done, so drain it in a colander and place it into a medium-sized baking dish • Spoon the sauce over the cauliflower, and sprinkle over another 1 cup of grated Cheddar, followed by your breadcrumbs • Place in the preheated oven for 45 minutes or until golden, crisp, and bubbling

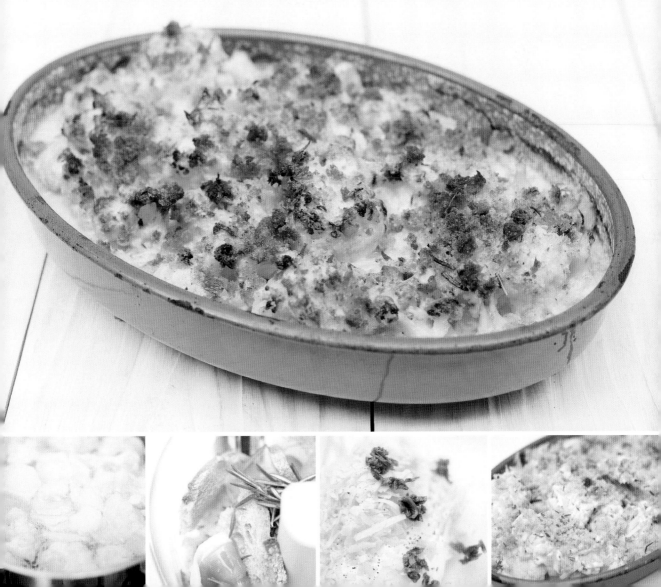

BRAISED BACON CABBAGE

serves 4–6

Strip all the leaves off 1 **Savoy, green, or spring cabbage** and wash them • Roll the leaves up together, like a cigar, and slice finely • Peel and finely chop 2 cloves of **garlic** • Slice up 6 slices of **smoked bacon, preferably free-range or organic** • Place the bacon in a large saucepan on a medium heat with a lug of **olive oil** and stir around for a few minutes until perfectly crisp and golden • Stir in the garlic and as it begins to color add 2 tablespoons of **Worcestershire sauce**, 2 pats of **butter,** and all your finely sliced cabbage • Stir well, give the pan a shake, and turn the heat to high • Drop 1 **chicken or vegetable bouillion cube** into 1¼ cups of boiling water, pour this broth into the pan, and give it all a good stir • Place a lid on top and cook for 5 minutes, then remove the lid and continue to cook for another 5 minutes • Taste, and season with **salt and pepper** if you think it needs it • Drizzle with a lug of **extra virgin olive oil** just before serving

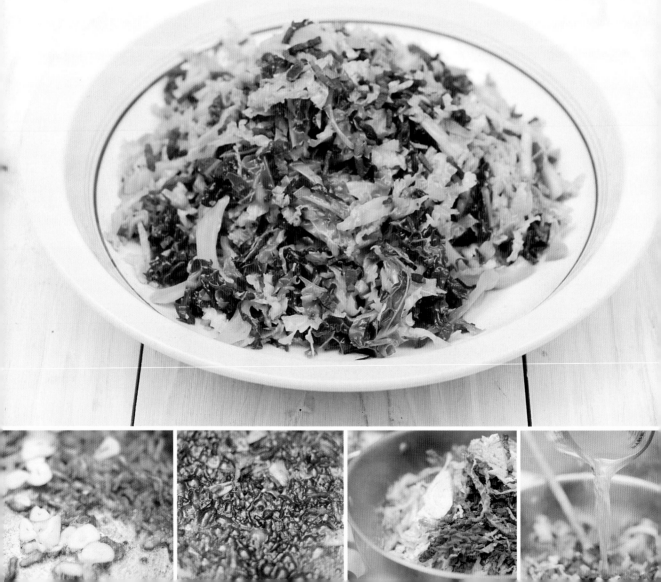

MEXICAN-STYLE CORN

serves 4

Boil 4 heads of **corn on the cob** in salted, boiling water for 8 to 10 minutes with a lid on the pan • When tender, drain in a colander • Grate ¾ cup of **Parmesan cheese** over the surface of a large serving platter or over 4 individual serving plates • Halve, seed, and finely chop 1 **fresh red or green chile** and sprinkle evenly over the cheese • Place a little pat of **butter** on each cob and brush over the corn to coat • When the butter has melted, roll each cob in the cheese and chile, so the flavors stick to the outside • Season with a good pinch of **salt and pepper** • Serve with **lime wedges** for squeezing over

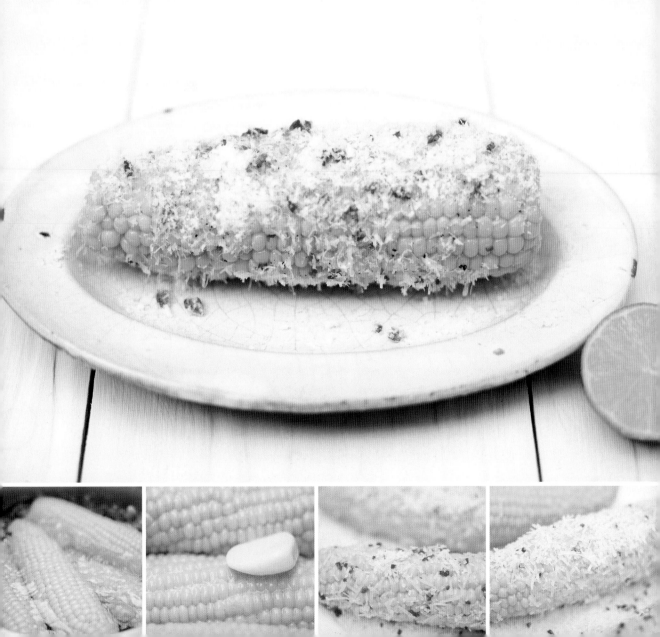

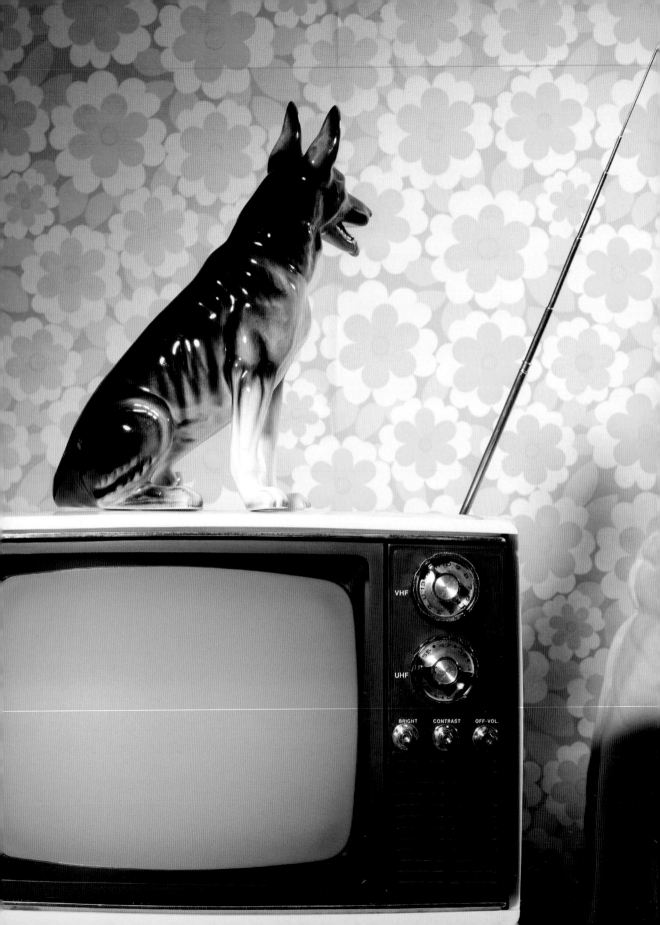

Quick-cooking meat and fish

This chapter concentrates on the most common cuts of meat and fish bought from butchers, fishmongers, and grocery stores. On the meat side, it's pork chops, lamb chops, steaks, and chicken breasts, and for fish it's salmon, cod or other white fish, tuna, and trout. I'm going to give you a couple of recipes for each of these that are exciting and quick, and ideal for beginners to have a go at making.

These days there's quite a lot of controversy over buying meat and fish. I must admit that some of this has been brought about by me! Of course I endorse free-range and organic foods — any food or animal lover would — but if budget is an issue, then I would suggest eating meat less often, but spending a bit more on the meat you do buy so it's as delicious and wonderful as it should be.

There's also a lot of controversy surrounding fishing and ethics. Due to over-fishing in certain areas, farmed fish seems to be the only sustainable option. If you're interested in finding out a bit more about endangered fish around the world, take a look at these websites: www.MSC.org or www.fishsource.org.

At the end of this chapter you'll find a section that includes some delicious and quick sauces, salsas, and flavored oils — they're great for serving with any of the meat or fish recipes.

PAN-FRIED GLAZED PORK CHOPS

It really is worth buying outdoor-reared meat. Basic pork is usually too lean and dry, so it's far better to spend a bit more on quality meat – you'll enjoy it much more. Try eating better pork, less often, and think of it as a treat. These glazed pork chops have a big, comforting flavor with a great combination of meat and sweet stickiness. It's a good idea to serve something fresh and green with them – try a crisp salad or some steamed veggies dressed with extra virgin olive oil and lemon juice.

serves 2

2 x 8-ounce pork chops, preferably
  free-range or organic
olive oil
sea salt and freshly ground black pepper

4 sprigs of fresh sage
optional: 1 lemon
applesauce, mango chutney, apricot jam, maple syrup,
  or honey, to glaze

To prepare your pork

Using a very sharp knife, or kitchen scissors, carefully trim the skin off the edges of each chop – you're going to turn this into crackling • Cut each strip of skin lengthways into 2 strips, so you end up with 4 strips in total • Use a sharp knife to make cuts every ¼ inch along the fat remaining on the chops – this will help it render and crisp up while cooking • Rub both sides of the chops with olive oil and season really well with salt and pepper • While you're at it, season your strips of skin • Pick the sage leaves off their stalks, toss them lightly in a little olive oil, and put to one side

To cook your pork

Put a frying pan over a high heat and add your strips of skin • Move them about in the hot pan and remove when golden, crisp, and crackling • Lay both chops flat in the pan and give them 4–5 minutes on each side, turning every minute • When they're looking golden, add a few sage leaves to the pan • Let them crisp up and cook for about 30 seconds, then remove them to a plate • Spoon a large tablespoon of applesauce (or other chosen glazing ingredient) over each chop • Keep turning the chops over so they get nicely coated • Have the confidence to cook them until almost a dark reddy-golden color and wonderfully thick and sticky • Remove the chops to a plate and let them rest for a minute or two, squeezing over a little lemon juice if you want to balance out the sweetness a bit

To serve your pork

Serve your chops on a plate, with the crackling and the crispy sage leaves • Lovely with some dressed veggies, a fresh salad, plain rice, or mashed potatoes

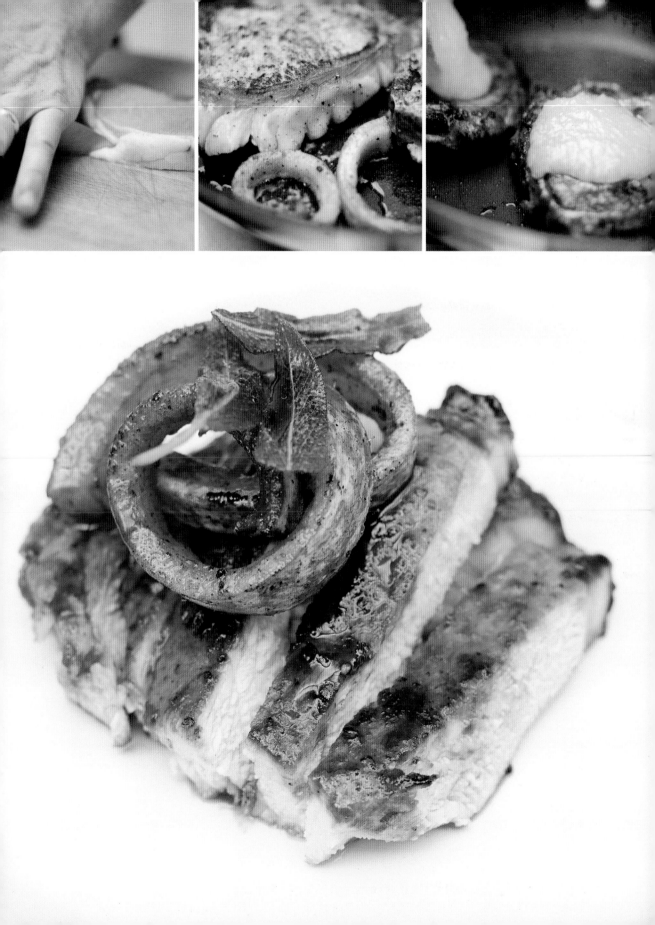

GRILLED FILET MIGNON WITH HORSERADISH SAUCE

Meat cooked this way is quick, simple, and totally delicious. Rubbing the top of the meat with a garlic clove as it cooks is a little trick I've learned from the American barbecue king, Adam Perry Lang. You're standing there watching the meat cook anyway, so you may as well keep busy and give it some love! It's such a small thing but it really makes the meat taste great – give it a try, you'll never go back.

serves 2

a small bunch of fresh rosemary
sea salt and freshly ground
  black pepper
olive oil
2 ½-pound filet mignon steaks
1 large clove of garlic

For the dressing
2 tablespoons crème fraîche or sour cream
1 tablespoon grated horseradish, fresh or jarred
sea salt and freshly ground black pepper
1 lemon
extra virgin olive oil

To prepare your beef and sauce

Put a grill pan on a high heat and let it get screaming hot • Pick the rosemary leaves off the woody stalks and finely chop • Mix with a good pinch of salt and pepper and scatter over your clean board • Drizzle olive oil over both sides of the steaks and roll them in the rosemary and seasoning • Put the crème fraîche (or sour cream) and horseradish into a small bowl with a pinch of salt and pepper • Halve your lemon and add a squeeze of juice to the bowl • Add a splash of extra virgin olive oil and mix well • Taste and add a little more horseradish if you think it needs to taste more fiery

To cook your beef

Lay the steaks in your hot pan and press them down gently • Wait a minute, then turn them over • Cut the tip off the garlic clove and discard • Rub the hot, charred side of the meat with the garlic • Flip the steaks again after another minute, repeat the garlic rub, and press down again • For medium-rare meat, cook for around 4 to 5 minutes on each side • For well-done meat, cook for a few minutes more • Remove the steaks from the grill to a plate to rest for a few minutes • Drizzle with a little olive oil to keep them from drying out

To serve your beef

Place your steaks on clean plates and spoon a good dollop of the horseradish sauce on top or next to them • Drizzle some of the lovely resting juices on top, and a little extra virgin olive oil • Alternatively you can slice the steaks in half at an angle and serve them on a bed of something light and fresh, like a watercress salad, with the horseradish sauce

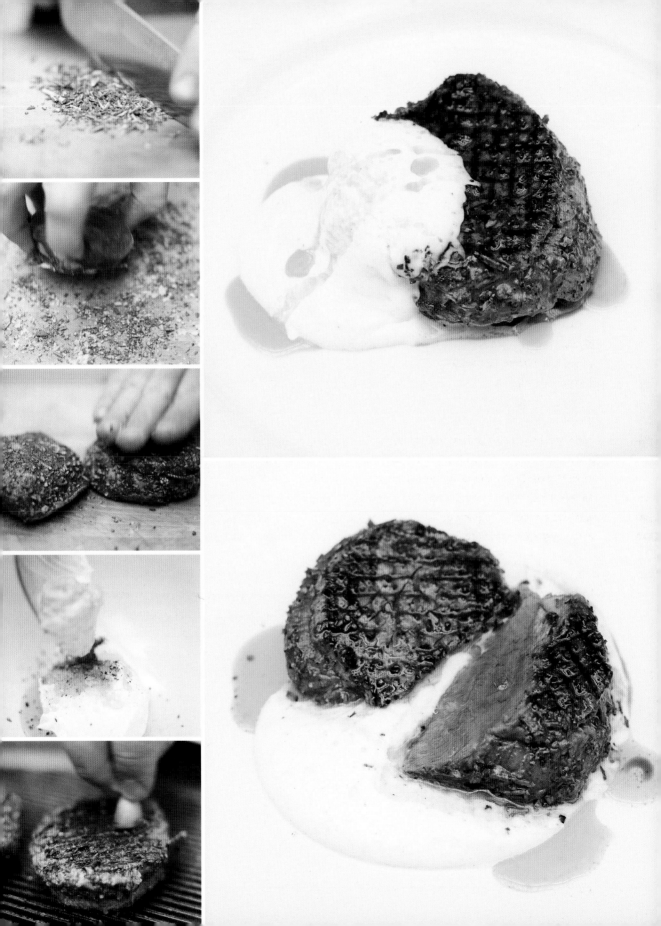

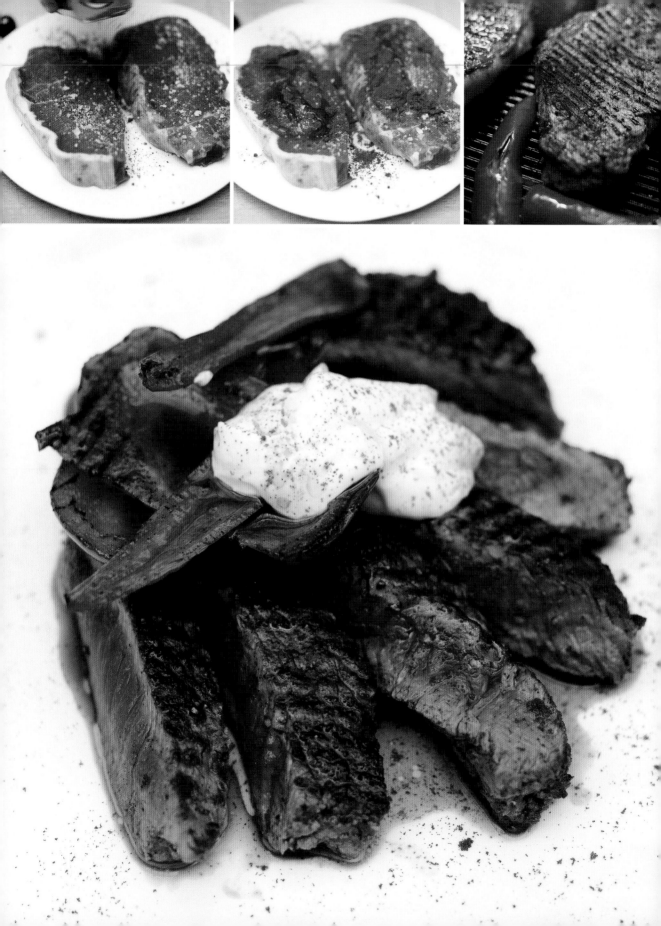

SPANISH-STYLE GRILLED STEAK

This is just a delicious, simple combination of great steaks, with all their fantastic juices, given a slightly Spanish twist using paprika and grilled chiles and bell peppers. Lovely served with a nice refreshing dollop of crème fraîche or sour cream, the meat is also wonderful served just on its own. It's also good inside some pita bread with salad, or with some rice.

serves 2

2 fresh red or green chiles
1 red bell pepper
2 x 8-ounce beef top loin steaks
sea salt and freshly ground black pepper
a good sprinkling of normal or smoked paprika
olive oil

1 large clove of garlic
extra virgin olive oil
1 lemon
1 cup crème fraîche or sour cream

To prepare your steaks

Put a grill pan on a high heat and let it get screaming hot • Halve and seed your chiles and bell pepper, then cut both bell pepper halves in two • Season your steaks really well with salt, pepper, and paprika • Drizzle with a good lug of olive oil and give the steaks a rub on both sides, making sure they are well coated in the seasoning

To cook your steaks

Lay the steaks in your hot pan with the chiles and bell peppers • Cut the tip off the garlic clove and discard • Your steaks should take 5–8 minutes in total to cook, depending on how you like them – every minute, turn them over, rub the hot, charred side of the meat with the garlic, and press down again • Don't forget to flip your bell peppers and chiles over too • Remove the steaks from the grill to a plate to rest for about 5 minutes • Cook the bell peppers and chiles for another 2 minutes, or until slightly charred, then remove to another plate and drizzle with extra virgin olive oil • Halve your lemon and squeeze the juice from one half over the steaks

To serve your steaks

You can either leave the steaks whole or cut them into strips and serve them with the bell peppers and chiles piled on top • Lovely with a dollop of crème fraîche or sour cream • Drizzle with the amazing meat juices, sprinkle with a pinch of paprika, and finish with a nice drizzle of extra virgin olive oil and the juice from the other lemon half

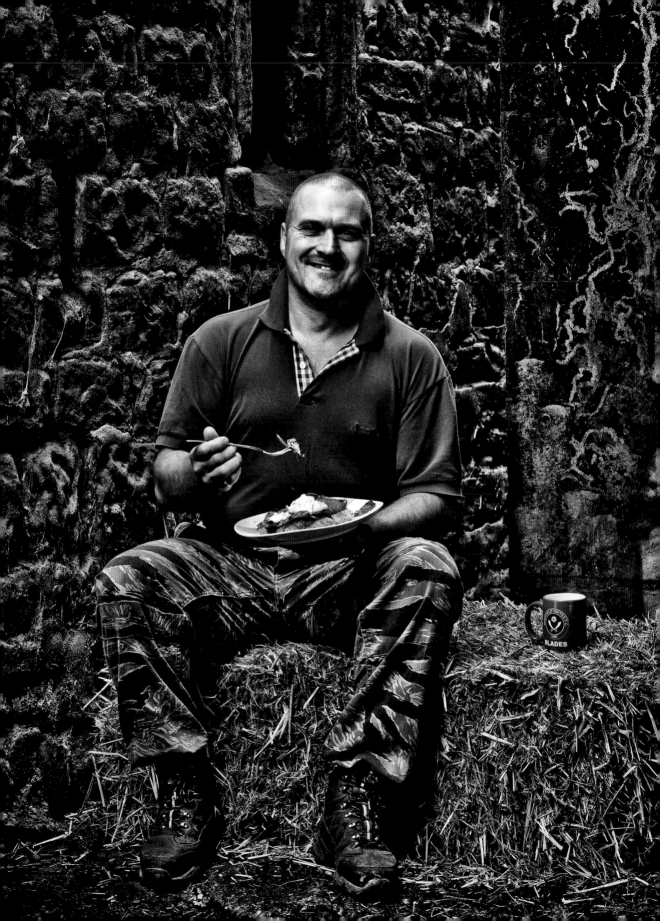

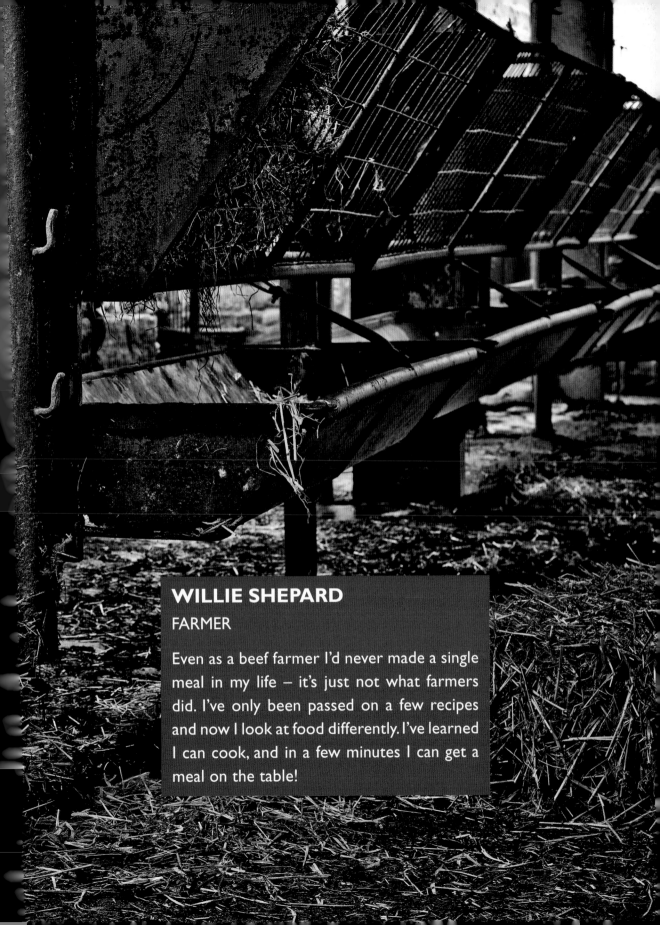

WILLIE SHEPARD

FARMER

Even as a beef farmer I'd never made a single meal in my life — it's just not what farmers did. I've only been passed on a few recipes and now I look at food differently. I've learned I can cook, and in a few minutes I can get a meal on the table!

PORK KABOBS

The key to making a good kabob is taking the time to ensure your ingredients are cut to roughly the same size and thickness. That way, everything cooks evenly and you get a lovely finished result. Kabobs are very versatile things to cook – they can be barbecued, grilled, or roasted. Have a go at trying out different combinations of meat and veggies. Things like mushrooms, onions, chiles, zucchini, and bell peppers all work really well with kabobs.

serves 2

1 pound pork tenderloin, preferably free-range or organic

16 small mushrooms

1 medium red onion

a small bunch of fresh rosemary

2 lemons

1 teaspoon ground cumin

sea salt and freshly ground black pepper

olive oil

1 teaspoon honey

To prepare your kabobs

If you're using wooden skewers, trim them down so they fit in your pan and soak them in water for at least 30 minutes so they don't burn • Preheat a grill pan on a high heat for 5 minutes and let it get screaming hot • Slice the pork into roughly ¾-inch pieces • Wipe the mushrooms and cut the stalks off • Depending on their size, either leave the mushrooms whole or cut them into chunks the same size as the meat • Peel and halve your onion, then quarter each half • Pull the rosemary leaves off the woody stalks • Zest one of the lemons and finely chop with the rosemary • Mix with the cumin and a good pinch of salt and pepper and scatter over your clean work surface • Drizzle the meat, mushrooms, and onions with olive oil and roll them in the rosemary, lemon zest, and cumin • Skewer a piece of pork, followed by a piece of onion or mushroom, and repeat until all the pieces have been used • Don't squeeze things too tightly on the skewers – if you leave little spaces, it means the steam and heat can get in there and cook everything • Drizzle the kabobs with oil and season well with salt and pepper

To cook your kabobs

Put your kabobs on the hot grill pan and push them down gently • Cook for about 8 minutes in total, turning every 2 minutes so that you cook all four sides, until everything is golden, slightly charred, and the pork is cooked through • Use a sharp knife to cut into the pork and check it's ready • If it's still a bit pink, continue cooking for a few more minutes • Once the pork's done, give the kabobs a tiny drizzle of olive oil, a little more salt, a good squeeze of lemon juice, and a tiny drizzle of honey • Cook for another 30 seconds, turning as you go

To serve your kabobs

Put your kabobs on a plate and drizzle them with the lovely juices from the pan • Serve with lemon wedges and anything from dips, salsas, sour cream, to salad or rice – you name it, it'll go well with these

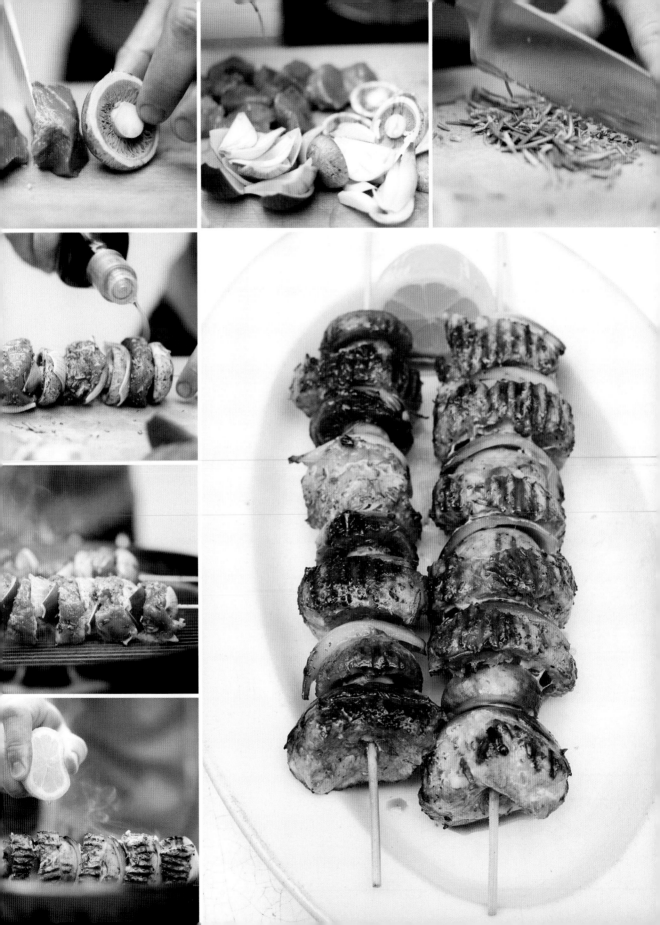

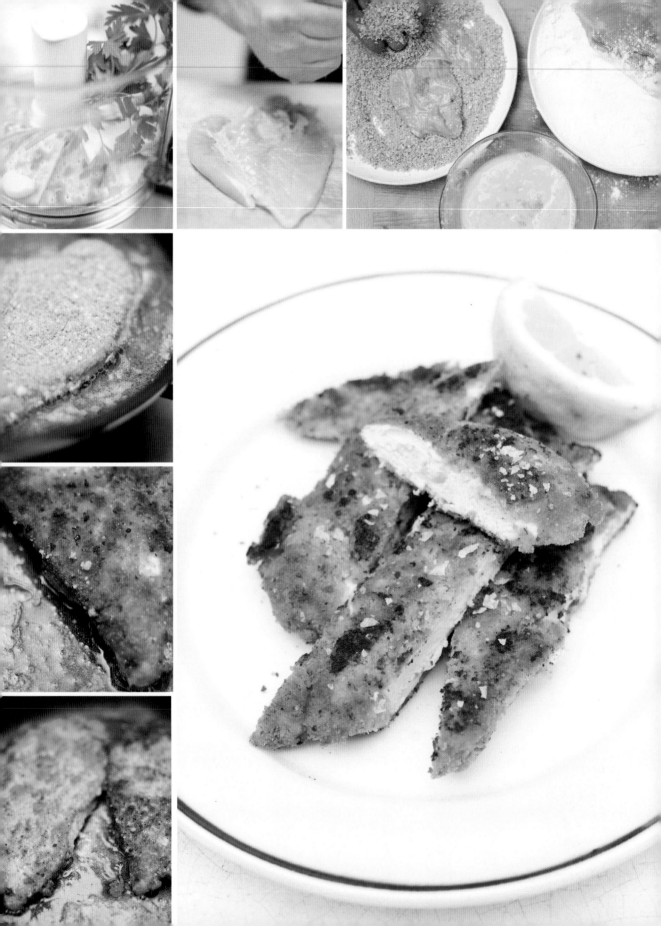

CRUNCHY GARLIC CHICKEN

This crumbing technique is so versatile – you can cook pork or even cod in exactly the same way. As there is butter in the crumb mixture, you can grill, fry, roast, or bake the meat dry in the oven and it will go lovely and golden.

serves 2

1 clove of garlic
1 lemon
18 unsalted saltine crackers
2 tablespoons butter
4 sprigs of fresh Italian parsley
sea salt and freshly ground black pepper

2 heaped tablespoons all-purpose flour
1 large egg, preferably free-range or organic
2 skinless chicken breast fillets, preferably free-range
* or organic*
olive oil

To prepare your chicken

Peel the garlic and zest the lemon • Put your crackers into a food processor with the butter, garlic, parsley sprigs, lemon zest, and a pinch of salt and pepper • Whiz until the mixture is very fine, then pour these crumbs on to a plate • Sprinkle the flour on to a second plate • Crack the egg into a small bowl and beat with a fork • Lightly score the underside of the chicken breasts • Put a square of plastic wrap over each one and bash a few times with the bottom of a pan until the breasts flatten out a bit • Dip the chicken into the flour until both sides are completely coated, then dip into the egg and finally into the flavored crumbs • Push the crumbs on to the chicken breasts so they stick – you want the meat to be totally coated

To cook your chicken

You can either bake or fry the chicken • If baking, preheat your oven to its highest temperature (475°), place your chicken on a sheet pan, and cook for 15 minutes • If frying, put a frying pan on a medium heat, add a few good lugs of olive oil, and cook the chicken breasts for 4 to 5 minutes on each side, until cooked through, golden, and crisp

To serve your chicken

Either serve the chicken breasts whole, or cut them into strips and pile them on a plate • Beautiful and simple served with a lemon wedge for squeezing over, and a tiny sprinkling of salt • Great with a lovely fresh salad or simply dressed veggies

PARMESAN CHICKEN BREASTS WITH CRISPY POSH HAM

This is a great way to prepare chicken breasts. The texture of the crisp cooked prosciutto goes brilliantly with the tender chicken. Bashing the chicken out thinly before you start cooking means it cooks much faster than a regular chicken breast. If you can't get hold of prosciutto, then any kind of thin ham, such as Parma ham, or even smoked streaky bacon, will work just as well.

serves 2

2 sprigs of fresh thyme

2 skinless chicken breast fillets, preferably free-range or organic

freshly ground black pepper

1 lemon

1 ¼ ounces grated Parmesan

6 slices of prosciutto

olive oil

To prepare your chicken

Grate your Parmesan • Pick the thyme leaves off the stalks • Carefully score the underside of the chicken breasts in a criss-cross fashion with a small knife • Season with a little pepper (you don't need salt as the prosciutto is quite salty) • Lay your breasts next to each other and sprinkle over most of the thyme leaves • Grate a little lemon zest over them, then sprinkle with the Parmesan • Lay 3 prosciutto slices on each chicken breast, overlapping them slightly • Drizzle with a little olive oil and sprinkle with the remaining thyme leaves • Put a square of plastic wrap over each breast and give them a few really good bashes with the bottom of a saucepan until they're about ½ inch thick

To cook your chicken

Put a frying pan over a medium heat • Remove the plastic wrap and carefully transfer the chicken breasts, prosciutto side down, into the pan • Drizzle over some olive oil • Cook for 3 minutes on each side, turning halfway through, giving the ham side an extra 30 seconds to crisp up

To serve your chicken

Either serve the chicken breasts whole or cut them into thick slices and pile them on a plate • Serve with some lemon wedges for squeezing over, and a good drizzle of olive oil • Lovely with mashed potatoes and green veggies or a crunchy salad!

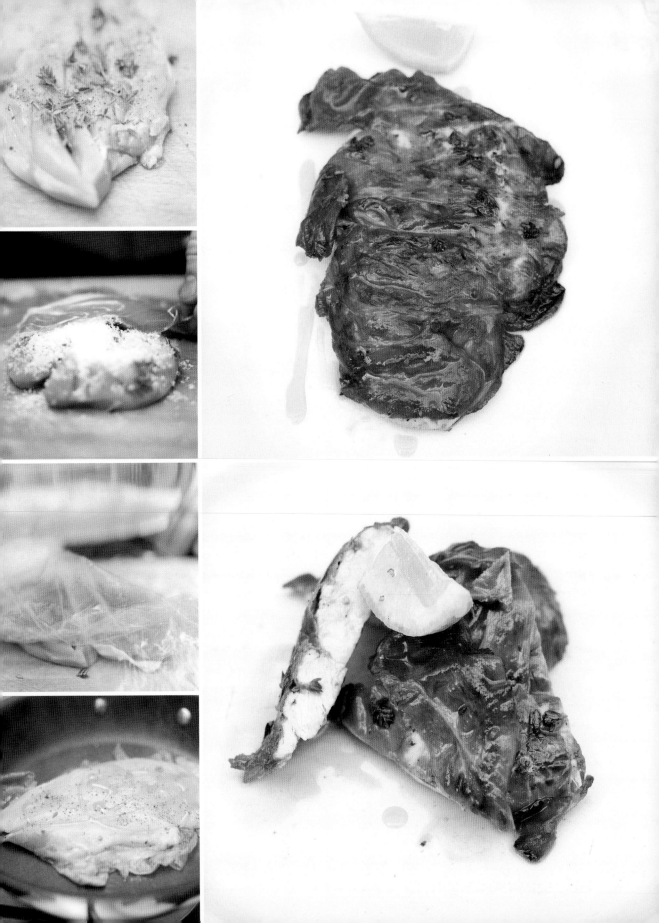

GRILLED LAMB CHOPS WITH CHUNKY SALSA

If you can get hold of some good-quality lamb, this is just a fantastic meal. When you cook a rack of lamb you want it to be blushing pink, but with chops you want them to be golden and really crispy on the outside and cooked all the way through for great flavor. I've served mine with a chunky salsa of tomatoes, chiles, and bell peppers. You can either cook the veggies first, or at the same time as the lamb, like I've done here. I prefer doing them together so all the flavors can benefit from each other. This is a dish you can cook in a frying pan or grill pan or on the barbecue.

serves 2

½–1 fresh red or green chile, to your taste

2 large ripe tomatoes

1 red bell pepper

a bunch of fresh basil

4–6 lamb rib chops, depending on their size

olive oil

sea salt and freshly ground black pepper

extra virgin olive oil

a splash of red wine vinegar

To prepare your chops and salsa

Put a grill pan on a high heat and let it get screaming hot • Halve your chile (seed it if you don't want your salsa too hot) • Cut your tomatoes in half • Halve and seed your bell pepper, then cut each half in two • Pick the basil leaves off the stalks and put them to one side • Drizzle both sides of your lamb chops with a little olive oil and season with salt and pepper

To cook your chops and salsa

Stand your chops upright in the hot pan so that the fatty edges are directly on the heat for about 1 minute until brown and crispy • Lay the chops flat in the pan and push them down gently for a minute or so • Add your chiles, bell pepper, and tomatoes – cut side down – around the sides of the pan • Cook your chops for about 4 to 5 minutes in total, turning them every minute or so and pushing the meat down each time • Turn your vegetables over halfway through • When the vegetables have softened and are nice and charred, transfer them to a chopping board • When the chops are golden and crisp, put them on a plate to rest for a minute or two while you prepare your salsa • Chop the chiles, tomatoes, bell pepper, and basil leaves (keeping a few smaller ones aside) until you get a nice chunky consistency • Put them into a bowl with a good lug of extra virgin olive oil and a pinch of salt and pepper • Add a little splash of red wine vinegar and stir in well • Taste, and add a touch more seasoning or vinegar if you think the salsa needs it

To serve your chops and salsa

Serve your chops on a bed of your lovely hot, chunky salsa • Finish by scattering the reserved basil leaves on top – fantastic

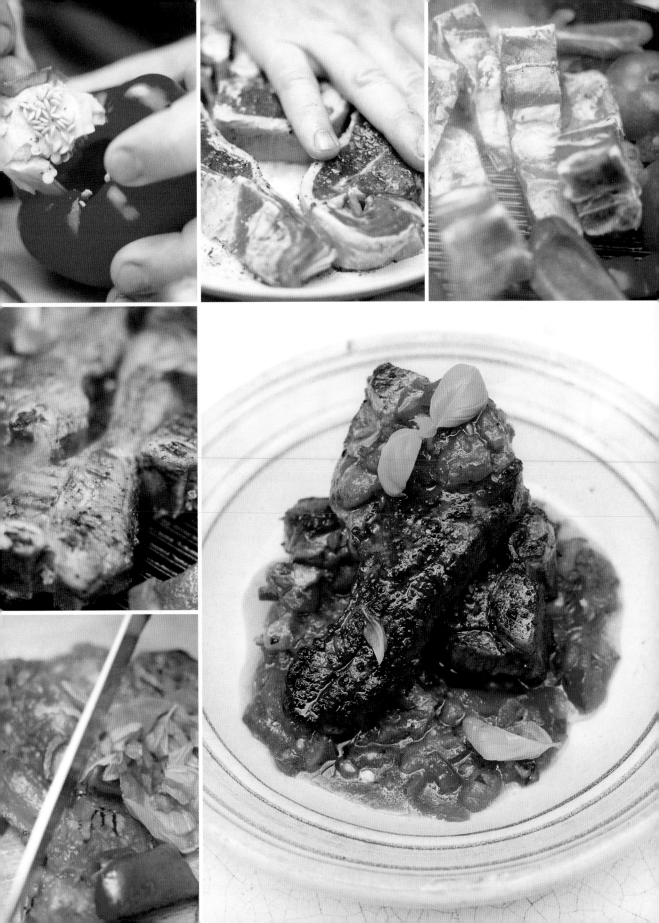

MOROCCAN LAMB WITH COUSCOUS

This is a lovely quick dish. Lamb leg steaks are good for this kind of quick cooking, and with a bit of attention they can be absolutely delicious. The trick is to cook them in a really hot pan until golden and crisp. The garbanzo beans add lovely texture to the sauce.

serves 2

1 medium red onion

3 ripe tomatoes

a small bunch of fresh Italian parsley

1 fresh red or green chile

8 dried apricots

olive oil

a small pat of butter

ground cumin

sea salt and freshly ground black pepper

a small handful of pine nuts

1 x 15-ounce can of garbanzo beans

1⅓ cups quick-cook couscous

1 lemon

1 tablespoon balsamic vinegar

½ pound lamb leg steak

⅔ cup natural yogurt, to serve

To prepare and cook your sauce and couscous

Peel, halve, and finely chop the onion and chop the tomatoes into chunks • Roughly chop the parsley, stalks and all, and halve, seed, and finely chop the chile • Finely slice your apricots • Put a frying pan on a high heat and add a lug of oil • Add your onions, chiles, apricots, and butter and cook until the onions soften slightly • Add 2 teaspoons of cumin, a pinch of salt and pepper, and the pine nuts, and stir • Add your tomatoes, most of the parsley, and the garbanzo beans, with all their juice and an extra ¼ cup of water • Leave the sauce to bubble away for about 5 minutes • While your sauce is simmering, put your couscous into a bowl and pour in just enough boiling water to cover (no more!) • Add a pinch of salt and pepper, a good squeeze of lemon juice, and a drizzle of olive oil, then cover the bowl with aluminum foil and set aside for 5 to 8 minutes • Then go back to your sauce and use a spoon to mash it up a bit • When it looks quite saucy, add a pinch more salt and pepper and the balsamic vinegar

To prepare and cook your lamb

Put a second frying pan over a high heat and let it get really hot • On a chopping board, cut the lamb into roughly 1-inch cubes • Sprinkle the board with a little cumin and a good pinch of salt and pepper • Move the meat around the board to coat it in the seasoning and push down with your hand to flatten the cubes into medallions • Add a few lugs of olive oil and your lamb to the hot pan • Cook for about 2 minutes on each side, until lovely and golden

To serve your lamb and couscous

Uncover the couscous, fluff it up a bit with a fork, and spoon onto your plates • Put a few lamb medallions next to it with a nice amount of sauce • Sprinkle with the remaining parsley and serve with a dollop of yogurt, a drizzle of olive oil, and any juices from the meat pan

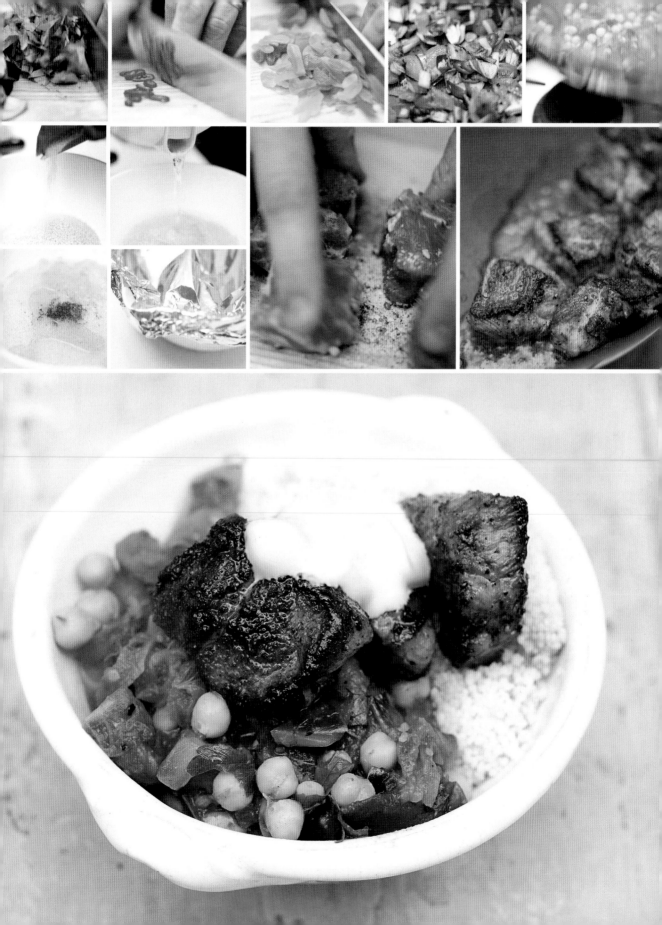

SALMON BAKED IN A FOIL PARCEL WITH GREEN BEANS AND PESTO

This is so simple to put together – a portion of salmon, a handful of green beans, a dollop of good-quality pesto, and a little squeeze of lemon juice. Such a great combination. Lovely with rice or baby potatoes or crusty bread. For a dinner party, feel free to use a whole fillet of salmon and treat it exactly the same way, just cook it for twice as long – it will look very dramatic when you open up the parcel at the table.

serves 2

2 handfuls of green beans
sea salt and freshly ground black pepper
2 lemons

2 x 7-ounce chunky salmon fillets, skin on, scaled and
  bones removed
2 heaped tablespoons green pesto
olive oil

To prepare your salmon
Preheat your oven to 400°F• Trim your beans by cutting off the stalk ends but leave the wispy tips on • Put the beans into a large pan of boiling water with a pinch of salt and cook for 3 to 4 minutes • Halve one of the lemons • Get yourself about a yard of aluminum kitchen foil and fold it in half to give you two layers • Put a handful of green beans in the middle of the aluminum foil • Lay a salmon fillet, skin side down, across the beans and spoon over a good tablespoon of green pesto • Drizzle with olive oil, squeeze over the juice from one of the lemon halves, and season with salt and pepper • Pull the aluminum foil edges together and scrunch them up to seal the parcel • Repeat these steps to make your second salmon fillet parcel and place both foil parcels on a sheet pan

To cook and serve your salmon
Put the sheet pan into your hot oven and cook for 15 to 20 minutes depending on the size of your fillets • Remove the pan from the oven and let it stand for a minute before carefully unwrapping and checking that the salmon is cooked through • Either serve the parcels on plates as they are, or carefully unwrap them before serving • Cut the remaining lemon in half and serve on the side for squeezing over • Nice served with new potatoes

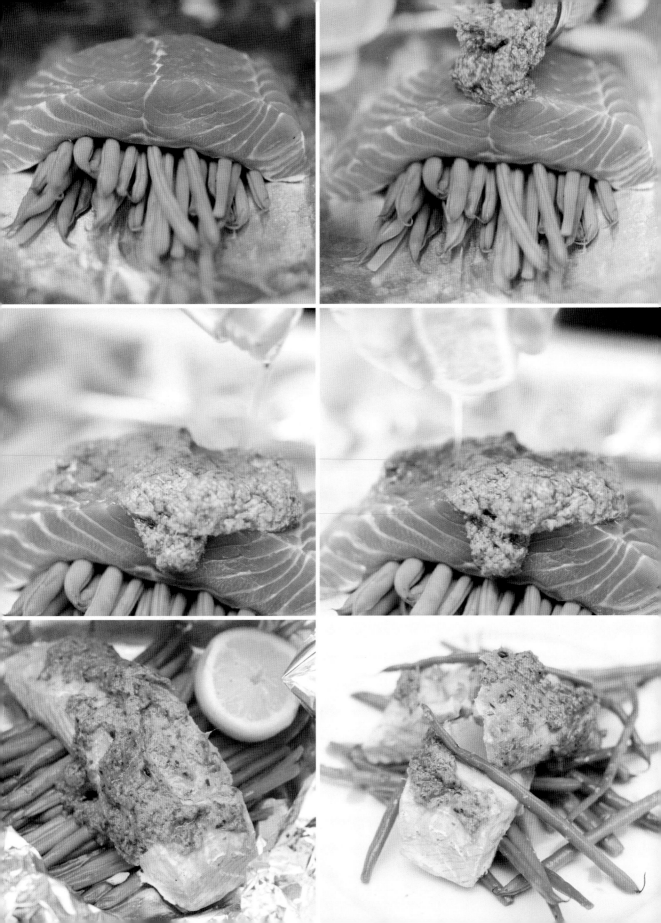

ASIAN-STYLE STEAMED SALMON

This dish works best if you have a proper steamer, but if you don't, a saucepan of water with a colander over it will do the trick. Because everything is steamed, the flavors are quite light. Water chestnuts add a nice crunch and flavor to the dish. I've also made a zingy little dressing to go with the fish and veggies. Feel free to use other fish and vegetables like cod and asparagus or asparagus, peas, and greens.

serves 2

a large handful of broccolini
  or broccoli rabe
1 x 8-ounce can of water chestnuts
a large handful of sugar snap peas
2 salmon fillets, skin on, scaled and bones removed
  (about 7 ounces each)

For the dressing
a thumb-sized piece of fresh root ginger
1 clove of garlic
½ a fresh red or green chile
1 scallion
2 tablespoons soy sauce
3 tablespoons extra virgin olive oil
1 lemon

To prepare your salmon

Fill a saucepan halfway up with water and put it on a high heat to boil • Trim the ends off the broccolini stalks • Drain your water chestnuts in a colander • Add the sugar snaps • Lay the salmon fillets, skin side down, on top of them, then scatter the broccoli over • Cover the colander with aluminum foil and scrunch it tightly around the edges to seal the steam in

To cook your salmon and make your dressing

Put the aluminum foil–covered colander over your pan of boiling water and let it steam for 8 to 10 minutes • While that's happening, peel and grate the ginger and half your clove of garlic into a small bowl • Finely slice your chile and scallion and add them to the bowl with the soy sauce and extra virgin olive oil • Squeeze the juice from half the lemon into the bowl • Mix everything together well with a spoon and put to one side • After your salmon and vegetables have been steaming for 8 minutes, peel back the foil and check the fish is cooked through – it should flake apart

To serve your salmon

Divide the salmon, water chestnuts, and veggies between your serving plates or bowls • Give the dressing a quick stir and drizzle it over • Serve with the remaining lemon half, cut into wedges, for squeezing over

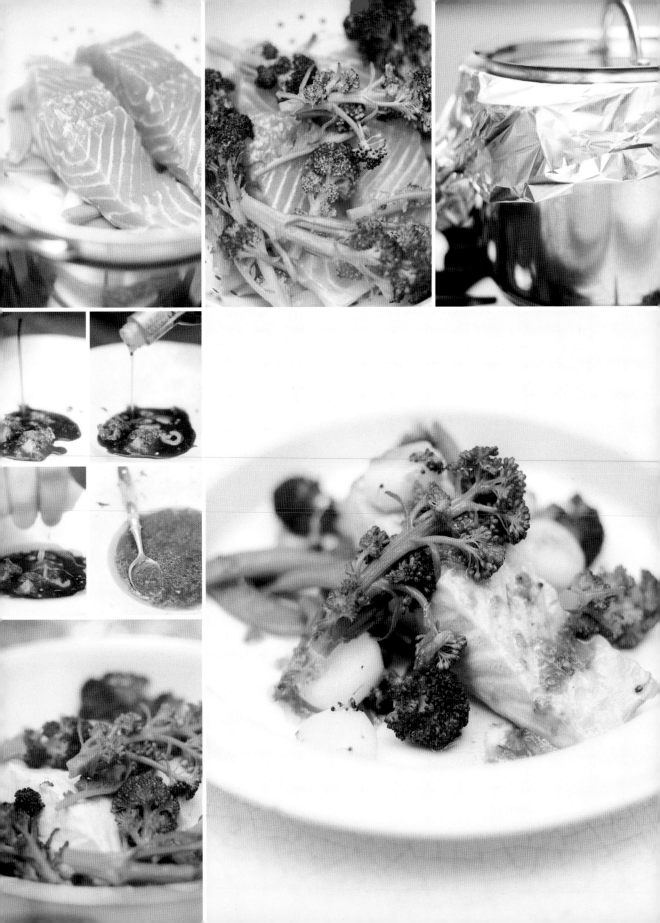

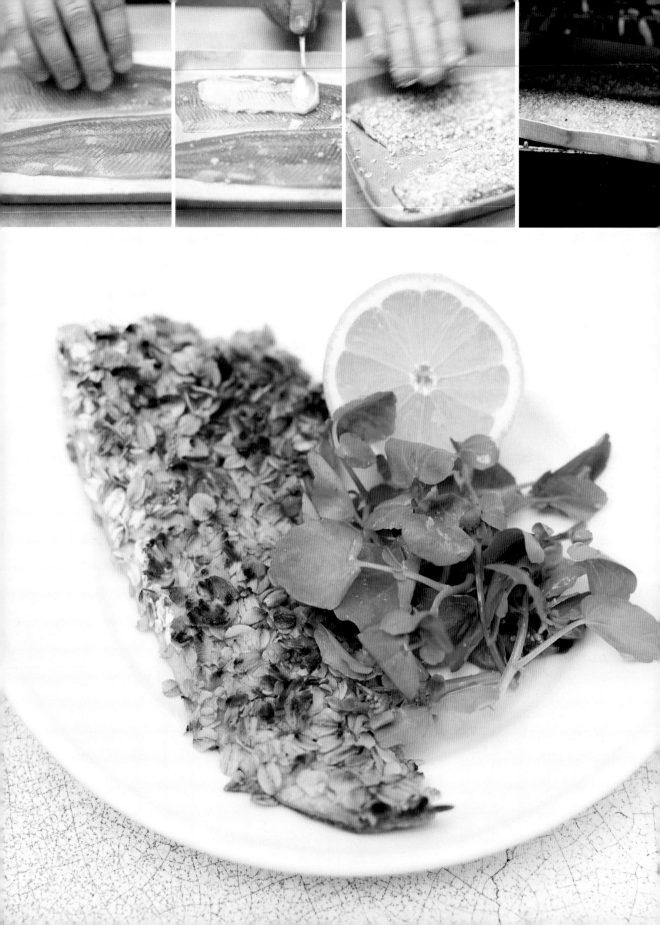

BROILED TROUT TOPPED WITH MUSTARD AND OATS

You've got to give this a try. It's quite an old English style of cooking, giving slightly oily fish, like trout, carp, mackerel, and sardines, a sense of texture using old-fashioned oats and mustard. As this dish is crunchy and rich, it's nice to offset it with a salad or with simple steamed vegetables and baby potatoes.

serves 2

olive oil
2 chunky trout fillets, skin on, scaled and bones
*   removed (about 7 ounces each)*
sea salt and freshly ground black pepper

2 teaspoons Dijon mustard
2 handfuls of old-fashioned oats
1 lemon

To prepare your trout
Preheat your broiler to the highest setting • Drizzle a sheet pan with some olive oil and rub all over • Lay the trout fillets, skin side down, on the pan and season well with salt and pepper • Smear a teaspoon of mustard over each fillet • Put the oats into a bowl, drizzle a little olive oil over them, and toss around to coat • Sprinkle a handful of oats over each fillet and gently pat down • Drizzle with a little more olive oil and give them another pat

To cook your trout
Put the sheet pan under the preheated broiler for about 10 minutes, until the oats are golden brown and crispy and the fish is cooked through

To serve your trout
Divide between your plates and serve with simple baby potatoes, some fresh watercress, and a lemon wedge for squeezing over

SIMPLE PAN-FRIED TROUT

What I like about pan-frying is that it's so visual. You can actually see the heat from the pan creeping up the sides of the fish and cooking it. When it comes to pan-frying, good contact with the pan is important – especially with fish. Most things shrink up as soon as they hit a hot pan, so make sure you push the fillets down gently with a spatula when you first put them in.

serves 2

2 chunky trout fillets, skin on, scaled, and bones
   removed (about 7 ounces each)
sea salt and freshly ground black pepper
olive oil

a pat of butter
a few big handfuls of fresh spinach
1 lemon

To prepare your trout
Put a non-stick frying pan on a medium to high heat • Sprinkle the trout fillets with some salt and pepper and drizzle with olive oil • Rub all over the fish until well coated

To cook your trout
When the pan is nice and hot, add your trout fillets, skin side down, and cook for 3 minutes until crisp • While cooking, shake the pan around a little • When the heat has crept up nearly to the top of the fish and you think they're ready, flick the fillets over for 30 seconds to cook the other side – this will give you a crisp skin and a soft flakiness to the insides • Remove from the heat and place on your serving plates, skin side up • Add the butter and the spinach to the pan with a sprinkling of salt and pepper and place back on the heat • Keep moving the spinach around for just a minute using a pair of tongs • When it has wilted it's ready to come off the heat

To serve your trout
Serve your fillets with the spinach, and lemon wedges for squeezing over • Some people don't like the idea of eating fish skin and that's fine – you certainly don't have to – but if you've never tried it, have a go, as the crispy skin is really delicious • Yum yum!

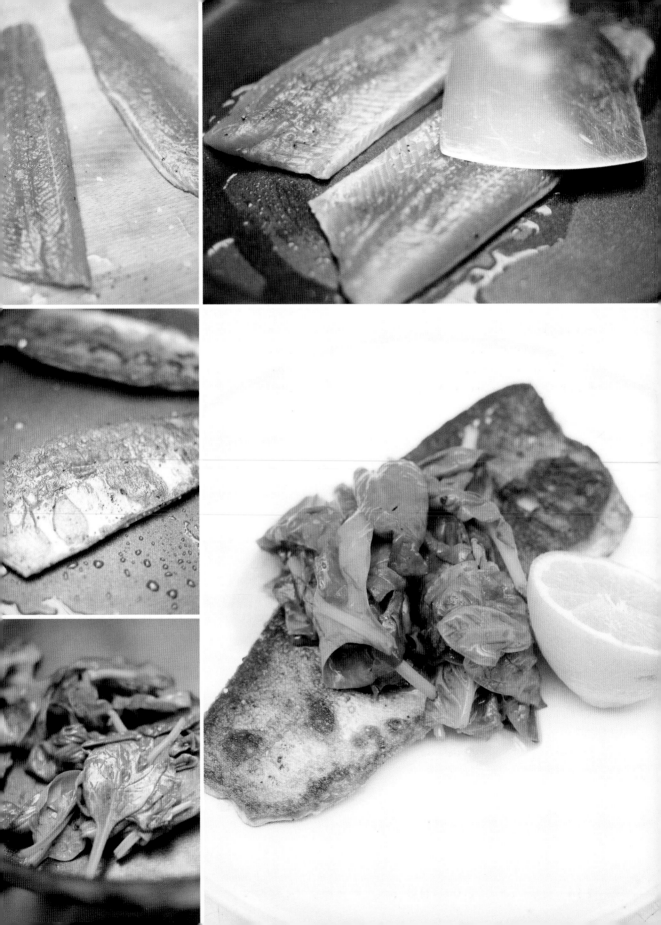

BAKED COD WRAPPED IN BACON WITH ROSEMARY

Surf and turf, man! The reason I love treating cod, or any other white fish, like this is because of the great flavor and texture you get from the smoked bacon. It goes crisp in the oven, in contrast to the lovely, flaky fish, which has, in turn, been protected from the harsh heat by the bacon. As far as herbs are concerned, you could also try using thyme or basil.

serves 2

4 sprigs of fresh rosemary

olive oil

sea salt and freshly ground black pepper

2 chunky cod fillets, skin on, scaled and bones
   removed (about 7 ounces each)

8 slices of smoked bacon, preferably
   free-range or organic

1 lemon

To prepare your cod

Preheat your oven to its highest temperature (475°) • Pick the leaves from 2 of your rosemary sprigs and finely chop on a chopping board • Drizzle the chopped rosemary with olive oil and sprinkle with salt and pepper • Season the cod fillets by rolling them around the chopping board until they're evenly coated in the herbs and seasoning • Lay half your slices of bacon on the board next to each other, letting them overlap • Flatten them out a little by running the edge of your knife along each slice – this will make them slightly thinner • Place a cod fillet across them and wrap the bacon around it • Repeat with the second cod fillet and the remaining bacon • Drizzle a sheet pan with some olive oil and rub all over • Lay the cod fillets in the pan, skin side down • Put a sprig of fresh rosemary on top of each fillet and drizzle with a little olive oil

To cook your cod

Place the sheet pan in the preheated oven for 10 to 12 minutes, until the bacon is golden and delicious and the fish is cooked through

To serve your cod

Serve straight out of the oven, with a lemon wedge for squeezing over • This is brilliant with mashed potatoes or baby potatoes and any freshly dressed boiled green vegetables or salad

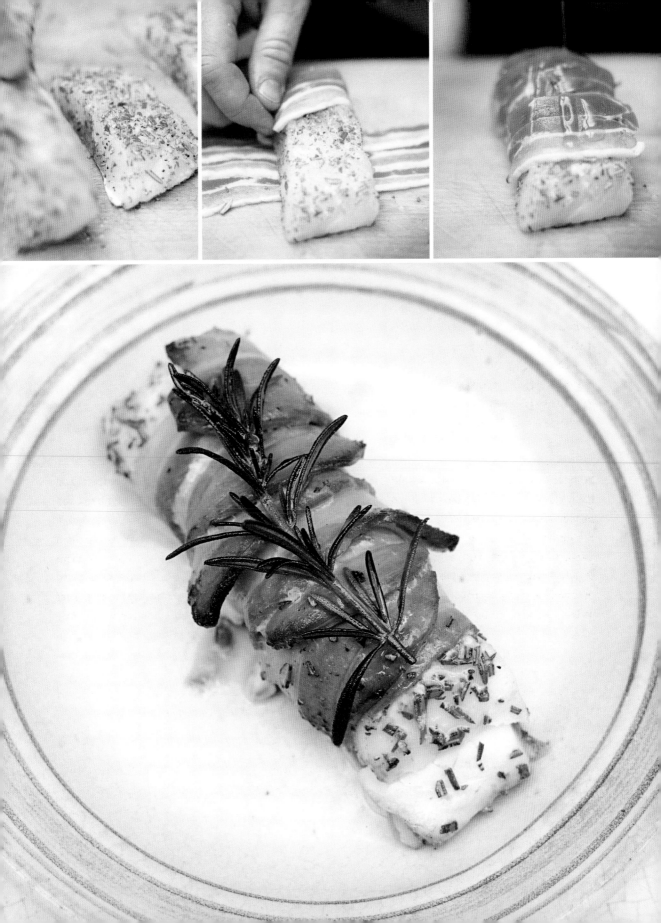

PAN-FRIED CURRIED COD

What I like about this method of cooking is the contrast in taste and texture you get with a thin layer of curry spices on a chunky fillet of white fish, as opposed to cooking meat with spices. When it's cooked in a little butter until golden you'll get a lovely richness alongside the fresh, delicate flavor of the fish. With a squeeze of lemon, it will definitely put a smile on your face!

serves 2

3 tablespoons mild curry powder
sea salt and freshly ground black pepper
2 chunky cod fillets, skin on, scaled, and bones
  removed (about 7 ounces each)

a few sprigs of fresh cilantro
a pat of butter
olive oil
2 cups natural yogurt

To prepare your cod
Sprinkle the curry powder with a good pinch of salt and pepper over a plate or chopping board • Roll the cod fillets in the powder, patting them until they are completely covered • Pick the cilantro leaves off the stalks

To cook your cod
Put a non-stick frying pan on a high heat and add your pat of butter and a lug of olive oil • Lay your fillets, skin-side down, in the pan • Keep spooning the hot oil over the fillets as they cook to get them nice and crisp – the easiest way to do this is by angling the pan to collect the oil • Cook them for 2 to 3 minutes on each side – this is about right for a 7-ounce fillet, so give them a little longer if you have a chunkier fillet – until they're cooked through and the flesh is flaking away from the skin

To serve your cod
This is lovely served up on a bed of fluffy rice (see pages 95–96), with a spoonful of natural yogurt and some cilantro leaves sprinkled on top

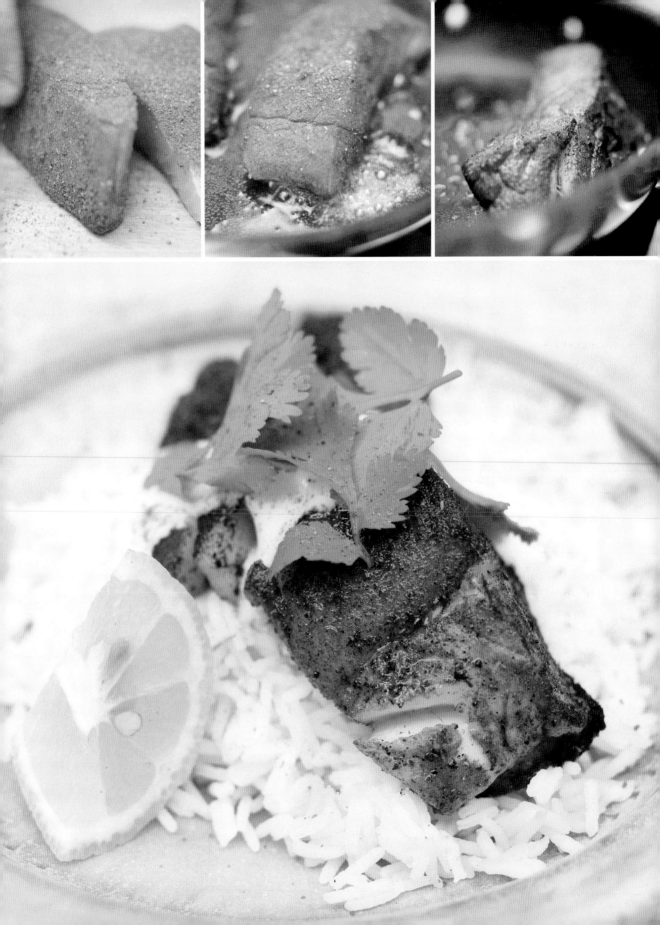

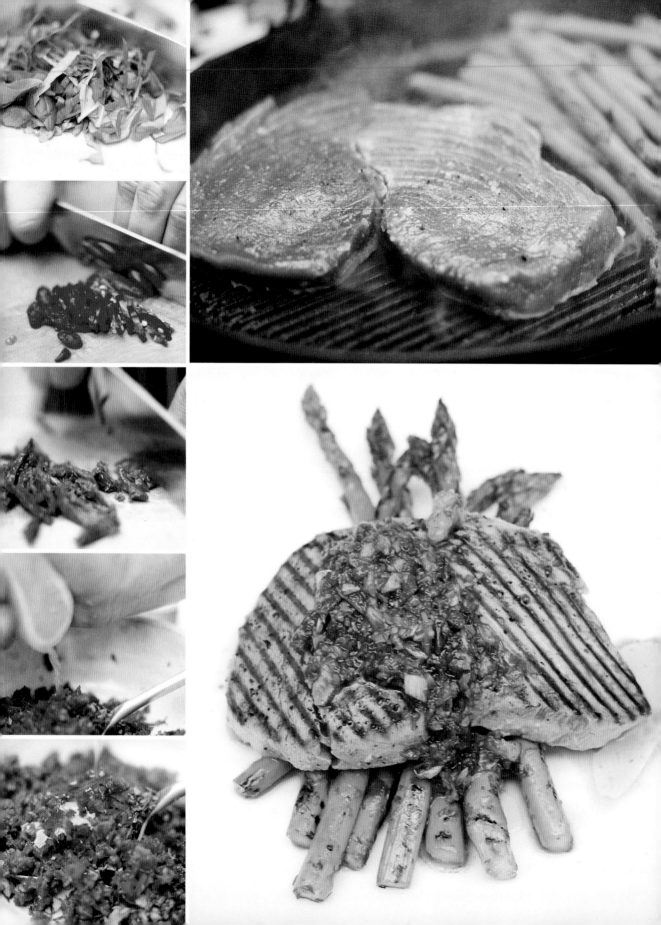

GRILLED TUNA AND ASPARAGUS

Another great, quick meal. In a screaming hot pan, a thin slice of tuna will cook at roughly the same time as your asparagus, and while the pan is heating you can get on with making up the amazing lemon dressing. Very zingy, very brilliant.

serves 2

a bunch of asparagus
olive oil
2 tuna steaks (about 7 ounces each, ½ inch thick)

For the dressing
a small bunch of fresh basil
½ a fresh red or green chile

a small handful of sun-dried tomatoes (the type
   packed in oil)
I lemon
extra virgin olive oil
balsamic vinegar
sea salt and freshly ground black pepper

To prepare your dressing and tuna
Put a large grill pan on a high heat and let it get screaming hot • Pick the basil leaves off the stalks and finely chop • Seed and finely chop the chile • Finely chop the sun-dried tomatoes and put into a bowl with the basil and chile • Halve the lemon and squeeze all the juice into the bowl • Add a lug of extra virgin olive oil and mix together • Add a splash of balsamic vinegar, season with salt and pepper, and put to one side • Bend the asparagus gently until the woody bottoms of the stalks break off • Discard these woody ends • Drizzle a little olive oil over the tuna, then season with salt and pepper and rub into the fish

To cook your tuna
Lay your asparagus tips on the hot, dry grill pan • Turn them every minute or two, letting them char a little but not burn – this will give them a wonderfully nutty flavor • After a few minutes, push them to one side and add the tuna to the pan • You will be able to see the heat cooking up the tuna from the bottom • After a minute or so, when the tuna has cooked halfway through, flip both steaks over • Cook for another minute or two • You may think it strange, as it's fish, but the tuna should actually remain slightly pink in the middle when you serve it – it will become too dry if you overcook it

To serve your tuna
Pile a few asparagus spears on each plate and spoon some of your tangy dressing over them • Lay the tuna fillets over the asparagus and spoon another dollop of the dressing on top • Drizzle with a little extra virgin olive oil before serving

ITALIAN PAN-SEARED TUNA

The great thing about this meal is that it all happens quickly, in one pan. Remember, tuna should be cooked hot and quickly so it's still a little blushing in the middle – don't be tempted to overcook it. I like to buy olives with the pits still in because the flavor is much better.

serves 2

2–3 cloves of garlic

1 pint ripe red and yellow cherry or grape tomatoes

a handful of black olives, pits in

a small bunch of fresh basil

1 lemon

2 tuna steaks (about 7 ounces each, ½ inch thick)

sea salt and freshly ground black pepper

1 teaspoon dried oregano

olive oil

4 anchovies

To prepare your tuna

Put a large frying pan over a high heat • Peel and finely slice your garlic • Halve your tomatoes and cut any larger ones into quarters • To remove the pits from your olives, press down firmly on them using the palm of your hand so they break open, and discard the pits • Pick the basil leaves off the stalks and put the smaller ones to one side for serving • Halve your lemon

To cook your tuna

Season your tuna steak with salt and pepper and sprinkle over the oregano • Put a lug of olive oil in the hot pan, followed by the tuna steaks • Cook for 1 minute on each side, then remove to a warm plate • Put the pan back on the heat with a little more olive oil • Add the garlic and olives and cook for 1 minute, then add the anchovies and tomatoes • Squeeze in the juice from one half of your lemon • Cook for 1 minute, stirring every so often • Just before you take the pan off the heat, throw in most of your whole basil leaves, tearing up any larger ones • Squeeze in the juice from the remaining lemon half, toss everything together and season to taste with salt and pepper

To serve your tuna

Divide the sauce on to your plates • Slice up your tuna steaks into ¾-inch-thick pieces and lay over the top • Sprinkle with the remaining basil leaves and serve with some lovely crusty bread and fresh salad

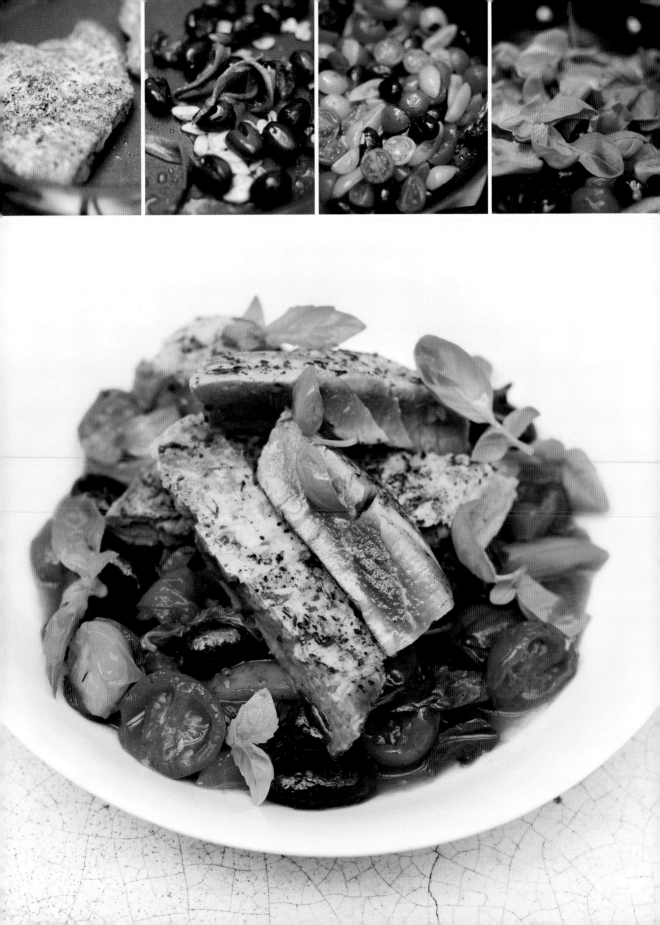

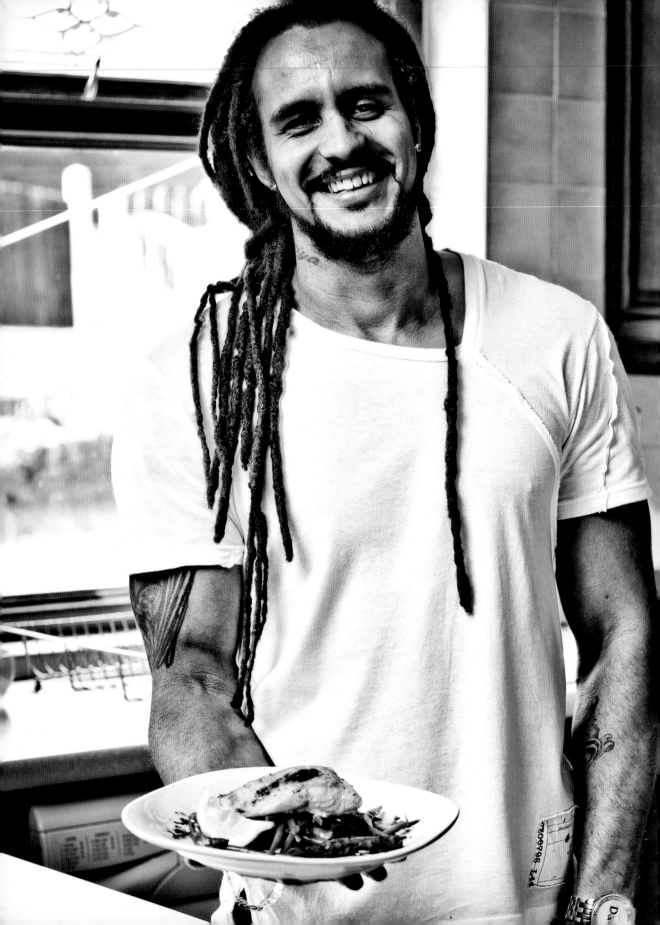

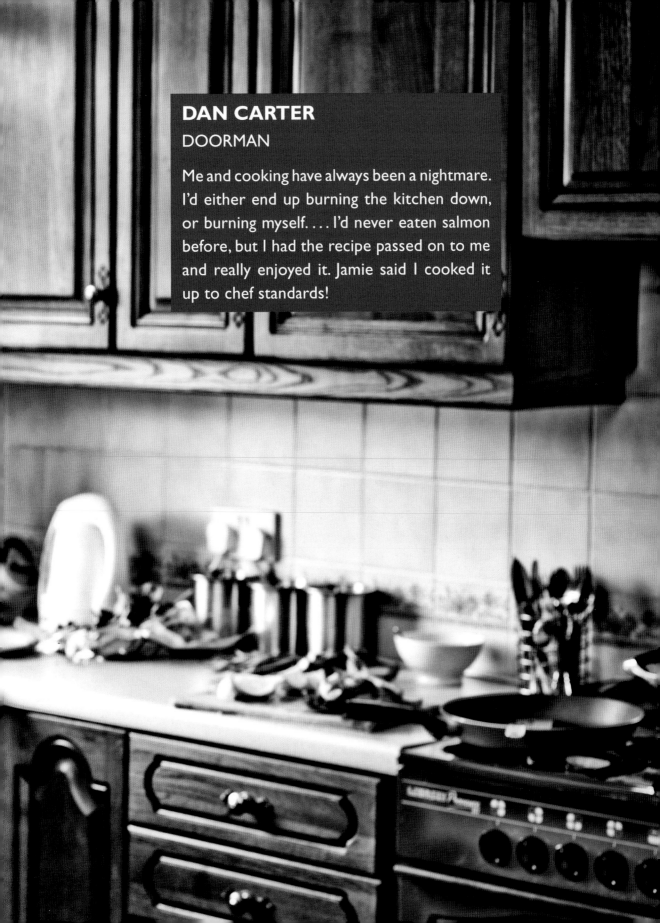

DAN CARTER

DOORMAN

Me and cooking have always been a nightmare. I'd either end up burning the kitchen down, or burning myself. . . . I'd never eaten salmon before, but I had the recipe passed on to me and really enjoyed it. Jamie said I cooked it up to chef standards!

SAUCES

SIMPLE CHEESY MUSTARD serves 4

a small bunch of fresh Italian parsley / olive oil / 3 teaspoons English mustard / 3 tablespoons brandy / 1 ¼ cups heavy cream / a handful of freshly grated Parmesan or Cheddar cheese

Finely chop the parsley leaves and stalks • Get a frying pan on a high heat and add 2 lugs of olive oil and the mustard • Add the brandy • Now, you don't have to do this, but feel free to let it catch fire and flame – this will burn off the alcohol quickly • Add most of the parsley and the cream and bring to a boil • Remove from the heat and stir in the cheese, then sprinkle with a little extra parsley • Drizzle with olive oil and serve immediately with your chosen fish or meat (this sauce will split if left to stand for too long) • Absolutely delicious on a portion of cod

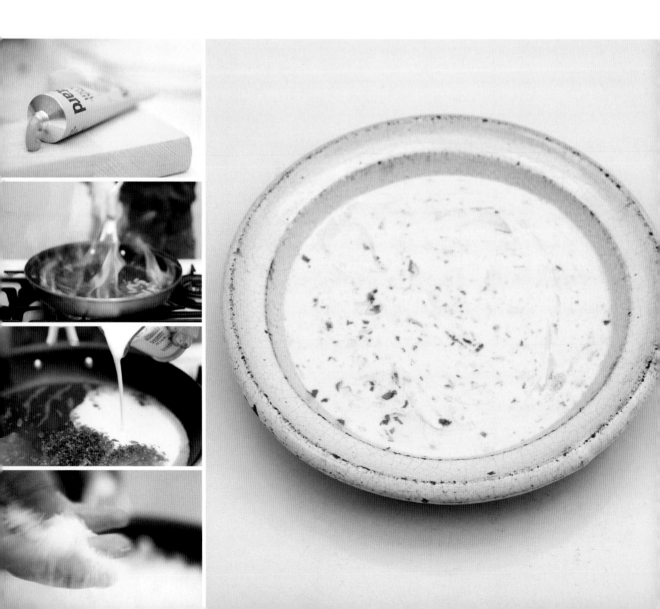

CHERRY TOMATO, CAPER, AND BALSAMIC serves 4

4 cloves of garlic / about 25 (1pint) cherry or grape tomatoes, mixed colors if possible / olive oil / dried oregano / 2 tablespoons capers, drained (from a jar, in brine) / sea salt and freshly ground black pepper / a pat of butter / balsamic vinegar

Peel and finely slice the garlic • Halve the tomatoes • Put a frying pan on a medium heat and add 2 good lugs of olive oil • Add your garlic, a big pinch of oregano, and the capers • When lightly golden, add your tomatoes • Season to taste with salt and pepper, and stir • Add the butter and 2 big splashes of balsamic vinegar and stir again • Leave the sauce to bubble away for around 3 to 5 minutes • The tomatoes will soften and make a lovely rich sauce • Serve hot, with your chosen fish or meat, or stir into hot cooked pasta

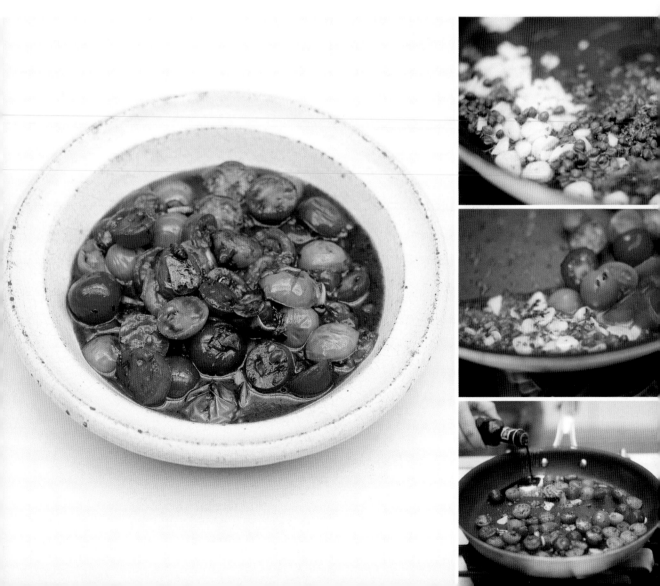

MUSTARD, CRÈME FRAÎCHE, AND WHITE WINE
serves 4

6 heaped teaspoons wholegrain mustard / 1 cup white wine / ¼ cup crème fraîche or heavy cream / sea salt and freshly ground black pepper / optional: a small handful of fresh Italian parsley

Get yourself a frying pan on a high heat • As soon as it's nice and hot, add your mustard and white wine – it will steam and bubble • Let it boil for a minute to reduce the liquid slightly, then add your crème fraîche (or heavy cream) • Bring to a boil, then simmer for 7 to 8 minutes until you've got a good consistency happening – it should pour like half and half • Add a good pinch of salt and pepper • Feel free to add a little chopped parsley at this point • Serve hot, with your chosen fish or meat

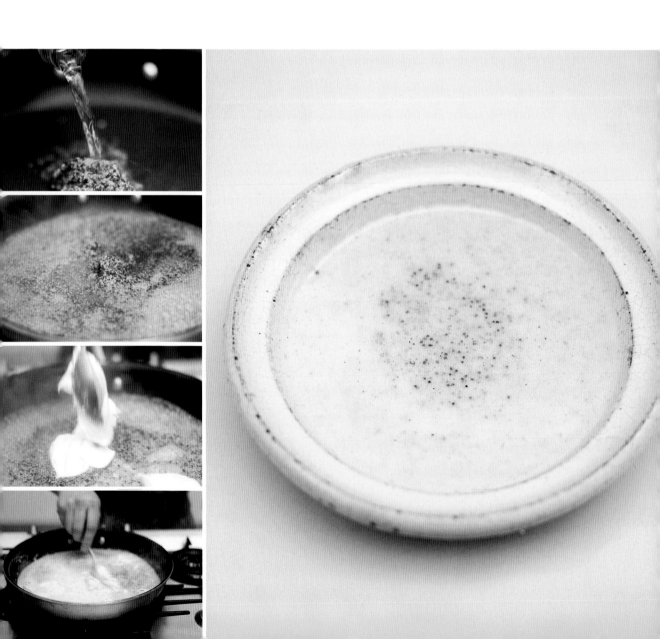

TOMATO, OLIVE, BASIL, AND CHILE
serves 4

2 cloves of garlic / a small handful of black olives / a few sprigs of fresh basil / 1 fresh red or green chile / olive oil / 1 14-ounce can of diced tomatoes / sea salt and freshly ground black pepper

Peel and finely slice your garlic • Squash the olives, using the base of a jar or something heavy, and remove the pits • Roughly chop the olives • Pick the basil leaves off their stalks, ripping up any larger leaves • Seed and finely slice the red chile • In a frying pan on a high heat add a good lug of olive oil followed by the garlic, olives, and chile • When the garlic is lightly golden, add your basil leaves and give the pan a shake • Add the tomatoes, stir, and bring to a boil • Season with just a small pinch of salt (as the olives can be quite salty) and pepper • Serve at once with your chosen fish or meat, while still hot

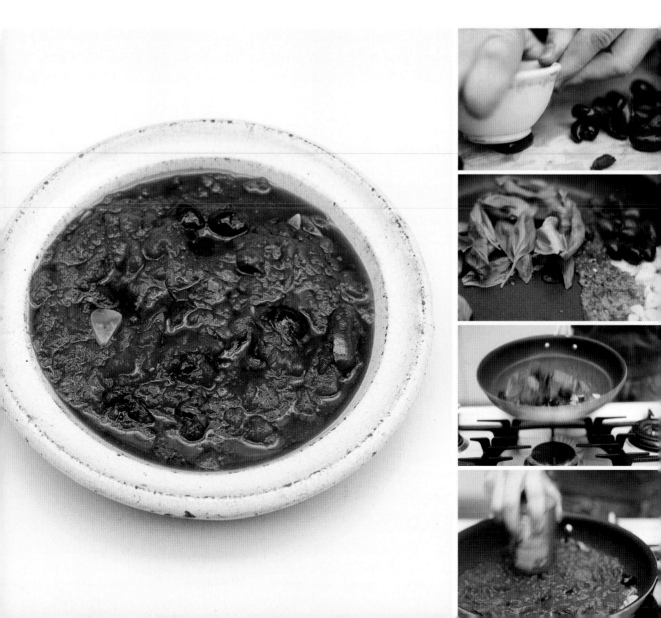

BACON AND MUSHROOM CREAM serves 4

olive oil / 4 slices of smoked bacon, preferably free-range or organic / ½–1 fresh red chile, to your taste / ½ pound portobello mushrooms / 4 sprigs of fresh thyme / sea salt and freshly ground black pepper / ⅓ cup crème fraîche or heavy cream

Put a large pan on a medium heat and add a good lug of olive oil • Slice the bacon into small pieces and add to the pan • Fry for a couple of minutes until golden and crispy • While the bacon is cooking, seed and finely slice the chile, thinly slice the mushrooms, and pick the thyme leaves off the stalks • Add the chile, mushrooms, and thyme leaves and continue to fry for a couple of minutes • Season carefully to taste with salt and pepper • Add the crème fraîche, bring the sauce to a boil, and let it bubble and simmer for a minute or so • Serve hot, to top a piece of fish, like skate, or with some roast chicken, or stir into hot cooked pasta

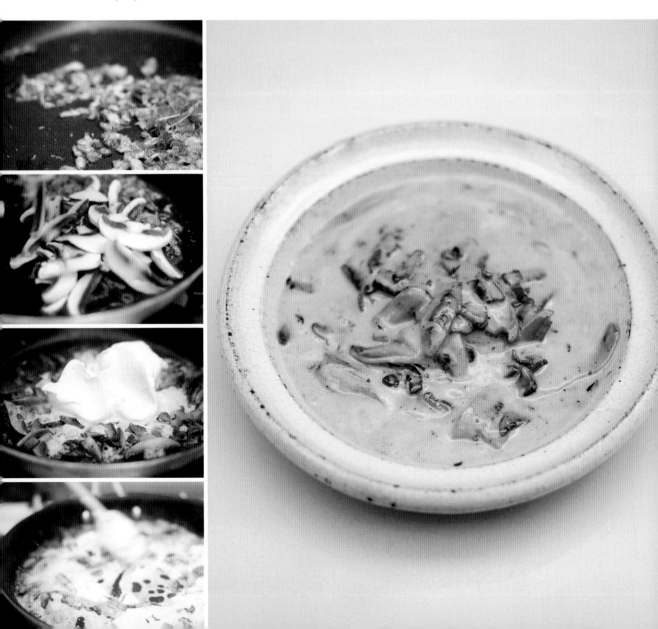

VERY SIMPLE CURRY serves 4

6 scallions / a large bunch of fresh cilantro / olive oil / 5 heaped teaspoons curry powder / 1 tablespoon of butter / 2 x 14-ounce cans of coconut milk / sea salt / juice of 1 lemon

Trim and finely slice your scallions • Finely chop your cilantro • Put a pan on a low heat and add 2 good lugs of olive oil • Sprinkle in the curry powder and add the scallions • Stir around and add the butter • Cook for 20 to 30 seconds and when it's all bubbling nicely, add your coconut milk • Bring to the boil, then turn the heat down and simmer for 2 minutes • To finish, season to taste with salt and stir in the cilantro and lemon juice • Serve hot, with your chosen fish or meat

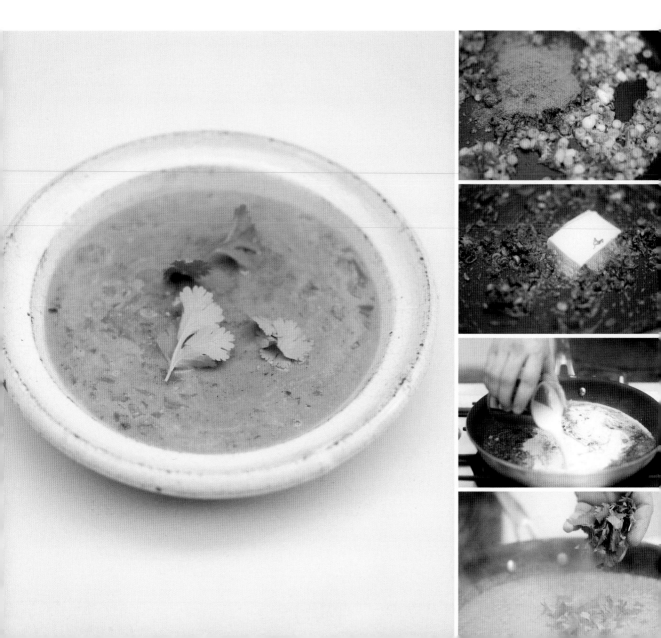

SALSAS

MANGO, CUCUMBER, AND CHILE serves 4

1 ripe mango / ½ a cucumber / 4 sprigs of fresh mint / 2 scallions / 1 fresh red or green chile / extra virgin olive oil / 2 limes / sea salt and freshly ground black pepper

Remove the skin from the mango using a speed peeler • Slice the fruit away from the pit and roughly chop • Put into a bowl • Peel and chop the cucumber to the same size as the mango and add to the bowl • Pick the mint leaves and finely chop with the scallions • Halve, seed, and finely chop the chile • Stir the mint, scallions, and chile into the mango and cucumber mixture, and add enough extra virgin olive oil to cover everything lightly • Add the juice from the limes and season with salt and pepper before serving

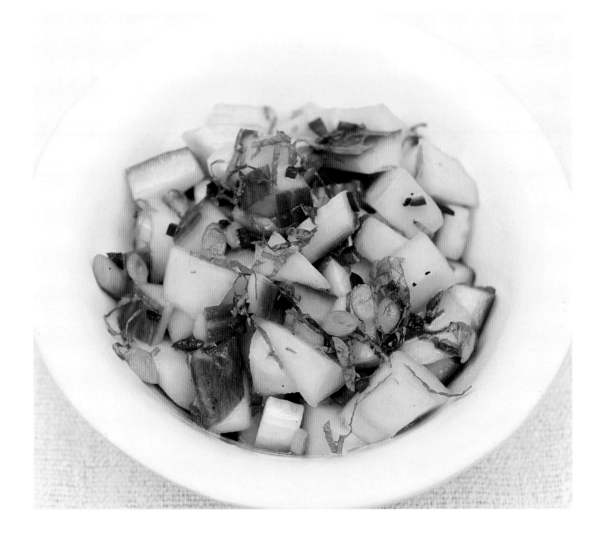

TOMATO serves 4

1 clove of garlic / 2 scallions / ½ a fresh red or green chile / 6 ripe tomatoes / a small handful of fresh cilantro / juice of 1–2 limes / extra virgin olive oil / sea salt and freshly ground black pepper

Peel the garlic • Trim the scallions • Seed the chile • Finely chop all these together on a board • Add the tomatoes to the board and continue chopping and mixing everything together • Lastly, add the cilantro leaves and stalks and chop these into the mix • Scrape the salsa into a bowl and add the juice from 1 lime, tasting and adding more if needed • Add about the same amount of extra virgin olive oil, then stir and season to taste • Serve with wedges of lime

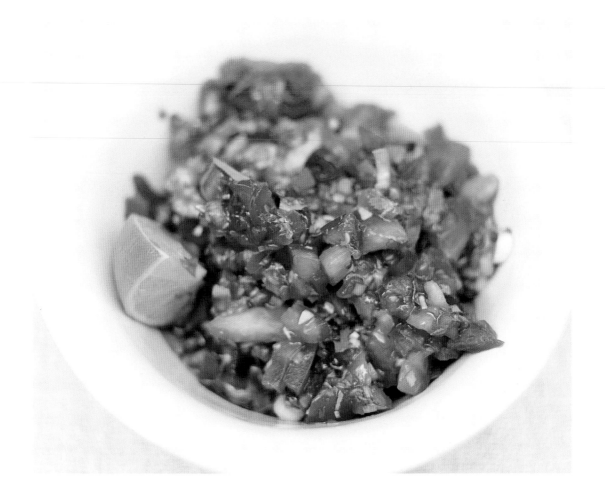

CHOPPED PESTO serves 4

1 clove of garlic / a large bunch of fresh basil / a handful of pine nuts or almonds / a large handful of freshly grated Parmesan cheese / extra virgin olive oil / juice of ½ a lemon / sea salt and freshly ground black pepper

Peel the garlic and pick the basil leaves from the stalks • Chop up the garlic first, then add the nuts and all the basil leaves, plus some of the finer basil stalks, and continue chopping until fine • Put into a bowl with the grated Parmesan and enough extra virgin olive oil to loosen to a wet paste • Add a small squeeze of lemon juice and have a taste • If you think it could do with some salt and pepper, feel free to add some

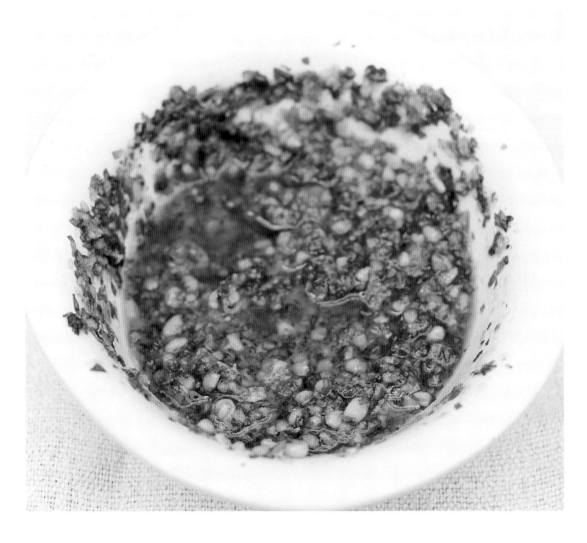

BLACK OLIVE, SUN-DRIED TOMATO, AND CELERY
serves 4

3 celery stalks / 2 handfuls of pitted black olives / a handful of sun-dried tomatoes (from a jar, in oil) / 2 tablespoons balsamic vinegar / extra virgin olive oil / sea salt and freshly ground black pepper

Tear the yellow leaves off the celery stalks and put to one side • All on the same board, roughly chop your olives, sun-dried tomatoes, and celery and mix together well • When you have a consistency that you like, scrape into a bowl with all the juices • Add your celery leaves, balsamic vinegar, and a good lug of extra virgin olive oil, and give it a good stir • Add a pinch of pepper – you probably won't need to add any salt (as the olives can be salty), but have a taste and decide • You may also want to add a little splash of water, as this can help the flavors to combine • This salsa can be served straightaway, or it can be left to rest for an hour before serving

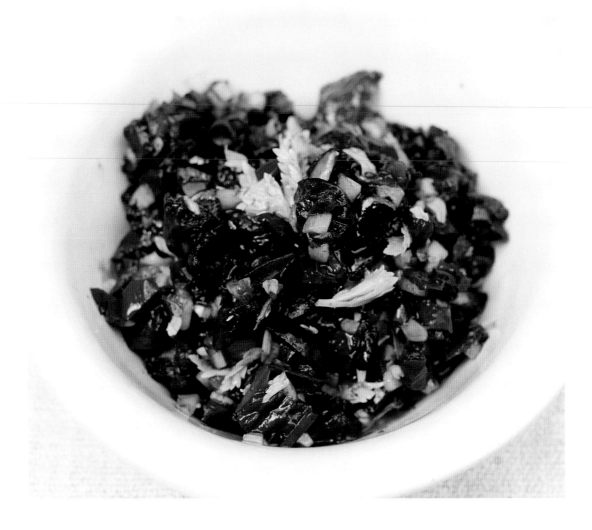

OILS

Flavored oils can be knocked up in minutes and are perfect with any type of meat or shellfish. One or two tablespoons drizzled over a steak, or a lamb chop or a fish fillet, will make such a difference. They're also really good with mozzarella cheese. The ones in this chapter are like a cross between a flavored oil and a dressing. So you can also use them over salads.

ASIAN OIL

a thumb-sized piece of fresh root ginger / 1 tablespoon soy sauce / juice of 1 lime / 4 sprigs of fresh cilantro / ½ a fresh red chile / 6 tablespoons extra virgin olive oil

Peel the ginger and finely grate into a bowl • Add the soy sauce and squeeze in the lime juice • Finely chop the cilantro leaves and chile and add to the bowl • Pour in enough extra virgin olive oil just to cover, then mix well • You can either serve the oil like this or you can strain it, really squeezing the flavors through to give you a lovely, smooth oil

BASIL AND LEMON OIL

8 tablespoons extra virgin olive oil / juice of 1 lemon / a few sprigs of fresh basil / sea salt and freshly ground black pepper

To make this you can use a pestle and mortar, a food processor, or a blender • Add the extra virgin olive oil, lemon juice, and basil to the blender and add a good pinch of salt and pepper • Whiz together until you have a smooth oil • You can serve it like this or pass it through a strainer to give you a much smoother oil • It can be kept in the fridge for a couple of days • Give it a quick shake before serving

CHOPPED HERB OIL

a small handful of mixed fresh soft green herbs (use one type or a mixture of basil, parsley, and mint) / 8 tablespoons extra virgin olive oil / red wine vinegar / sea salt and freshly ground black pepper

Finely chop the herbs • Put them into a bowl with the extra virgin olive oil, a swig of vinegar, and a good pinch of salt and pepper • Mix well before serving

CHILE AND MINT OIL

1 fresh red or green chile / a few sprigs of fresh mint / 8 tablespoons extra virgin olive oil / juice of ½ a lemon / sea salt and freshly ground black pepper

Halve the red chile and seed it if you don't want your oil to be too spicy • Finely chop the chile • Pick the mint leaves and finely chop • Put the chile and mint into a bowl with the extra virgin olive oil, lemon juice, and a good pinch of salt and pepper • Mix well before serving

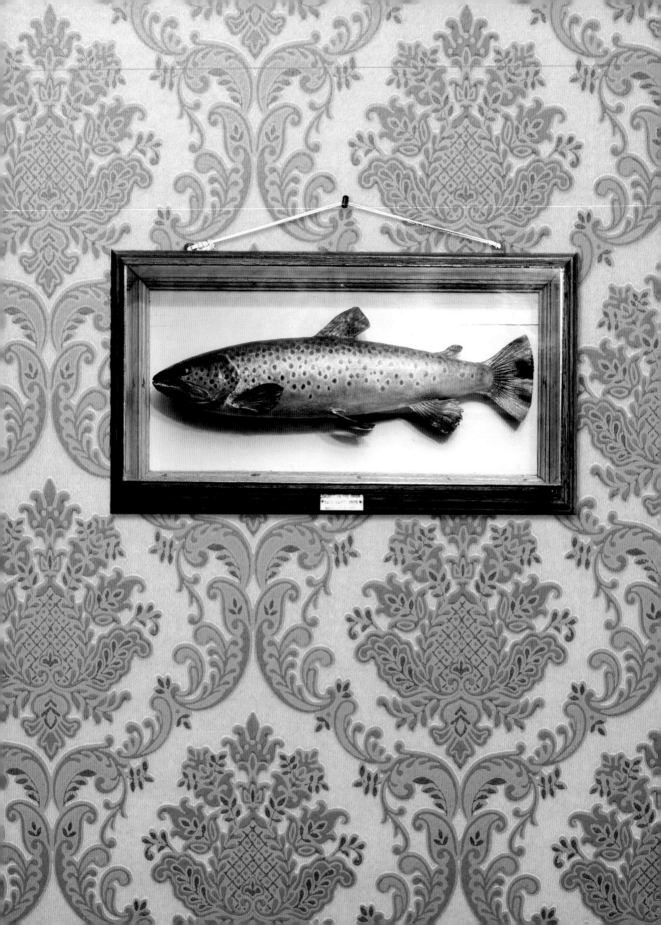

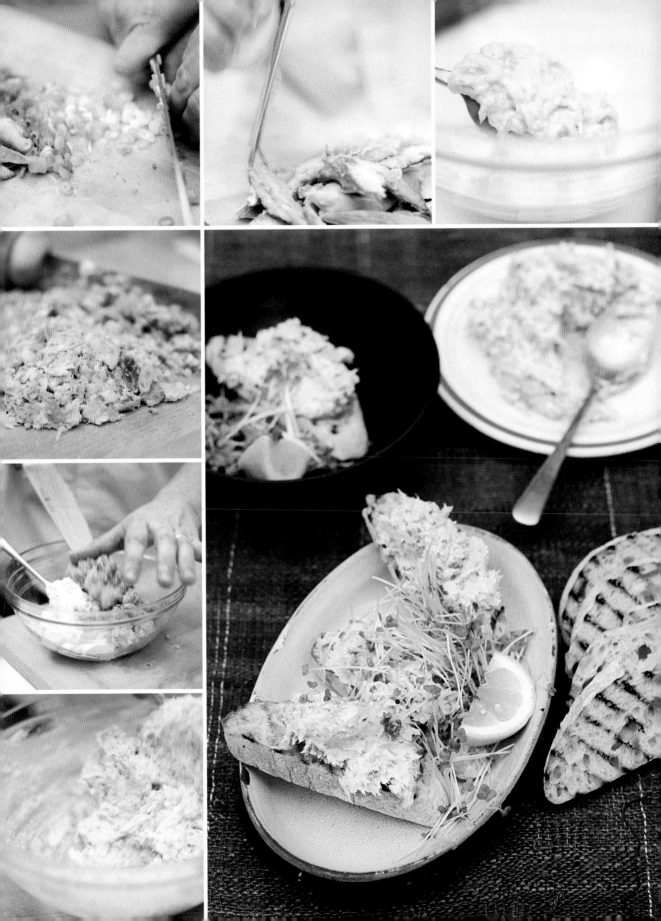

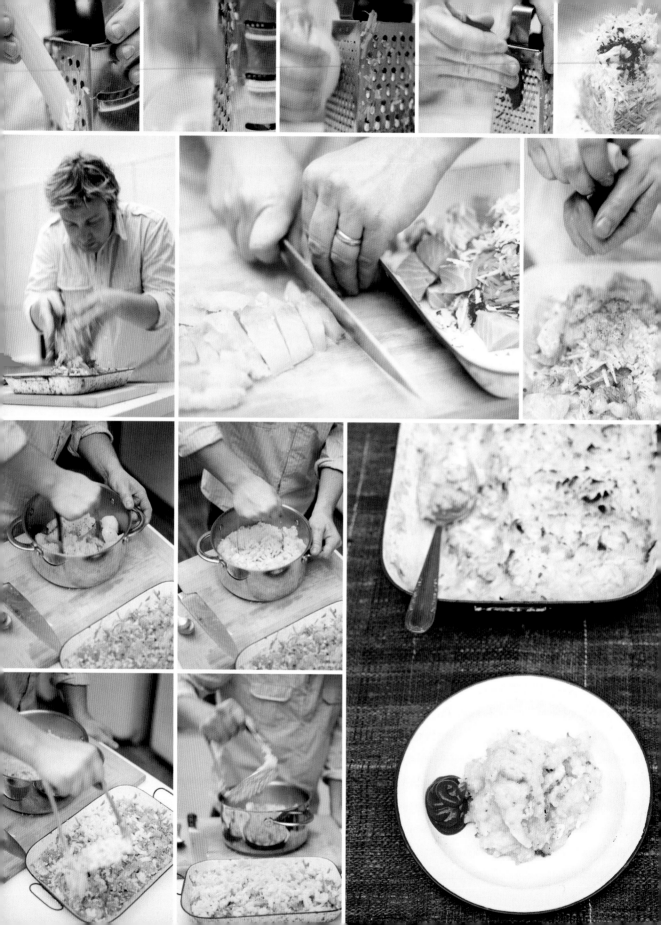

FISH PIE

This is a fantastically simple fish pie which doesn't involve poaching the fish or making a tedious béchamel sauce. Loads of good, fragrant vegetables are added quickly by grating them in. You can use whatever fish you like, making this as luxurious as you want it to be. If you like your fish pie to be creamy, feel free to add a few tablespoons of crème fraîche or heavy cream to the fish.

serves 4–6

sea salt and freshly ground black pepper

2¼ pounds potatoes

1 carrot

2 celery stalks

6 ounces grated good Cheddar cheese

1 lemon

½ a fresh red or green chile

4 sprigs of fresh Italian parsley

10 ounces salmon fillets, skin off and bones removed

10 ounces finnan haddie or cod fillets, skin off and
   bones removed

¼ pound large shrimp, raw, peeled

olive oil

optional: a good handful of spinach, chopped

optional: a couple of ripe tomatoes, quartered

To prepare your fish pie

Preheat the oven to 400°F and bring a large pan of salted water to a boil • Peel the potatoes and cut into ¾-inch chunks • Once the water is boiling, add your potatoes and cook for around 12 minutes, until soft (you can stick your knife into them to check) • Meanwhile, get yourself a deep baking pan or earthenware dish and stand a box grater in it • Peel the carrot • Grate the celery, carrot, and Cheddar on the coarse side of the grater • Use the fine side of the grater to grate the zest from the lemon • Finely grate or chop your chile • Finely chop the parsley leaves and stalks and add these to the pan

To cook and serve your fish pie

Cut the salmon and finnan haddie or cod into bite-size chunks and add to the pan with the shrimp • Squeeze over the juice from the zested lemon (no seeds please!), drizzle with olive oil, and add a good pinch of salt and pepper • If you want to add any spinach or tomatoes, do it now • Mix everything together really well • By now your potatoes should be cooked, so drain them in a colander and return them to the pan • Drizzle with a couple of good lugs of olive oil and add a pinch of salt and pepper • Mash until nice and smooth, then spread evenly over the top of the fish and grated veggies • Place in the preheated oven for around 40 minutes, or until cooked through, crispy, and golden on top • Serve piping hot with tomato ketchup, baked beans, steamed vegetables, or a lovely green salad

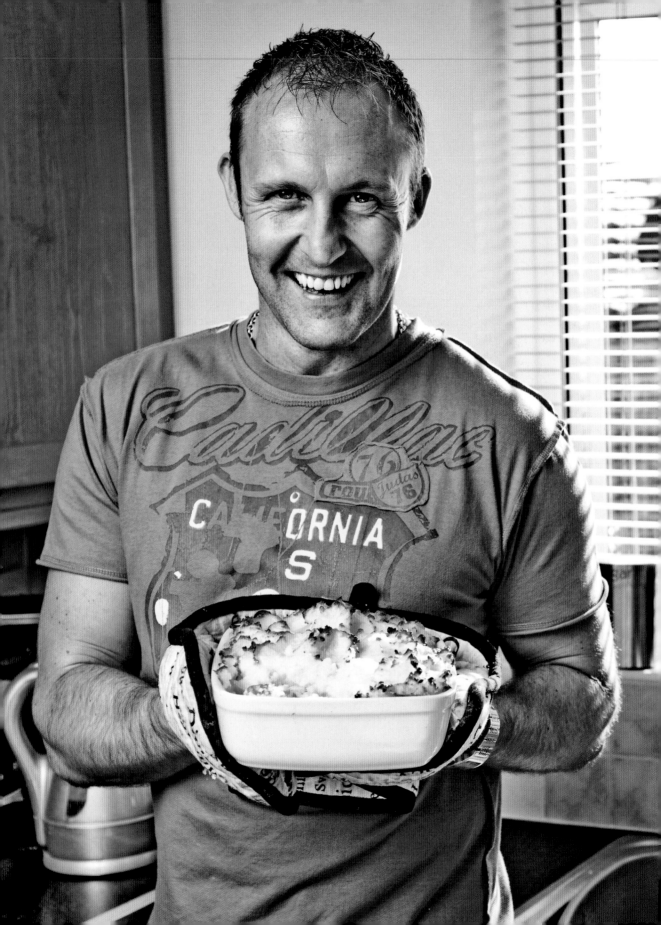

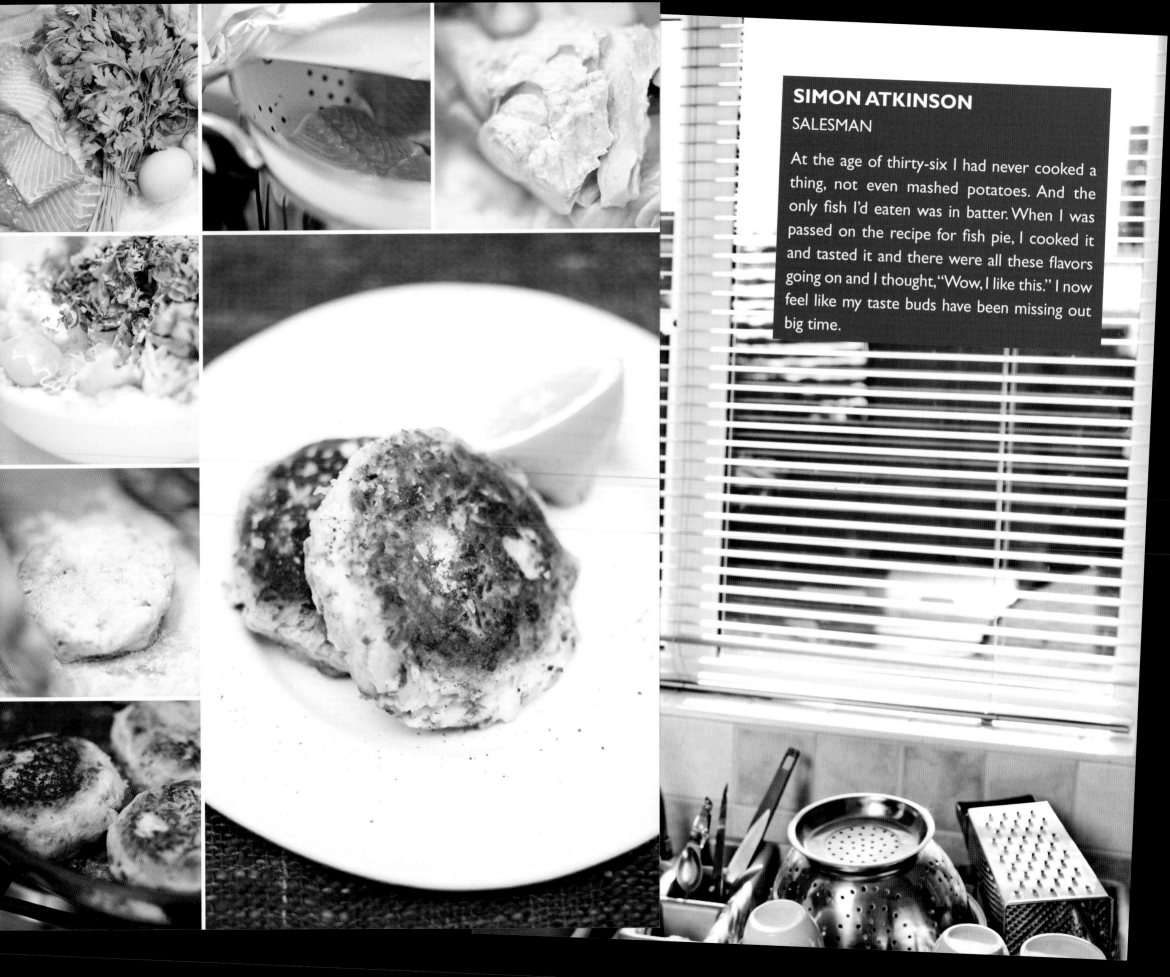

SIMON ATKINSON
SALESMAN

At the age of thirty-six I had never cooked a thing, not even mashed potatoes. And the only fish I'd eaten was in batter. When I was passed on the recipe for fish pie, I cooked it and tasted it and there were all these flavors going on and I thought, "Wow, I like this." I now feel like my taste buds have been missing out big time.

KEDGEREE

This is a delicious dish which I like to eat for breakfast or dinner. Don't be put off because you have to poach the fish, peel the hard-boiled eggs, and cook the rice – yes, it's a bit of a bother, but it should only take you 20 minutes to do.

serves 4

sea salt and freshly ground black pepper
1¼ cups basmati rice
¾ pound finnan haddie or cod fillets
4 large eggs, preferably free-range or organic
2 bay leaves, fresh or dried
optional: ½ a fresh red or green chile
a small bunch of fresh cilantro
1 medium onion

2 lemons
olive oil
2 tablespoons Madras or hot curry paste, such as
  Patak's
¼ pound smoked trout or whitefish, skin removed
  and flaked.
a large handful of fresh or frozen peas
natural yogurt, to serve

To prepare your kedgeree

Bring 2 large pans of salted water to a boil • Add the rice to one of the pans and the fish, eggs, and bay leaves to the other • Bring both pans back to a boil, then turn down to a simmer • Cook the rice according to the package timings and the finnan haddie or cod and eggs for about 6 minutes • Finely slice the chile, if using • Pick the cilantro leaves and put them in the refrigerator until required later, then roughly chop the stalks • Peel, halve, and finely slice the onion • Cut one of the lemons in half

To cook your kedgeree

Put a large casserole-type pan on a medium heat with a couple of lugs of olive oil • Add the onion, chile (if using), and cilantro stalks and cook gently for 5 minutes • Stir in the curry paste, smoked trout, and peas and season with salt and pepper • After the finnan haddie and eggs have had their 6 minutes, use a slotted spoon to remove them from the pan to a plate – the fish will flake up nicely into big chunks as you do this and you will easily be able to remove any skin and bones from the fish • Let the eggs cool down a little, then peel the shells away • Drain the rice in a strainer, then add to the onion mixture followed by the flaked finnan haddie and a good squeeze of lemon juice • Cut the eggs into quarters and add to the pan • Gently stir everything together, using a wooden spoon • Season with a little more lemon juice, salt, and pepper

To serve your kedgeree

Sprinkle over the cilantro leaves and serve at the table with a pot of natural yogurt and a lemon cut into wedges for squeezing over

ED MACKEREL PÂTÉ

ly thing to eat. There's loads of goodness in the skin of the mackerel, so try to leave it
e this – you won't really notice it once the fish is all chopped up. However, if you don't
n you can remove it.

mackerel or smoked trout fillets

delphia cream cheese

2 tablespoons creamed horseradish
sea salt and freshly ground black pepper
1 large ciabatta or other crusty loaf
2 large hand fulls sprouted cress or alfalfa

pâté

e skin off each piece of mackerel, do this now and discard it • Trim and finely slice the
mackerel into chunks • Finely grate over the zest of one of your lemons, then cut it
m cheese into a large bowl with the creamed horseradish • Chop up the mackerel,
zest on a chopping board, mixing everything together as you chop until you have a
his to the bowl with the cream cheese and horseradish, season to taste with salt and
e juice of your zested lemon, and mix again

té

oast the slices • Serve the mackerel pâté on the hot toasted bread, with a little
e second lemon, cut into wedges for squeezing over – delicious!

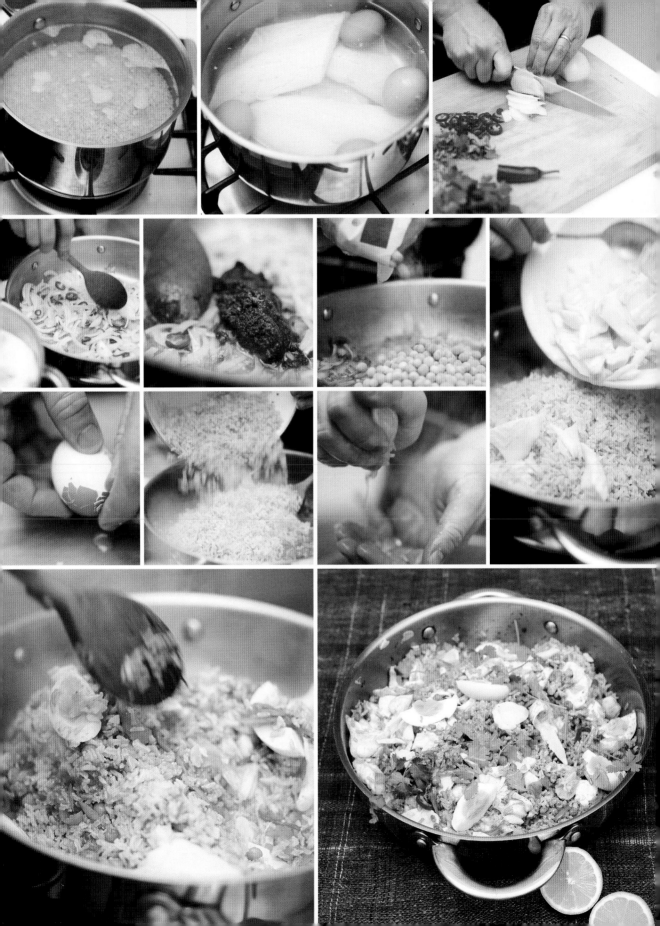

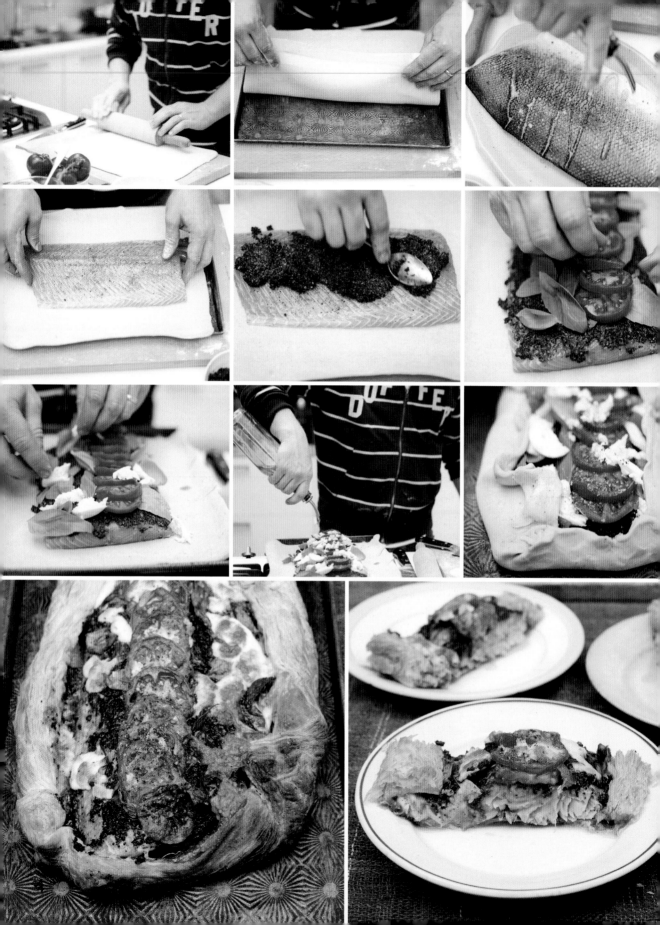

SALMON EN CROÛTE

This term "en croûte" describes food that is wrapped up in pastry and baked. It's good to have an evenly shaped piece of salmon for this, so ask your fishmonger for a fillet from the top and not a tail-end piece. Feel free to try this out using other fish like trout, haddock, or sustainable cod.

serves 4–6

all-purpose flour, for dusting

2 sheets puff pastry, preferably made with all-butter

1 x 1¾ pounds salmon fillet, bones removed

olive oil

sea salt and freshly ground black pepper

¼ cup black olive tapenade paste

a small bunch of fresh basil

2 ripe tomatoes

¼ pound ball of fresh mozzarella cheese

1 large egg, preferably free-range or organic

To prepare your salmon en croûte

Preheat the oven to 400°F • Get yourself a large, flat sheet pan and dust it with flour • Dust a clean work surface and a rolling pin with flour. Lay the puff pastry sheets one on top of the other. Roll out your puff pastry, dusting as you go, until it's the same size as the sheet pan (about 12in x 6in) • Place the pastry on your floured pan • Drizzle the salmon fillet with olive oil and season with a pinch of salt and pepper • Transfer to the pastry, skin-side down, then spoon the black olive paste over the top, spreading it out into a thin layer • Pick the basil leaves and place them over the fish • Slice the tomatoes and place them over the basil • Tear the mozzarella into pieces and scatter these on top • Sprinkle with salt and pepper and drizzle with olive oil • Gather up the sides of the pastry and pinch and push them together • Crack the egg into a cup and beat it with a fork, then use a pastry brush to paint this egg wash all around the pastry edges

To cook and serve your salmon en croûte

Place the sheet pan at the very bottom of the preheated oven, with an empty sheet pan or cookie sheet on the shelf above to protect the top of it from getting too much heat • Cook for 35 minutes, then remove from the oven and serve in the middle of the table so that everyone can cut themselves a slice • Great served with any steamed vegetable or a lovely green salad (the usual story!)

PAELLA

This is a traditional dish from Spain that works like a dream. Mixing meat and fish is absolutely brilliant – and the spicy flavors of the chorizo bring the dish together and make it something really special. Feel free to use whatever fish or shellfish you fancy – paella is always amazing regardless of whether you're using cheaper or more expensive fish.

serves 6

1 pound mixed seafood (mussels, peeled shrimp, clams, squid, white fish)

a small bunch of fresh Italian parsley

4 skinless and boneless chicken thighs, preferably free-range or organic

¼ pound chorizo sausage

4 slices of smoked bacon, preferably free-range or organic

1 medium onion

2 cloves of garlic

1½ quarts chicken broth, preferably organic

olive oil

optional: a pinch of saffron

2 cups paella rice

sea salt and freshly ground black pepper

2 handfuls of frozen peas

2 lemons

To prepare your paella

Scrub the mussels or clams • If you're using squid or white fish, slice into 1-inch pieces • Pick and chop your parsley leaves and roughly chop the stalks • Cut the chicken thighs into bite-size pieces • Slice up the chorizo sausage and bacon • Peel, halve, and roughly chop your onion and garlic • Put the chicken broth into a saucepan and bring to a boil.

To cook and serve your paella

Place a large casserole-type pan on a high heat and drizzle in some olive oil • Add the parsley, chicken, chorizo, and bacon to the pan and stir together • Cook for about 5 minutes, until the chicken turns golden • Add your onion and garlic to the pan and cook for 5 minutes • Add the saffron (if using) and rice to the pan with a pinch of salt and pepper, giving it a good stir • Pour in your hot broth and bring to a boil, stirring and scraping all the goodness off the bottom of the pan as you go • Put a lid on the pan, turn the heat down to a simmer, and cook the rice according to the package instructions • When the rice is nearly done, stir in the seafood and peas, then squeeze in the juice of 1 lemon • Cook for a further 5 minutes, have a taste, and add more salt and pepper and a little extra water if you think it's needed – you don't want the rice to become too dry • Serve in the middle of the table with some lemon wedges for squeezing over and let everyone help themselves

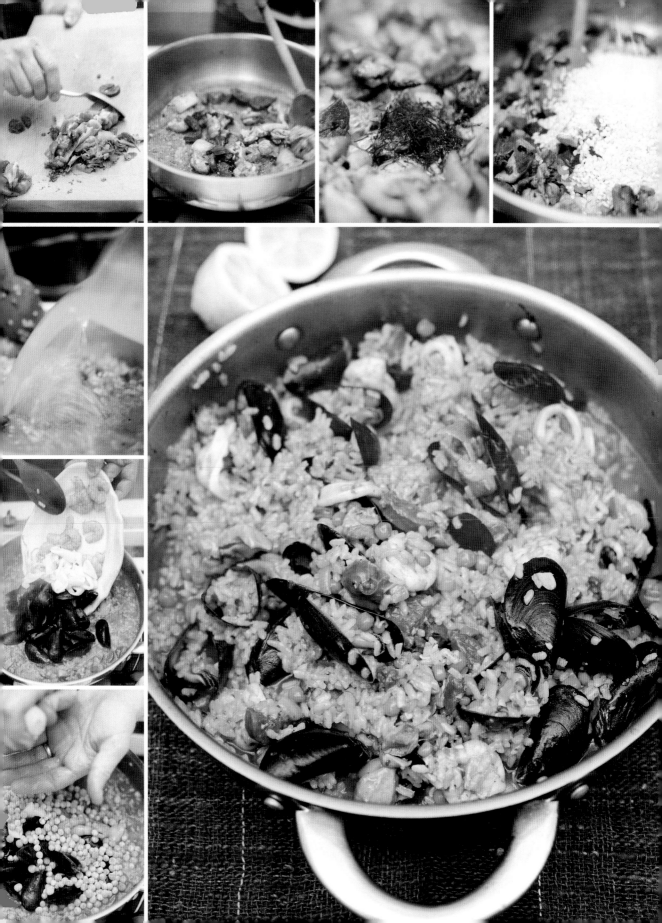

SHRIMP AND SWEET CORN CHOWDER

This is inspired by a great classic American soup, clam chowder. In this version I use shrimp, but in America clam chowder is made using whole jars of pre-cooked clams, so you could also have a go at using these.

serves 4–6

1 large leek

1 pound potatoes

1 quart chicken broth, preferably organic

olive oil

6 rashers of smoked streaky bacon, preferably free-range or organic

1⅔ cups frozen corn

½ pound large shrimp, raw, peeled

1¼ cups heavy cream

sea salt and freshly ground black pepper

a small bunch of Italian parsley

crackers to serve

extra virgin olive oil

To prepare your chowder

Cut the ends off the leek, quarter lengthways, wash under running water, and slice across thinly • Peel your potatoes and chop them into 1-inch chunks • Pour the chicken broth into a saucepan and bring to a boil

To cook your chowder

Put a large casserole-type pan on a high heat and add a drizzle of olive oil • Slice your bacon and add to the pan • Cook until golden and really crispy, letting all the fat and flavor cook out into the pan • Using tongs, remove and transfer the bacon to a plate, leaving the fat in the pan • Add the leek and potatoes to the pan and give them a good stir • Cook for 3 to 5 minutes, until the leek has softened • Add the corn and shrimp • Pour the hot broth into the pan with the cream • Add a good pinch of salt and pepper and stir • Bring to the boil and simmer for 10 minutes • Meanwhile, roughly chop the parsley • Roughly break up the crackers and place them on the plate next to your bacon • Take the soup off the heat and use a hand blender to gently whiz it up until you have a smooth but slightly chunky texture • Season once more to taste

To serve your chowder

Pour into a large serving bowl and drizzle with extra virgin olive oil • Serve at the table, sprinkle with the bacon, crackers, and chopped chile, and tuck in!

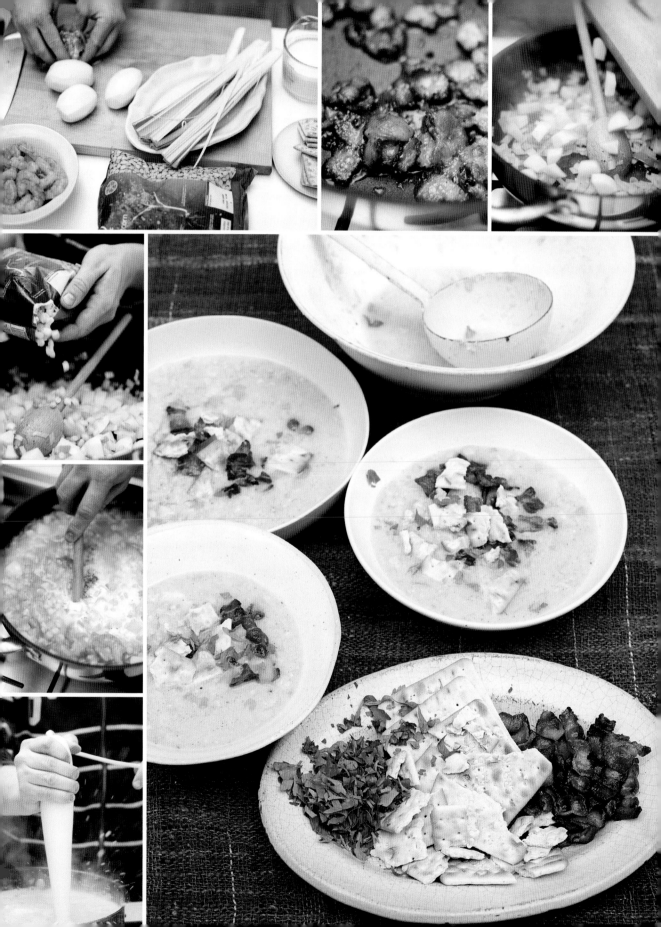

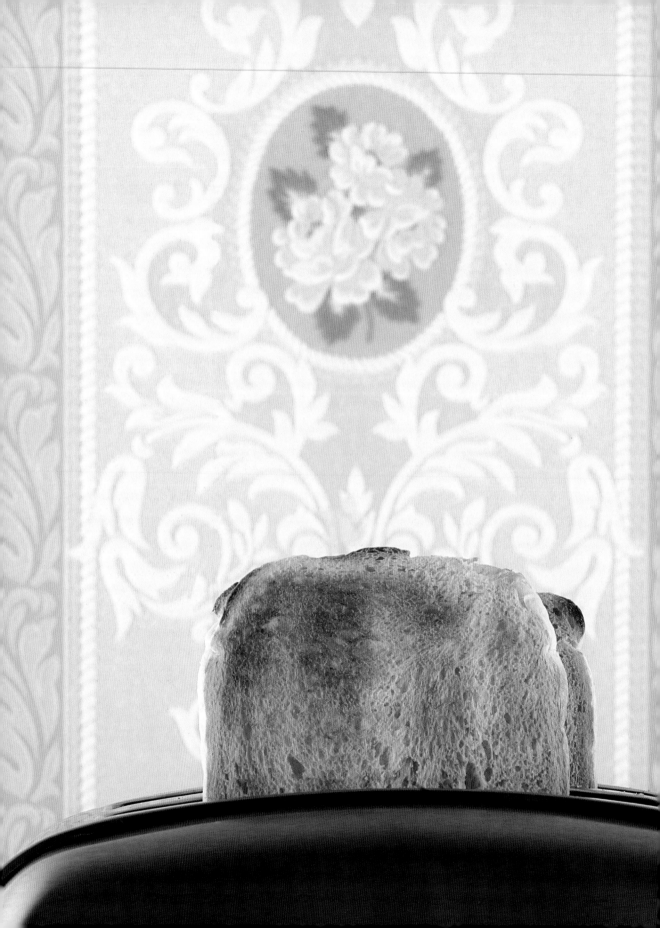

Kick-start breakfasts

Lots of recent studies have shown that having breakfast in the morning sets you up for the day. Not only does it help you to concentrate better and retain more information – which is great for work and school – but also, if you're watching your weight, people who eat breakfast are more likely to maintain their weight or steadily lose weight than people who avoid eating breakfast and binge later. You know, and I know, that since kids we have always been told to eat a good breakfast. Our parents knew what they were talking about, didn't they? You only have to look at the Scots, who eat oatmeal, to see what a good breakfast can do. If you go there in the winter you'll never see any underpants under those kilts, and only a good bowl of oatmeal can protect you from the windchill of the Scottish Highlands!

Anyway, enough of the worthy and the silly, I'm bringing this chapter straight back to what puts a smile on our faces, and that's taste. Here you'll find a handful of reliable breakfasts that are quite healthy but also taste bloody good; the sort of things that I feed my kids on a regular basis. You'll find a great recipe for oatmeal, with different ways to flavor it. I've looked at all the different methods of cooking eggs, and also given you a recipe for a fantastically simple but tasty omelet, plus lots of ideas for how to vary it. There's a healthier full Monty English breakfast (can you believe it?), a pancake recipe that you don't have to weigh any of the ingredients for (fantastic!), and a recipe to show you the simple, brave art of making regular everyday fruit look really attractive on a plate. Last but not least, I've given you some of my wife Jools's bloody marvelous smoothies.

Just a little thought … if you spend a bit of time teaching your kids, say at the age of eight or ten or whenever you feel's appropriate (I was about eight), to make great pancakes or good eggs, this will be a really good investment, because once they've mastered it you can get them cooking breakfast for you. Payback time!

A HEALTHIER FULL MONTY

I think everyone's trying to make a bit of an effort to have a healthier breakfast these days. However, while yogurt, fruit, and oatmeal are delicious and convenient, come a Saturday or a Sunday Brits still love a full English breakfast. It's fair to say that a lot of fry-ups aren't necessarily healthy, but if you remove the fat from the bacon, use high-meat-content sausages, and leave out buttering your toast, you'll be amazed how healthy they are in comparison to things like muffins, pastries, and croissants, which can be very calorific. You can get a full Monty coming in at under 500 calories if you do the things I suggest below.

serves 2

2 ripe tomatoes

2 portobello mushrooms

4 slices of smoked Canadian bacon, preferably free-range or organic

2 good-quality sausages, preferably free-range or organic

sea salt and freshly ground black pepper

olive oil

½ x 15-ounce can of low salt and sugar baked beans

4 slices of whole wheat bread

2 super-fresh eggs, preferably free-range or organic

To prepare your full Monty

Preheat your broiler to high • Get yourself a wire rack and pop it on top of a sheet pan • Halve your tomatoes • Trim the stalks from the mushrooms • Remove any fat from the bacon • Score the sausages lengthways and open them out so they're flat – this way, they'll cook at the same time as everything else and also it will help to cook the fat out • Put the tomatoes, mushrooms, and sausages on the wire rack, with the tomatoes cut side up and the mushrooms stalk side up • Sprinkle a little salt and pepper over the tomatoes and mushrooms • Very lightly rub them with a little olive oil – you don't need much (an olive oil spray is great for this job)

To cook your full Monty

Place the sheet pan and wire rack under the hot broiler for 5 minutes and put a pan of water on to boil • After 5 minutes, add the bacon to the wire rack and turn the sausages over • Put back under the broiler and cook for a further 4 to 5 minutes (depending on the speed of your broiler), until the bacon is golden and crispy • Meanwhile, put the beans into a small saucepan over a medium heat to warm through • Pop your slices of bread into the toaster • Crack the eggs into the pan of simmering water and poach for 2 to 3 minutes • To test if they're ready, carefully remove one of them from the water using a slotted spoon and touch it gently with your finger – common sense will tell you if it's really runny or quite solid in the center • If it feels too soft, give it a minute or so more in the water • Once the eggs are done to your liking, remove them from the pan with your slotted spoon and drain them on paper towels

To serve your full Monty

Divide everything between your two serving plates and sprinkle a tiny bit of salt and pepper over the eggs

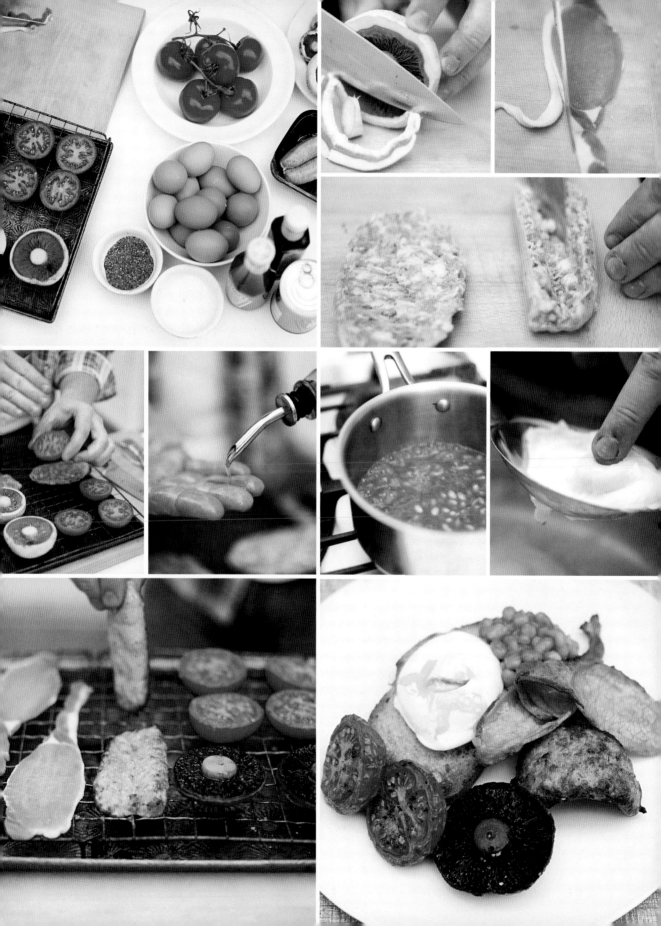

GET INTO OATMEAL

Oatmeal is an absolute classic breakfast, made with either milk or water. You can buy the most delicious packs of oats these days, called quick cooking oats. There are loads of things besides milk and sugar you can add to oatmeal before serving to make it extra tasty. Here's a basic recipe for how to make oatmeal, followed by four of my favorite flavor combinations.

serves 4

2 cups quick cook oats (not instant)
3 cups milk, soy milk, or water
sea salt

To make your basic oatmeal

Place the oats and the milk or water in a saucepan with a small pinch of sea salt and put it on a medium heat • Bring to a steady simmer for 5 to 6 minutes, stirring as often as you can to give you a smooth, creamy oatmeal • While it's blipping away in the pan, choose one of the flavor combinations below and prepare the ingredients • 1 or 2 minutes before the oatmeal is ready, add your flavoring (see below) • If you like your oatmeal runnier, simply stir in a splash more milk or water until you've got the consistency you're after

Banana and cinnamon

2 ripe bananas, finely sliced
½ teaspoon ground cinnamon
2 tablespoons poppy seeds
2–4 tablespoons maple syrup or runny honey, or to taste
a small handful of toasted sliced almonds or unsweetened shredded coconut

Blackberry and apple

2 apples, cored and diced
a tablespoon of butter
a small extra handful of uncooked oats
1 tablespoon honey, plus extra to taste
2 handfuls of fresh or frozen blackberries
Fry the apples in a pan with the butter until soft and golden • Add the uncooked oatmeal and honey, and cook for 1 minute • Squash the blackberries into the cooked oatmeal • Serve with the apple mixture on top

Banana, whisky, and nutmeg

2 ripe bananas, mashed
2 shots (¼ cup) of whisky (for grown-ups only, not for the kids!)
¼ of a nutmeg, finely grated
honey, to taste

Dark chocolate and Seville orange marmalade

2 ounces good quality bittersweet (60% cocoa solids minimum) chocolate, finely grated
heaped ¼ cup Seville orange marmalade

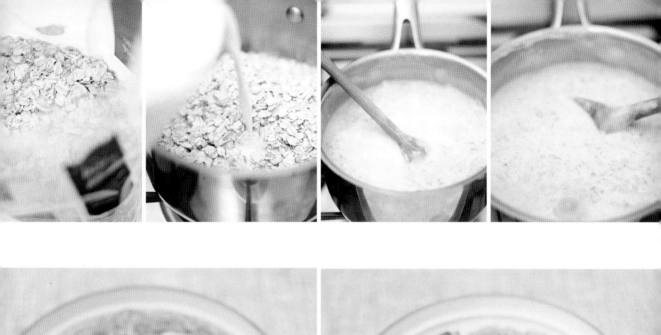

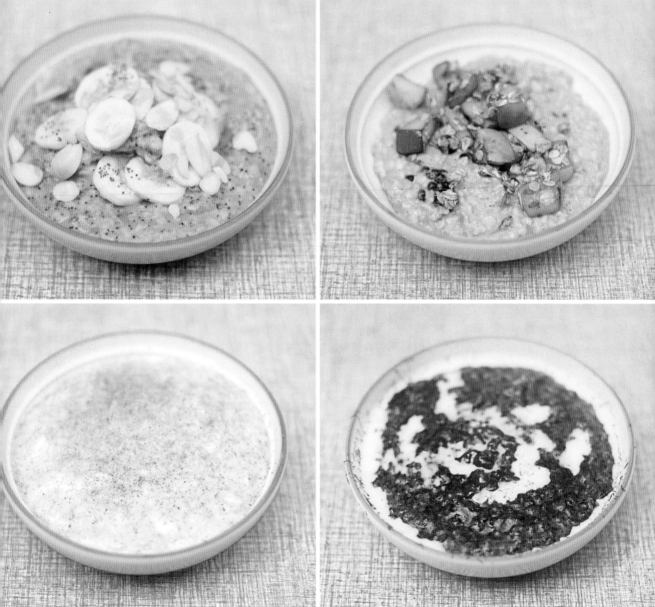

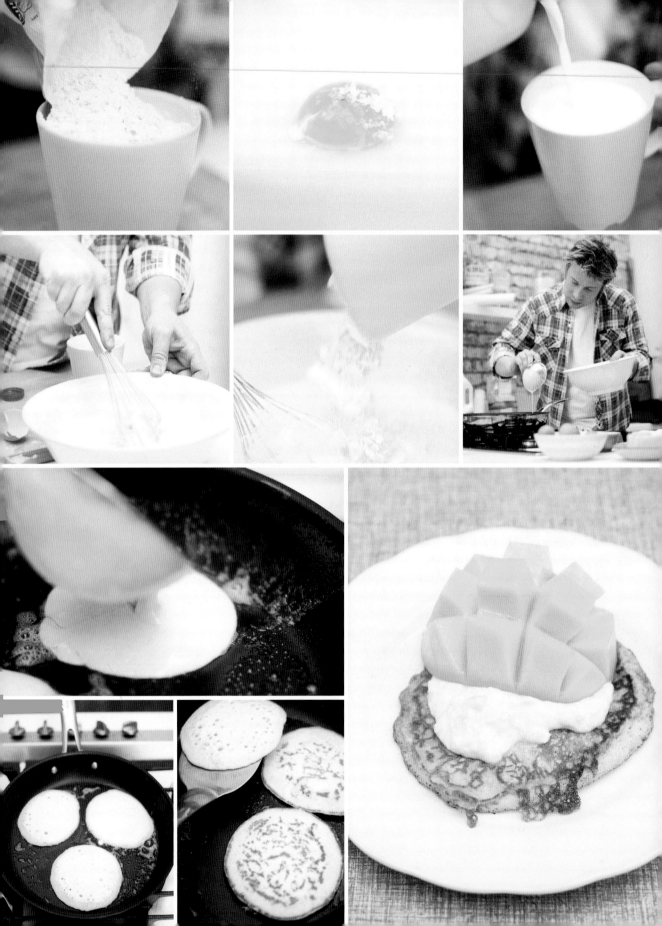

ONE-CUP PANCAKES, TROPICAL YOGURT, AND MANGO

These are the easiest pancakes to make – you don't even need scales to weigh your ingredients. All you need is a cup or a mug. As long as you use the same cup for measuring both the flour and the milk, you'll be laughing! These are great with a sprinkling of sugar and a squeeze of lemon juice (very old school!), or drizzled with maple syrup and served with crispy bacon. A handful of blueberries in the batter makes the most wicked blueberry pancakes. I also love eating them with coconut-flavored yogurt, which is delicious. I've given you a recipe here for making your own similar tropical-flavored yogurt. It actually gets better if you let it stand in the fridge for a few hours, as the coconut will soften.

serves 4

For the flavored yogurt
2 ripe bananas
a handful of unsweetened shredded coconut
I cup natural yogurt

For the pancakes
I egg, preferably free-range or organic

I cup of all-purpose flour (see above)
I cup of milk (see above)
I teaspoon baking powder
sea salt
2 ripe mangoes
2 tablespoons butter
I lime

To make your yogurt and your pancake batter

Peel your bananas, put them into a large bowl, and mash them with a fork • Add the coconut and the yogurt and mix well • Put this to one side until needed and get started on your pancakes • Crack your egg into a large mixing bowl • Add your flour, milk, baking powder, and a pinch of sea salt • Whisk everything together until you've got a lovely, smooth batter • Slice the mangoes away from their pits, score the flesh across, and push outward so that you can slice it off the skin to give you diced mango

To cook your pancakes

Put a large frying pan on a medium heat and add half the butter • When the butter has melted and the pan is nice and hot, use a ladle to spoon the batter into the pan • Each ladleful will make I pancake – they're quite small, so you can cook several at a time • Cook for 1 to 2 minutes and use a turner to flip them over when they start to brown on the bottom and get little bubbles on the top • When cooked on both sides, transfer them to a plate, carefully wipe the pan clean with paper towels, add the rest of the butter, and start again • Keep going until all the batter is used up

To serve your pancakes

Serve straight away, topped with a dollop of flavored yogurt, the diced fresh mango, and wedges of lime for squeezing over

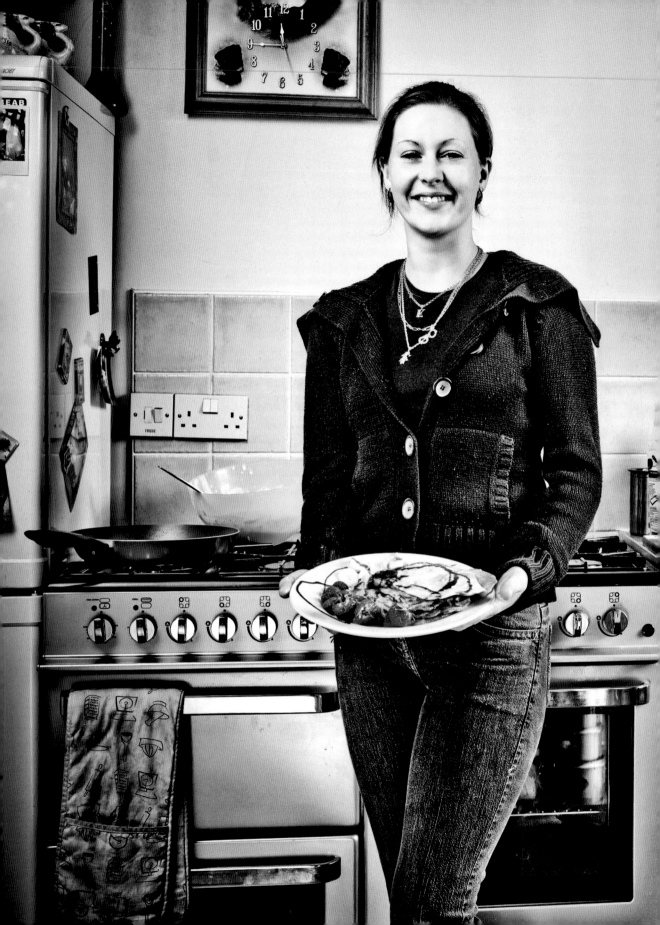

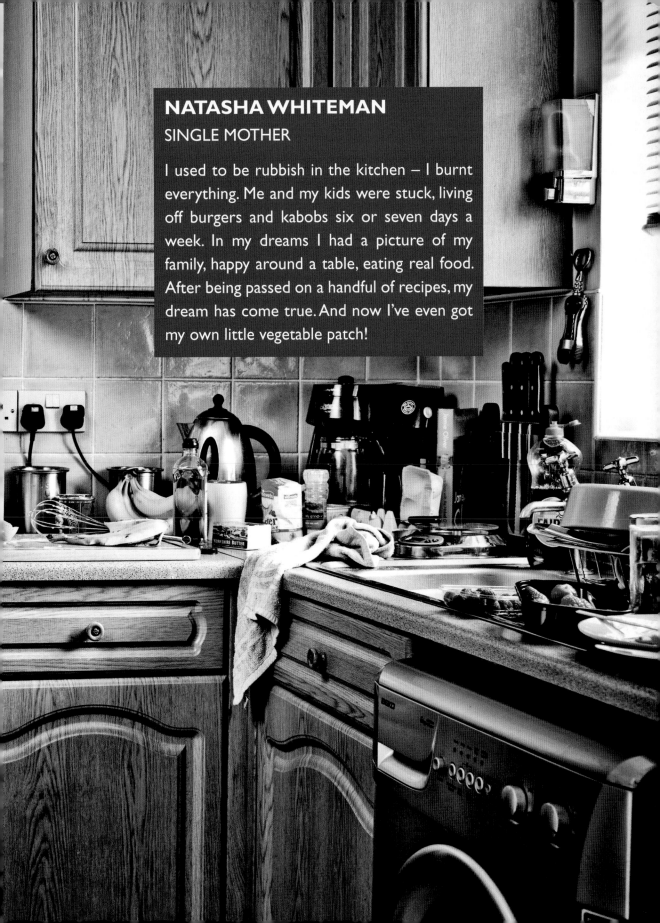

NATASHA WHITEMAN
SINGLE MOTHER

I used to be rubbish in the kitchen – I burnt everything. Me and my kids were stuck, living off burgers and kabobs six or seven days a week. In my dreams I had a picture of my family, happy around a table, eating real food. After being passed on a handful of recipes, my dream has come true. And now I've even got my own little vegetable patch!

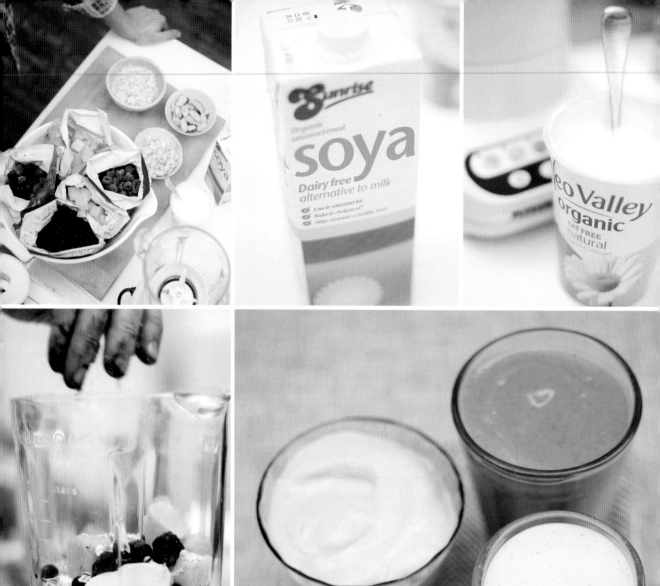
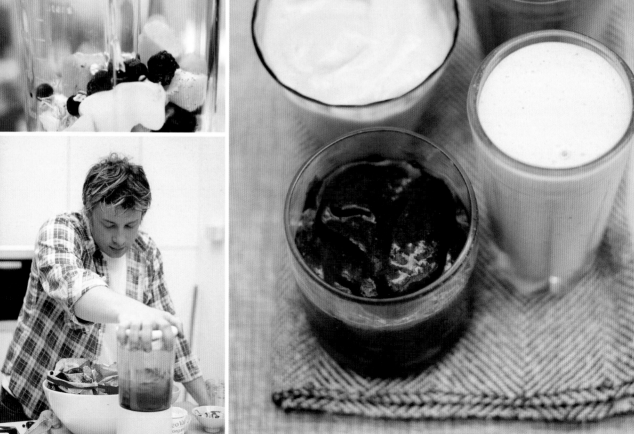

FROZEN FRUIT SMOOTHIES

Smoothies are not only deliciously tasty but they're also perfect to have for breakfast, as they're full of goodness. Adding quick cook oats and nuts to them is great, because it helps slow down the absorption of the sugar from the fruit into your bloodstream, which gives you more energy for longer. The great thing about frozen fruit is that it's been picked at its best, at the right time, and hasn't been forced to grow out of season, like so much of the "fresh" fruit on offer to us these days. It's also cheaper and far more convenient – it will keep happily in your freezer for months on end, so any time you fancy a smoothie, you can have one!

These smoothies are best made in a blender, as opposed to a food processor, as this will give your smoothies a lovely silky texture. And feel free to use any fruit you like, either one type or a mixture. Raspberries are really tasty and you can use them here, but I tend to stay away from them because of the seeds.

makes 2 glasses

1 ripe banana
1 glass of frozen fruit of your choice: mango,
   blackcurrants, or strawberries
2 heaped tablespoons natural yogurt

1 small handful of quick cook oats (not instant)
1 small handful of mixed nuts
1 glass of soy milk, fat free milk, or apple juice
optional: honey, to taste

Peel and slice your banana and put it into a blender with your frozen fruit and the yogurt • Whiz it up and add the oats and nuts • Add the soy milk, fat free milk, or apple juice and whiz again, until nice and smooth • If it's a bit too thick for you, just add a splash more milk or juice and whiz around again • Give it a good stir, then have a taste • Rarely with a frozen fruit smoothie should you need to sweeten it, but if you think it needs a bit of extra sweetness you can add a little honey to taste – you won't need much

BOILED EGGS serves 2

Boiled eggs and "soldiers" (fingers of toast) are one of the best things ever. Whether you like them hard-boiled or soft-boiled, it's easy to get your eggs just right simply by varying the cooking time. A good tip to remember is that if you add a small pinch of salt to the water it will help to prevent the eggs from cracking.

Get yourself a small saucepan, fill it three-quarters full with **water**, and bring it to a fast boil • Add a good pinch of **salt** and, using a spoon, dip in and out (dipping helps prevent the shock of the change in temperature from fridge to boiling, which sometimes makes them crack open) and then lower **4 large free-range or organic eggs** into the water, slowly, so the shells don't crack on the bottom

Cook for the following times, depending on how you like your eggs:
• **5 minutes** for runny
• **7½ minutes** for semi-firm
• **10 minutes** for hard-boiled

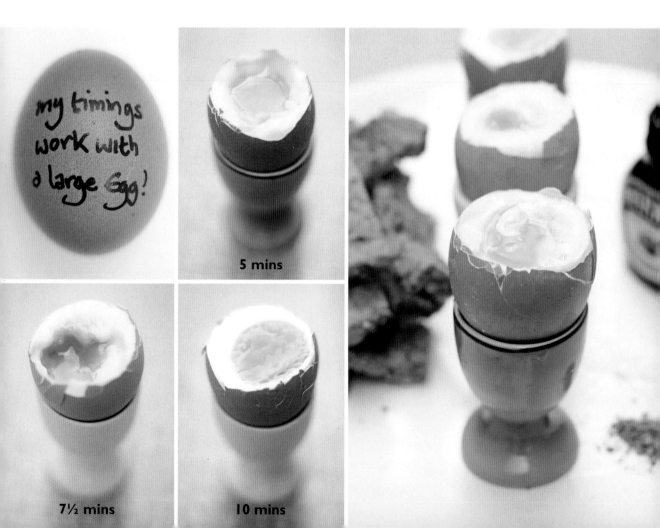

my timings work with a large egg!

5 mins

7½ mins

10 mins

FRIED EGGS   serves 2

Fried eggs are delicious and simple. There are different ways in which to fry them, but this is my favorite method. It does involve using ½ inch of olive oil in the pan, but by the time you've removed the egg from the pan with a slotted spoon and patted it dry with paper towels, most of the oil will have disappeared, leaving you with a perfect egg.

Get your frying pan on a medium to low heat and add ½ inch of **olive oil** • Crack 4 large **free-range or organic eggs** into the pan • As the oil gets hotter you'll see it start to change the color of the eggs • When they turn white, spoon some of the hot oil over the eggs as this will help to cook them through evenly • If the oil starts to spit it's because it's too hot, so turn the heat right down • You want this to be a gentle method of cooking – if the oil gets too hot too fast, you'll end up with crispy, bubbly eggs, but you want them to be soft and silky • When they're ready, remove the pan from the heat and take the eggs out using a slotted spoon • Place on a plate and dab them with some paper towels to soak up any excess oil • Serve on **toast** – no need to butter it – with a sprinkling of **sea salt and freshly ground black pepper**

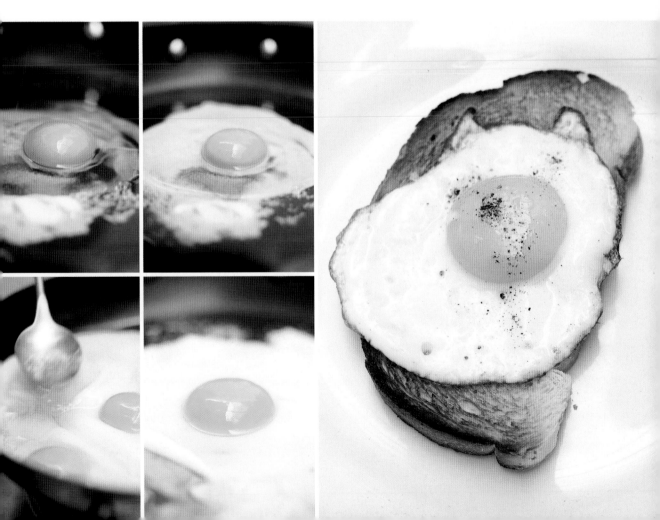

SCRAMBLED EGGS serves 2

Scrambled eggs can be one of the most fantastic, luxurious breakfasts around if you remember a few key things: always use really fresh free-range or organic eggs and good-quality butter, and always keep the eggs moving slowly over a low heat. Do this and you'll get luscious, buttery, creamy eggs every time.

Crack **4 large free-range or organic eggs** into a bowl, add a pinch of **sea salt and freshly ground black pepper**, and beat them together using a fork • Put a small saucepan over a low heat and add a good pat of **butter** • Melt it slowly until it's frothy • Pour the eggs into the pan and stir them slowly – use a wooden spoon or a spatula if you have one, so you can get right into the sides of the pan • While you're doing this, pop some **bread** into the toaster • Your eggs are done when they still look silky and slightly runny and underdone, as the heat will continue to cook the eggs to perfection • Even when you've served them, they'll still be cooking • Serve on your buttered toast

PS You can chop soft fresh herbs like chives or basil into the beaten egg mixture to add a little extra flavor • In Italy they like to add a little teaspoon of finely grated Parmesan cheese, and in Mexico you'll often find some chopped fresh chile added

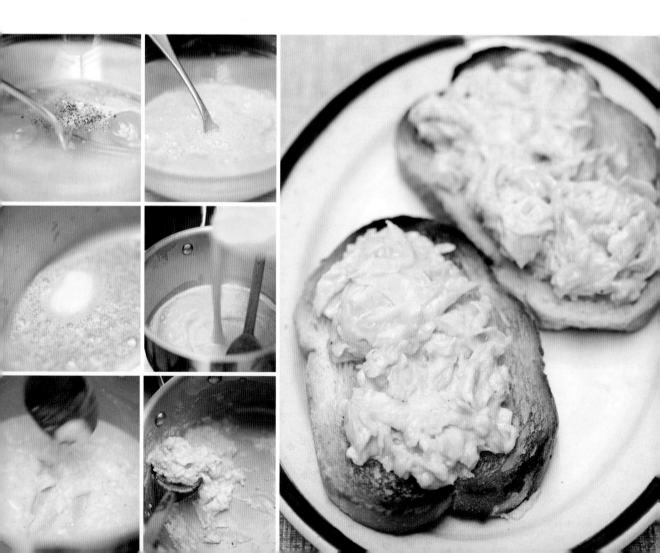

POACHED EGGS serves 2

A perfectly cooked poached egg is one of the most brilliant things in the whole world! They can be a little tricky to get right, but if you make sure you use the freshest eggs you possibly can you shouldn't have any problems. You can tell whether an egg is fresh by cracking it on to a saucer. If the yolk stands up and the white isn't watery, it's fresh as a daisy.

Get yourself a wide, casserole-type pan, fill it with water, and put over a medium heat • Bring it to a light simmer, add a pinch of **sea salt**, then crack one of your 4 **large free-range or organic eggs** into a cup and gently pour it into the water in one fluid movement • Repeat with the rest of the eggs • You'll see them begin to cook immediately – don't worry if the edges look a little scruffy • Depending on your pan, a really soft poached egg should take around 2 minutes and a soft to firm one will need 4 minutes (it depends on the size of the eggs and whether you're using them straight from the refrigerator) • To check whether they're done, remove one carefully from the pan with a slotted spoon and give it a gentle push with a teaspoon • If it feels too soft (use your instincts), put it back and give the eggs a minute or two more in the water to firm up • When they're ready, remove them to some paper towels to dry off and serve with **buttered toast** and a sprinkle of **sea salt and freshly ground black pepper**

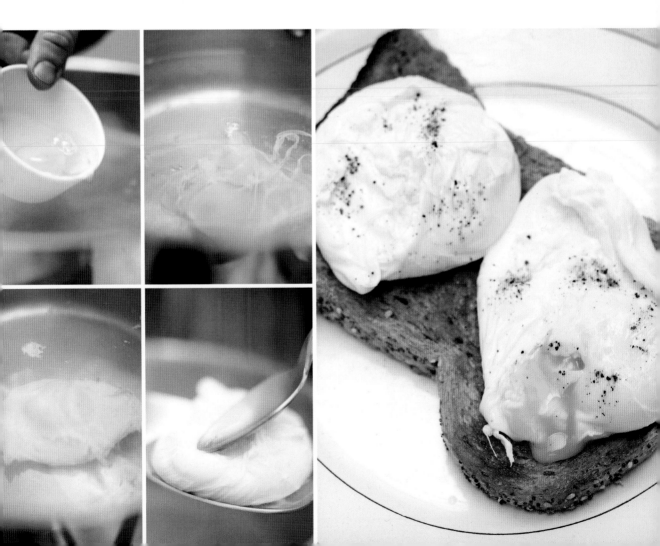

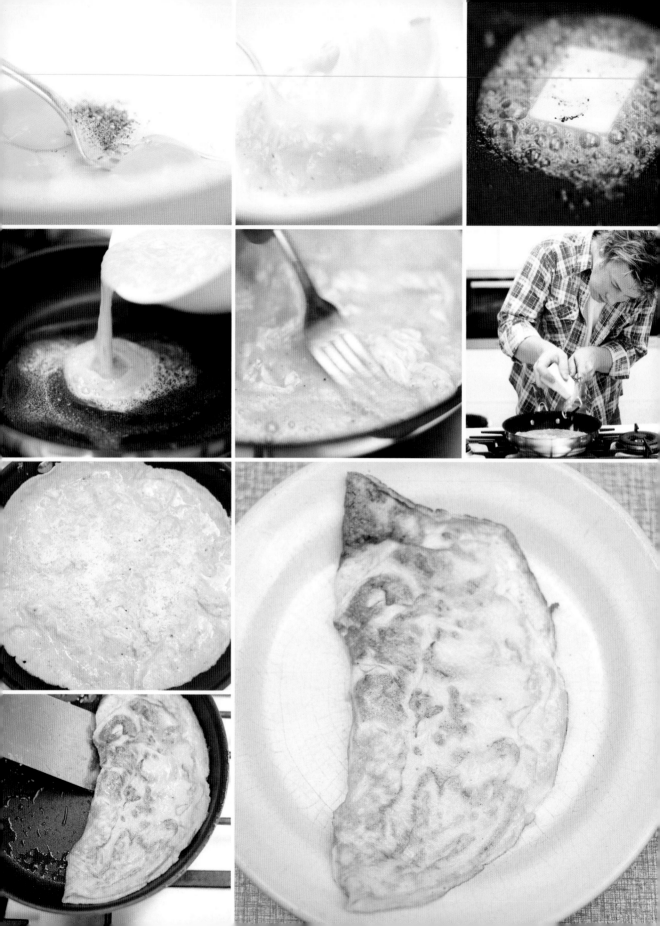

OMELETS

Omelets are tasty and super-quick to knock together. A simple omelet is delicious, but if you like to mix things up, some of the other flavor combinations I've given you on the next page are really good, whether you're eating your omelet for breakfast, lunch, or even dinner on those nights when you don't want to be in the kitchen for long.

serves 1

For each omelet you'll need:

2–3 large eggs, preferably free-range or organic

sea salt and freshly ground black pepper

a pat of butter

a small handful of grated Cheddar cheese

To make your simple, basic omelette

Crack the eggs into a mixing bowl with a pinch of salt and pepper • Beat well with a fork • Put a small frying pan on a low heat and let it get hot • Add a pat of butter • When the butter has melted and is bubbling, add your eggs and move the pan around to spread them out evenly • When the omelet begins to cook and firm up, but still has a little raw egg on top, sprinkle over the cheese (I sometimes grate mine directly on to the omelet) • Using a spatula, ease around the edges of the omelet, then fold it over in half • When it starts to turn golden brown underneath, remove the pan from the heat and slide the omelet on to a plate

Bacon omelet

Crack the **eggs** into a mixing bowl with a pinch of **salt and pepper** • Beat well with a fork • Finely chop 2 slices of **smoked bacon, preferably free-range or organic**, and fry in a hot frying pan with a tiny drizzle of **olive oil** • When crisp and brown, turn the heat down to medium and add your eggs • Move the pan around to spread them out evenly • When the omelet begins to cook and firm up, but still has a little raw egg on top, sprinkle over the **Cheddar** • Using a spatula, ease around the edges of the omelet, then fold it over in half • When it starts to turn golden brown underneath, remove the pan from the heat and slide the omelet on to a plate

---

Hangover omelet!

Crack the **eggs** into a mixing bowl with a pinch of **salt and pepper** • Beat well with a fork • Finely slice ½ a **fresh red or green chile** • Squeeze the meat out of 1 **good-quality sausage, preferably free-range or organic**, and crumble it into a hot frying pan with a tiny drizzle of **olive oil** and a pinch of salt and pepper • Fry until golden for a few minutes and, once browned, turn the heat down to medium and add ½ a teaspoon of **crushed fennel seeds**, the chile, and the eggs • Move the pan around to spread them out evenly • When the omelet begins to cook and firm up, but still has a little raw egg on top, sprinkle over the **Cheddar** • Using a spatula, ease around the edges of the omelet, then fold it over in half • When it starts to turn golden brown underneath, remove the pan from the heat and slide the omelet on to a plate

---

Tomato and basil omelet

Crack the **eggs** into a mixing bowl with a pinch of **salt and pepper** • Beat well with a fork • Pick the leaves off 2 or 3 sprigs of **fresh basil** and roughly tear them • Cut a handful of **cherry or grape tomatoes** in half and add to a hot frying pan with a small pat of **butter**, a drizzle of **olive oil**, and a pinch of salt and pepper • Fry and toss around for about 1 minute, then turn the heat down to medium • Add your eggs and move the pan around to spread them out evenly • When the omelet begins to cook and firm up, but still has a little raw egg on top, sprinkle over the **Cheddar** and the basil leaves • Using a spatula, ease around the edges of the omelet • When it starts to turn golden brown underneath, remove the pan from the heat and slide the omelet on to a plate

---

Mushroom omelet

Crack the **eggs** into a mixing bowl with a pinch of **salt and pepper** • Beat well with a fork • Quarter or roughly chop 2 or 3 nice **portobello mushrooms** and add to a hot frying pan with a small pat of **butter**, a drizzle of **olive oil**, and a pinch of salt and pepper • Fry and toss around until golden, then turn the heat down to medium • Add your eggs and move the pan around to spread them out evenly • When the omelet begins to cook and firm up, but still has a little raw egg on top, sprinkle over the **Cheddar** • Using a spatula, ease around the edges of the omelet, then fold it over in half • When it starts to turn golden brown underneath, remove the pan from the heat and slide the omelet on to a plate

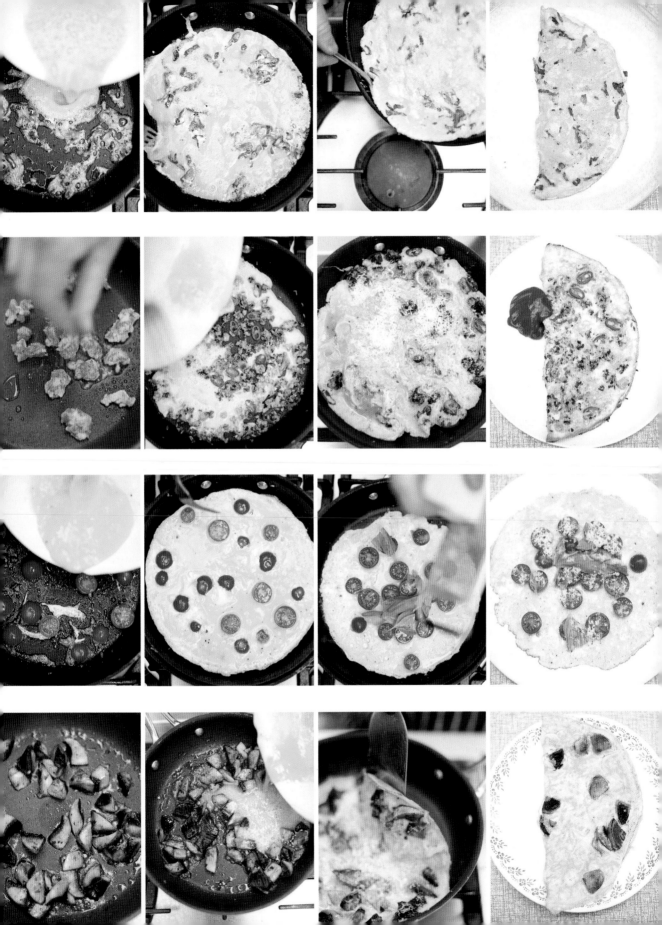

GRANOLA

Granola is a great way of enjoying all different types of dried fruits, nuts, and seeds that you might not otherwise eat in your diet. Because of the variety of ingredients, it has a great texture and it's so tasty, especially with the hit of cinnamon. It's brilliant with cold milk for breakfast.

makes enough to fill a large jar

2 cups quick cook oatmeal (not instant)

1 heaped cup mixed nuts (hazelnuts, almonds, walnuts, brazil nuts)

¼ cup mixed seeds (sunflower, poppy, pumpkin, sesame)

¾ cup unsweetened shredded coconut

1 teaspoon ground cinnamon

1½ cups dried fruit (raisins, cranberries, apricots)

5 tablespoons maple syrup or honey

5 tablespoons olive oil

To prepare your granola

Preheat the oven to 350°F • Put your dry granola ingredients, including the coconut and cinnamon but not the dried fruit, on a sheet pan • Stir well and smooth out • Drizzle with the maple syrup and a little olive oil and stir again • Place the pan in the preheated oven for 25 to 30 minutes • Every 5 minutes or so, take the granola out and stir it, then smooth it down with a wooden spoon and put it back into the oven • While it's toasting, roughly chop up any large dried fruit • When the granola is nice and golden, remove it from the oven, mix in the dried fruit, and let it cool down

To serve your granola

Once cooled, serve the granola in individual bowls with some milk or a dollop of natural yogurt • You can keep any leftover granola in an airtight container for about 2 weeks, but it's so delicious I'll be surprised if it lasts that long!

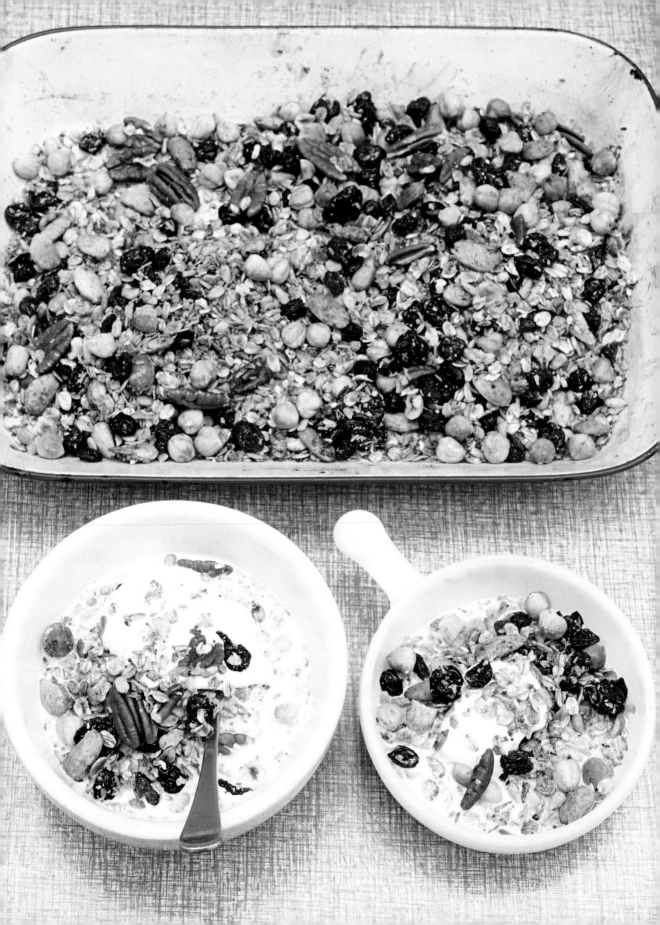

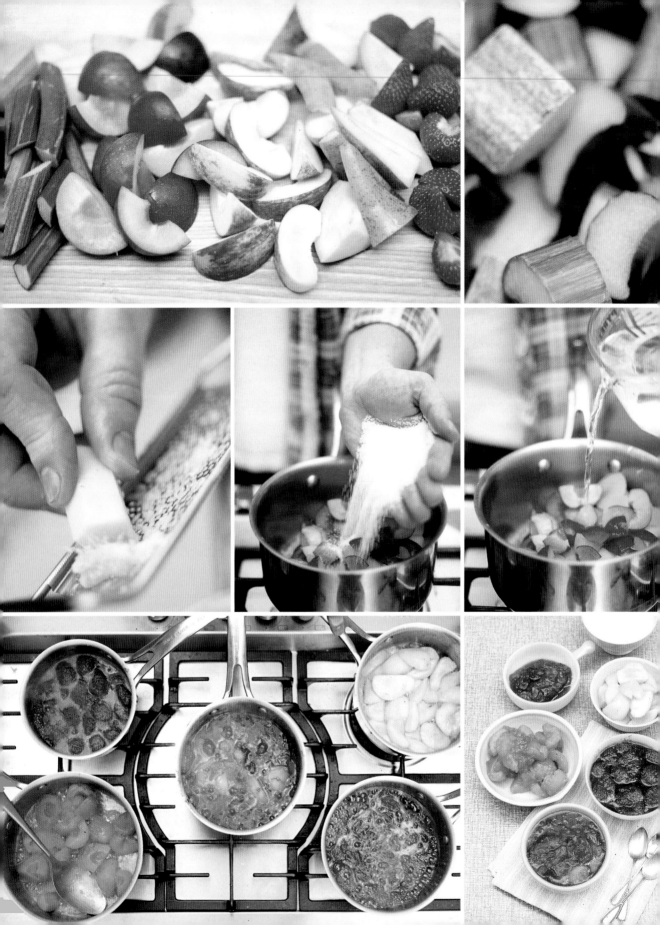

STEWED FRUIT

The really important thing to remember when you are stewing fruit is that it's best to decide for yourself how much sugar to add – I'll give rough amounts here to guide you but if, for example, your fruit is really ripe and sweet, you'll need less than I'm suggesting. Just have a taste as you go along and add more if you think you need to.

serves 4

1 ¾ pounds rhubarb, plums, apricots, strawberries, or pears

if using rhubarb: a 1 inch piece of fresh root ginger

sugar, to taste

Chop up all the fruit, discarding any pits • Place the fruit in a saucepan • If using rhubarb, peel the ginger and finely grate it into the pan • Add the sugar – I usually add 3 heaped teaspoons to rhubarb and 2 heaped teaspoons to any other fruit, but just taste as you go along and add more if you think it needs it • Add 2 tablespoons of water and cook on a medium heat with the lid on • Once the fruit has softened, remove the lid and let the liquid reduce – you want to end up with a fairly thick consistency • Serve over cereal, yogurt, pancakes, granola, muesli, or even with roast pork! • Also great as a crumble filling

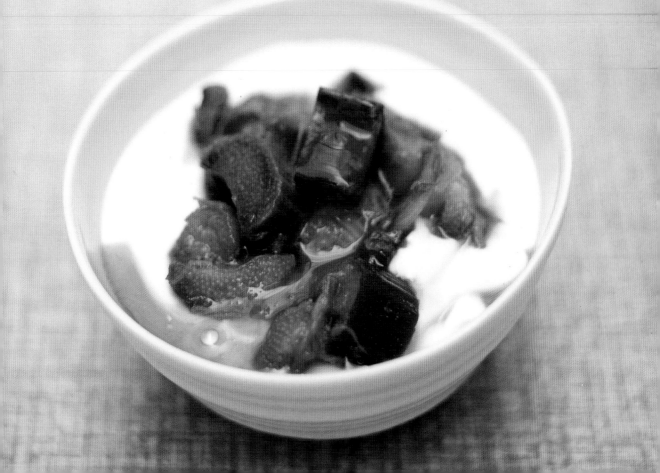

FRESH FRUIT PLATTER

This is great to serve for breakfast but is equally good as a dessert at lunch or supper time. Because everything is ready to eat, it's an easy way to encourage kids (and reluctant adults) to eat some lovely fresh fruit. If you wind up with leftovers you can pop them into the refrigerator to have next morning as a fruit salad, or whizzed up as a smoothie (see page 307).

serves 4

2 clementines

1 orange

½ a honeydew melon

a handful of strawberries

a small bunch of red grapes

3 ripe bananas

1 ripe pear

1 apple

a handful of blueberries

2 cups natural yogurt

Peel your clementines and halve them crossways • Cut the oranges into segments, leaving the skin on • Halve and seed your melon and scoop out the flesh from one half with a spoon • Remove the stalks from the strawberries and halve them if large • Peel the bananas and slice lengthways • Place all your prepared fruit on a large serving platter • Core the pears and apples, slice them into wedges, and add to the platter • Scatter over your blueberries • Serve with a bowl of natural yogurt and let everyone help themselves

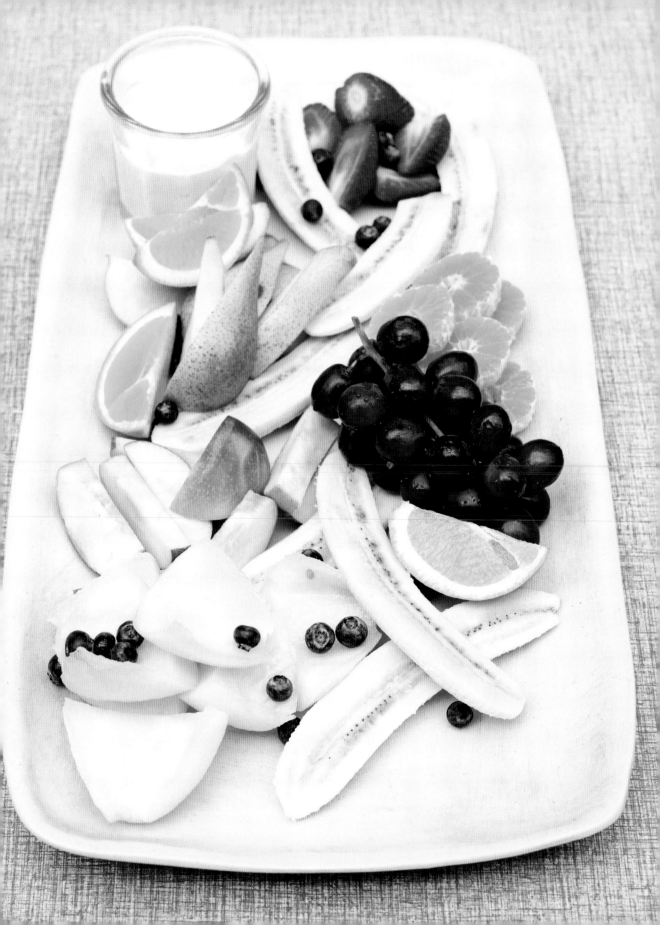

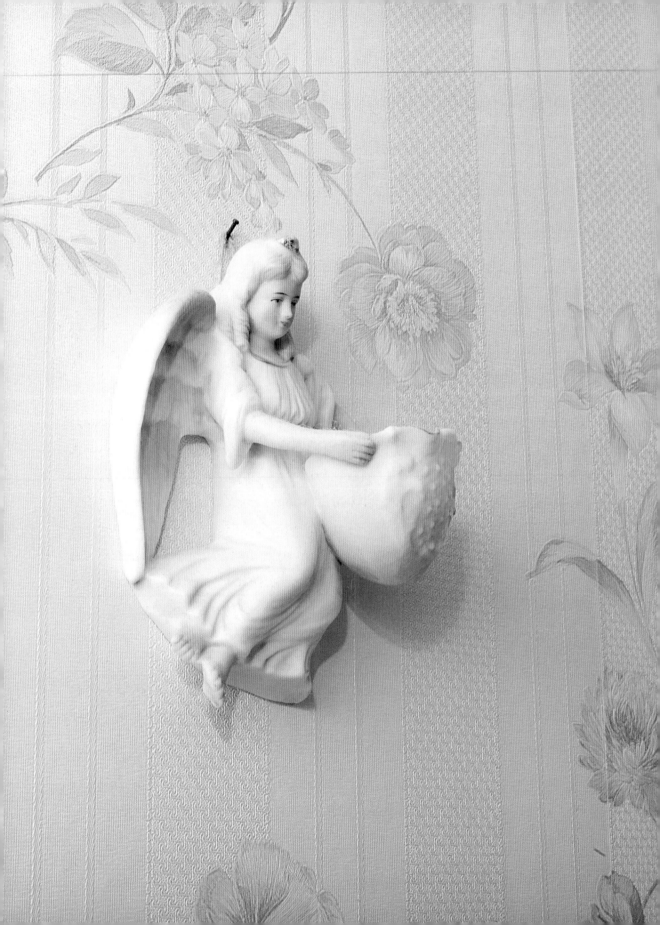

Sweet things

Of all the chapters in this book, baking is by far the most involved and time-consuming thing to try. As you have to stick to measurements very accurately, it's also more open to disaster than other areas of cooking. Which is why I find it interesting that most people who can't cook will have a little go at baking every now and again!

What I've come up with for this chapter is a whole range of classic sweet things that I've made incredibly easy, to help you along the way. If you fancy desserts, cakes, or cookies you'll find them here. From six ways to big up plain old ice cream, a real quickie, to brilliant old-school scones with clotted cream and jam. And I've included a fruit and nut chocolate tart that's so simple to make but very impressive – if you like fruit and nut chocolate bars you'll love it! You must try the banana tarte tatin: again, it looks amazing but is so easy to put together. And to top the chapter off, a great all-occasion sponge, fruit, and cream cake that you can make for birthdays or Mother's Day – the secret is using a panettone as the sponge base (panettone is largely a Christmas thing, so it's a good idea to stock up with a few then as they'll keep happily for about six months). So the emphasis in this chapter is that everything is very easy to make, but also very delicious. They'll serve you well if you're a beginner and need to get your confidence up a bit.

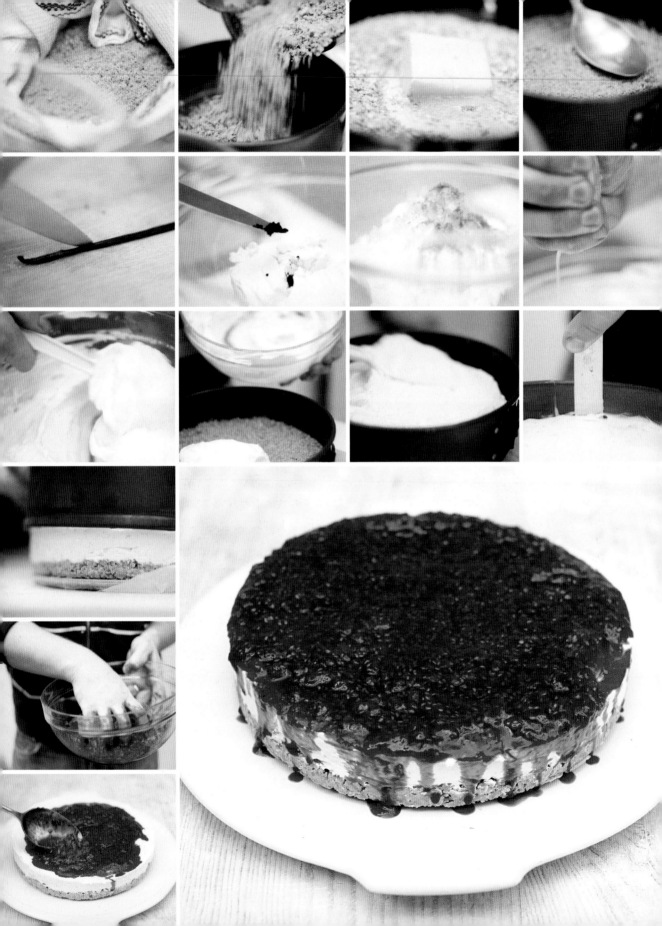

VANILLA CHEESECAKE WITH A RASPBERRY TOPPING

My family absolutely love this dessert. It works every time, and has a lovely hint of lemon. The graham crackers add a fantastic crumbly richness – God bless them! It's a solid vanilla cheesecake recipe that you can make without the addition of the raspberries, but if they're in season and at their best, make the sauce to drizzle over the cheesecake and you'll knock people's socks off! Other fruits that would work in place of raspberries are strawberries, cherries, blueberries, blackberries, and blackcurrants.

serves 8

13 tablespoons butter, plus an extra knob for
   greasing the tin
1 cup quick cook oatmeal (not instant)
2 cups graham cracker crumbs
1 vanilla bean or 1 teaspoon vanilla extract
3 × 8-ounce bars cream cheese
¾ cup superfine sugar

1 lemon
1 orange
1¼ cups heavy cream

For the raspberry topping
½ cup superfine sugar
4 cups raspberries

To make your base
Grease a 9-inch springform cake pan with the knob of butter • Put a saucepan over a low heat, add the oatmeal, and toast until it turns darker in color • Cut the butter into cubes and add it to the pan with your cracker crumbs • Gently stir with a wooden spoon until the mixture combines • Remove from the heat and spoon the mixture into your cake pan, smoothing it out evenly • Gently push down on the crumb base using the back of a metal spoon, or your hands – you want to pack it down flat and even • Put the base in the refrigerator to chill and set for 1 hour

To make your filling
If using one, cut your vanilla bean in half lengthways and gently drag the edge of your knife along the insides of the bean to scrape out the seeds • Put all the cream cheese into a mixing bowl, and add the vanilla seeds or the vanilla extract and the sugar • Grate over the zest of the lemon and orange, then squeeze in the juice from the lemon • Give it all a good stir until nice and smooth • In another bowl, whisk your cream until it gives you soft peaks • Add half of it to your cream cheese mixture and fold it in • Then fold the remaining cream in gently • Once everything is blended, spoon the mixture over the crumb base and use a spatula to smooth it out • Place your cheesecake in the refrigerator for at least an hour

To serve your cheesecake
Lift the cheesecake out of the cake pan by easing around it with a metal spatula • Place on a serving plate • Mix the sugar and raspberries in a bowl – use your hands and scrunch them together • Pour this mixture over the top of the cheesecake and smooth it out to the edges using the back of a spoon

ICE CREAM

It would be lovely if everyone had a go at making things like tarts, tortes, or pastry cases at home, but the reality is that most people won't make any of these things unless it's for a special occasion. Ice cream sales, however, are at an all-time high, so I've decided to include a few really tasty ideas for how to serve one of our favorite desserts.

each variation serves 1

Banana and dulce de leche with vanilla ice cream

Slice 1 **banana** and place in the bottom of your serving bowl • Drizzle with a tablespoon of **dulce de leche or condensed milk caramel** and top with a scoop of **vanilla ice cream** • Sprinkle with a crushed **graham cracker**

Rum and raisins with vanilla ice cream

Put a small pan on a low heat, add a handful of **raisins** and a good lug of **dark rum,** and warm through • Pour into the bottom of your serving bowl with a scoop of **vanilla ice cream** on top • Using a speed peeler, or very carefully using a sharp knife, shave a few curls of **good-quality bittersweet chocolate** over your ice cream

Sliced orange and malt with chocolate ice cream

Peel 1 **orange**, slice it into ½-inch rounds, and place these in the bottom of your serving bowl • Put a small pan on a low heat and melt a pat of **butter** in it • Add 1 tablespoon of quick cook oats, stir occasionally until nice and crunchy, then remove the pan from the heat • Dust a plate with a tablespoon of **malted milk powder** and quickly roll a scoop of **chocolate ice cream** in it until lightly coated • Place the ice cream on top of the orange slices and top with the crunchy oats

Strawberries and ginger snaps with vanilla ice cream

Crush a couple of **ginger snap cookies** in a serving bowl • Slice 2 or 3 **strawberries** and put these on top of the cookies, followed by a scoop of **vanilla ice cream** • Finely grate over some **good-quality bittersweet chocolate** to finish

Fresh raspberry sauce with vanilla ice cream

Put a large handful of **fresh raspberries** and one tablespoon of **superfine sugar** into a bowl • Use your hands to scrunch them up until you have a coarse raspberry sauce • Put a scoop of **vanilla ice cream** into your serving bowl and pour over the crushed raspberries

Pineapple and chile with chocolate ice cream

Cut the top off a **fresh pineapple** and slice off a piece ¾ inch thick • Cut the skin off with a small sharp knife and chop the flesh into cubes • Halve, seed, and very finely chop ½ a **fresh red chile** • Put the pineapple cubes into a serving bowl • Top with a scoop of **chocolate ice cream** and sprinkle over as much chile as you dare!

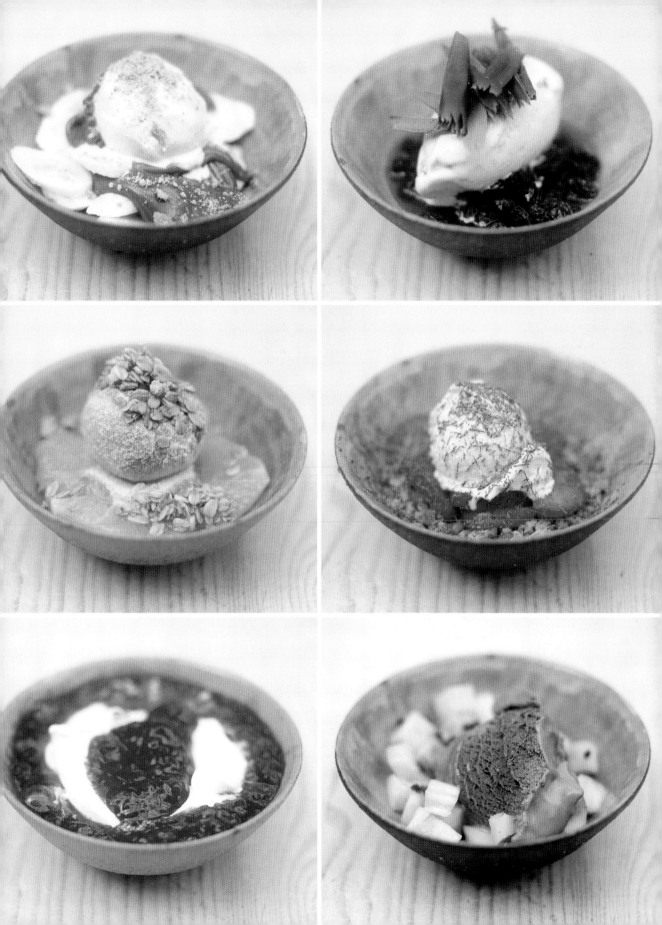

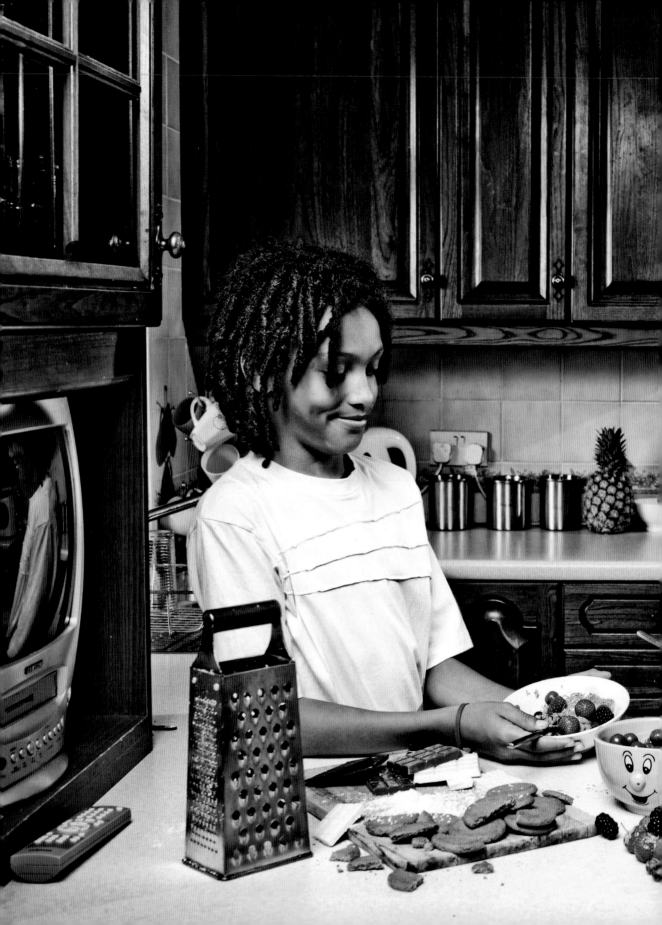

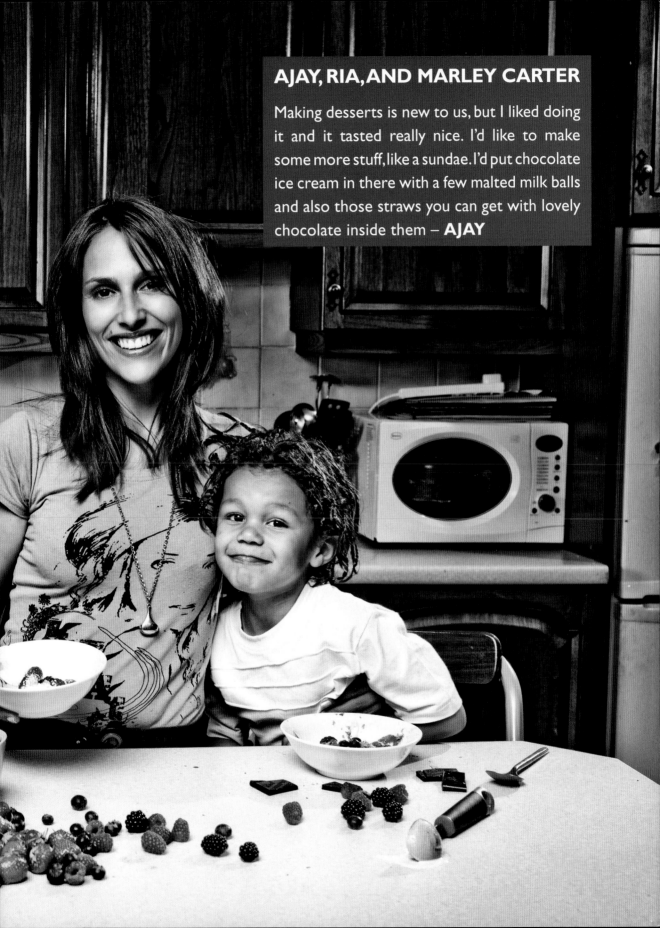

AJAY, RIA, AND MARLEY CARTER

Making desserts is new to us, but I liked doing it and it tasted really nice. I'd like to make some more stuff, like a sundae. I'd put chocolate ice cream in there with a few malted milk balls and also those straws you can get with lovely chocolate inside them – **AJAY**

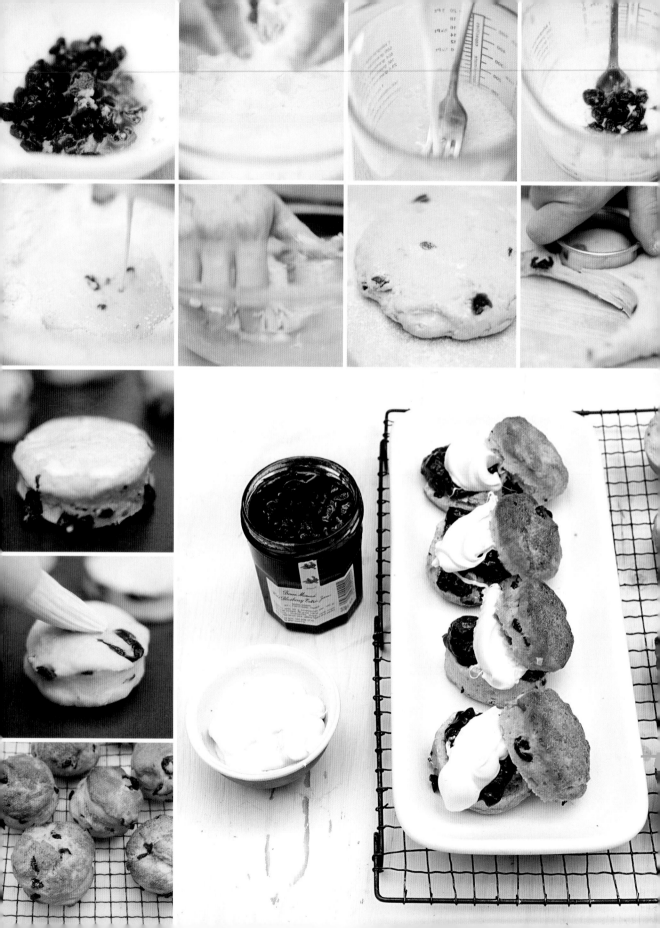

FRUIT SCONES

This is a cracking recipe for scones which uses dried cherries as well as the more traditional raisins. However, feel free to substitute any other dried fruit you like. Scones freeze really well, so you can make a batch of them, pop some into the freezer, and that way, if you have any unexpected visitors, you can always put them straight into the oven from frozen as a quick and delicious treat. Spread with jam and serve with clotted cream – nothing else will do!

makes 10 scones

Scant 1 cup mixture of dried cherries and/or raisins
orange juice, for soaking
4 cups self-rising flour, plus a little extra for dusting
2 teaspoons baking powder
½ cup butter

2 large eggs, preferably free-range or organic
⅓ cup milk, plus a little extra for brushing
salt
good-quality jam
⅔ cup clotted cream or heavy cream, whipped

To make your dough

Preheat the oven to 400°F • Soak the cherries and raisins in a little bowl with just enough orange juice to cover them • While they're soaking, you can either pulse the flour, baking powder, and butter in a food processor just until the mixture starts to look like breadcrumbs (don't be tempted to over-pulse!), or you can blend them together by hand • Transfer to a mixing bowl and make a well in the middle • In another bowl, beat the eggs and milk with a fork • Drain your cherries and raisins in a strainer and add them to the beaten eggs and milk with a good pinch of salt • Then pour your beaten eggs, milk, cherries, and raisins into the well in the flour mixture and stir well, adding a splash more milk if necessary, until you have a soft, dry dough • If your dough feels a little dry and doesn't come together, add an extra splash of milk

To make your scones

Dust a clean work surface and your rolling pin with flour • Roll out the dough until it's ¾ inch thick • Using a 2½-inch round biscuit cutter, or the rim of a glass, cut out 10 circles from the dough and place these on a non-stick cooke sheet (you may have to roll your dough out again in order to get all 10 rounds out of it, but try not to knead it too much, as you don't want to overwork it) • Dip a pastry brush into some milk and brush the top of each scone • Bake in the preheated oven for 12 to 15 minutes, until risen and brown • Take them out of the oven and trasfer to a wire rack to cool

To serve your scones

Cut each scone in half across the middle • Spoon a dollop of jam on to the bottom half of each one, followed by a dollop of clotted (or whipped) cream, and put the tops back on • Serve on a large plate in the middle of the table, or on individual plates – and don't forget a pot of tea!

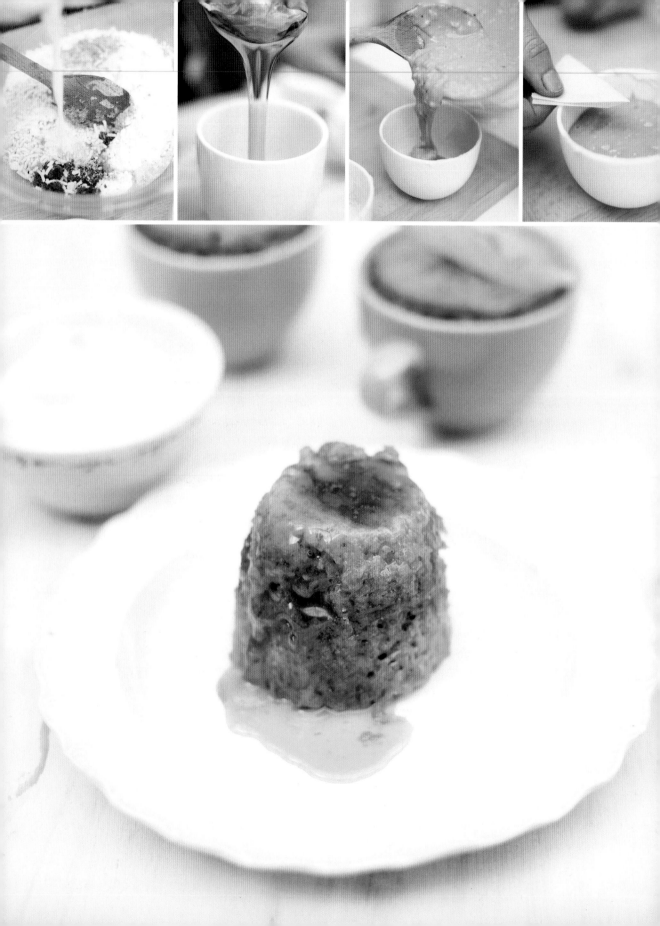

QUICK STEAMED MICROWAVE PUDDING CAKES

These little pudding cakes are great for serving up as a quick dessert. Usually you would make one large pudding cake in a bowl, but individual ones work just as well – you can use any type of small microwaveable dish. I used teacups for mine. You can also make these with a raspberry jam topping by putting 1 tablespoon of jam into the bottom of each cup instead of golden syrup. Once turned out, sprinkle with some unsweetened shredded coconut.

makes 6 individual puddings

butter, for greasing
1 small orange
1 ½ cups all-purpose flour, sifted
¼ cup packed, soft dark brown sugar
6 tablespoons butter
1 level teaspoon baking soda

2 teaspoons ground ginger
2 large eggs, preferably free-range or organic
juice and finely grated zest of 1 small orange
⅔ cup milk
11 tablespoons golden syrup (such as Lyle's) or maple syrup
crème fraîche or custard, to serve

To prepare your dishes

Grease the insides of 6 little microwaveable dishes, or 6-ounce ramekins, or teacups with butter until well coated • Finely grate the zest of the orange, then squeeze all the juice into a large bowl • Tip all the ingredients (except the golden syrup and the crème fraîche or custard) into a bowl • Add 1 tablespoon of golden syrup and mix together with a wooden spoon until well combined • Spoon 1 tablespoon of golden syrup into the bottom of each dish or ramekin and divide the cake batter between them

To make your puddings

Tear or cut out 6 circles of parchment paper a little larger in size than the diameter of the ramekins • Grease them with a little butter and place them gently, butter side down, on top of each ramekin, pressing down gently on to the pudding mix • Place all the dishes in the microwave and cook on a medium (50% power) setting for 7 ½ minutes, if using a 750W microwave (important – the microwave time will change if you decide to cook more or fewer puddings in one go, or if you have one with a different wattage) • Leave the cakes to stand in the microwave for a further 5 minutes before carefully removing the parchment paper

To serve your puddings

Warm ¼ cup of golden syrup in a microwaveable jug for a few seconds • Turn the cakes out on to serving plates (simply put a plate upside down on top of each cake and turn it over carefully) • Serve immediately, drizzling over some of the warmed golden syrup, and eat with a dollop of crème fraîche or some custard

BANANA TARTE TATIN

This is such a great recipe. The thing I love most about it is how simple it is. All you need to do is buy some ready-made puff pastry, split a few bananas in half, and get something magical happening in the oven! You just have to be extremely careful when you flip it out on to a board as hot caramel is one of the nicest things but can burn quite badly. It's best to cover your hand with a kitchen towel and make sure you concentrate on what you're doing. And if you don't like bananas, try using apples or pears.

serves 6

¼ cup unsalted butter

¾ cup superfine sugar

4 large bananas

¼ teaspoon ground cinnamon

1 orange

plain flour, for dusting

1 sheet puff pastry, defrosted if frozen

optional: crème fraîche

optional: vanilla ice cream and a few tablespoons of
  unsweetened shredded coconut

To make your caramel bananas

Preheat your oven to 350°F • Cut your butter into cubes and put into a sturdy deep-sided roasting pan approximately 7½ x 12in • Place the pan on a low heat, let the butter melt, add the sugar, and stir constantly until completely combined • Continue to cook for about 5 minutes, or until the sugar has dissolved and the mixture is golden and caramelized • Meanwhile, peel the bananas, halve them lengthways, and lay them carefully on top of the golden caramel • Remove from the heat, then sprinkle over the cinnamon and finely grate over the zest of half your orange

To make your pastry topping

Dust a clean work surface and rolling pin with flour • Rather than putting your pastry down flat and rolling it out, place it on its side (see the picture opposite) and roll it from there, as this will give you a lighter, crisper texture • Roll out the sheet of pastry until you have a rectangle shape about the same size as your pan and about ⅛ inch thick • Drape your pastry over your rolling pin and carefully lay it on the roasting pan, gently tucking it around the bananas to make sure they're well covered, with no gaps • Using a knife or fork, prick the pastry a few times • Place the tray at the top of the preheated oven for 25 to 30 minutes, until golden

To serve your tarte tatin

When your tarte tatin is ready you must turn it out at once or it will end up sticking to the pan • To do this, cover your hand with a folded kitchen towel, carefully hold the tray with a serving plate or board on top, and gently turn it over • Using the tip of a knife, pull a corner of the pastry up to check if it's all cooked underneath (if not, pop it back into the oven for another couple of minutes), then ease the whole thing out of the pan • If using crème fraîche or whipped cream, put it into a bowl, grate over the rest of your orange zest, and stir well • If using vanilla ice cream, sprinkle a few tablespoons of unsweetened shredded coconut on a plate and quickly roll a scoop of ice cream in it until coated • Serve your tarte tatin with a dollop of crème fraîche, whipped cream, or ice cream, and eat immediately!

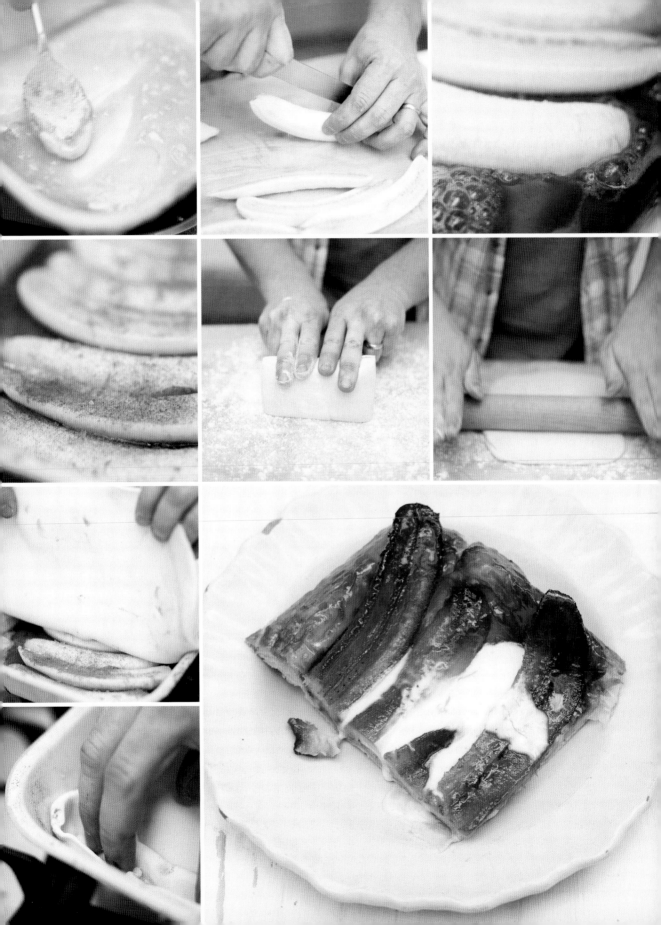

COOKIES

This is a basic refrigerator cookie dough recipe with a little added oatmeal to keep things healthy. I like to make it and just add the extras depending on what I'm in the mood for. If you fancy dried fruit and nut cookies instead of chocolate or citrus, feel free to use them, just keep the quantities the same as for the chocolate cookies.

makes about 15 cookies

For the basic cookie dough
2¼ sticks butter (1 cup plus 2 tablespoons)
1 cup superfine sugar
2 large eggs, preferably free-range or organic
scant 1 cup all-purpose flour
½ cup quick cook oatmeal (not instant)
¼ teaspoon baking powder
½ teaspoon salt

For the citrus cookies
2 oranges
2 lemons

For the double chocolate cookies
4 ounces white chocolate or ½ cup white chocolate chips
4 ounces bittersweet chocolate or ½ cup bittersweet chocolate chips

To make your basic cookie dough

Take your butter out of the refrigerator 15 minutes before you start so it has time to soften a bit first • If you've got a food processor, simply put your soft butter into it with the rest of the basic ingredients and whiz until smooth • Or you can put it into a mixing bowl with the sugar and mix with a wooden spoon until you get a thick, creamy consistency • Crack your egg into another bowl and beat it with a fork, then add it to the butter and sugar and mix well • Sift your flour into the bowl to remove any lumps, add the oats, baking powder, and salt, and mix until lovely and smooth

To flavor your cookie dough

Either finely grate your orange and lemon zest or roughly chop your chocolate • Stir the zest or chocolate into the cookie dough and mix together well • Spoon on to a piece of plastic wrap and roll into a sausage shape with a roughly 2-inch diameter • Pop the dough into the freezer for 30 minutes

To bake your cookies

Preheat the oven to 375°F • Get your chilled dough out of the freezer and cut it into ¼-inch-thick slices • Place these on two non-stick cookie sheets, making sure you leave a good bit of space between the slices because they'll spread while cooking • If you can't fit all your slices on the cookie sheets, just cook one batch after another • Place the cookie sheets in the middle of your preheated oven and bake for 8 to 10 minutes, until the edges of the cookies are golden brown • Let them cool down slightly before transferring to a wire rack to let cool completely and crisp up • Delicious with a glass of cold milk

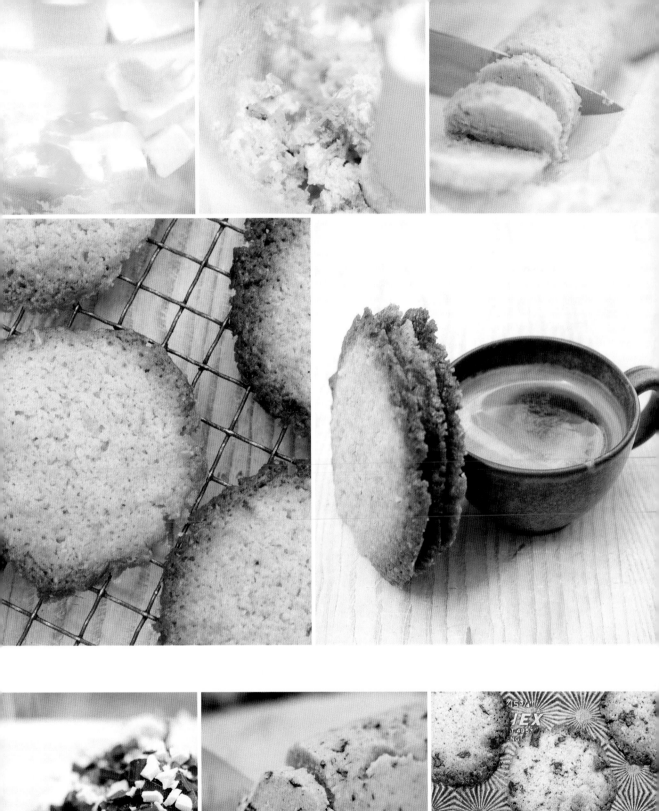
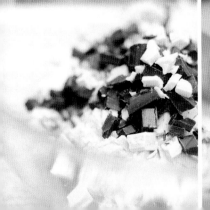
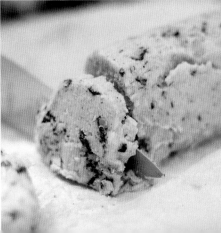
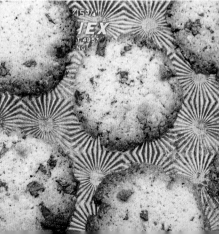

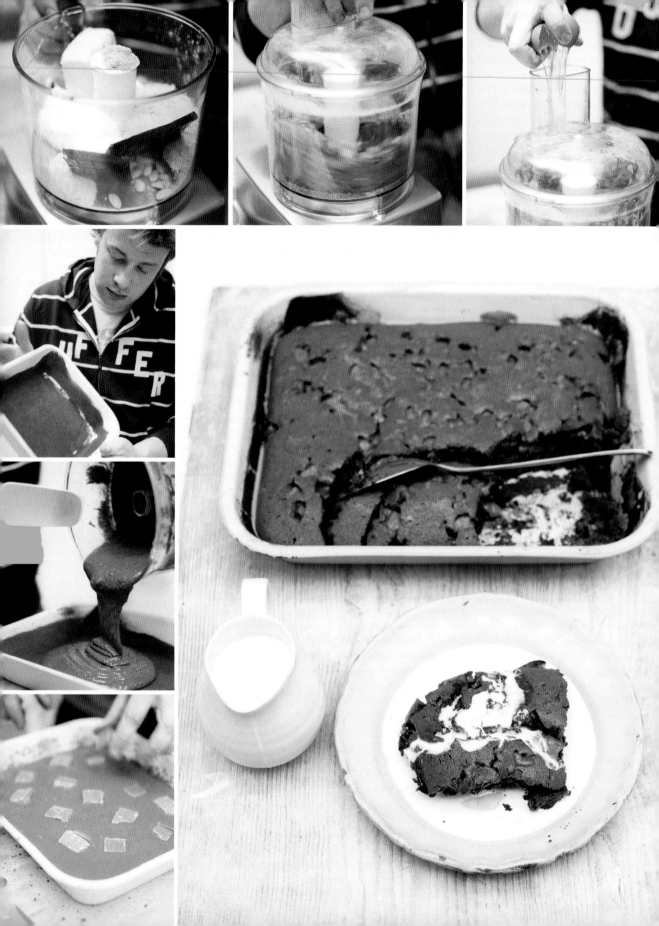

MEGA CHOCOLATE FUDGE CAKE

This cake is best made using a food processor, as you can simply add everything and blitz it up together, but you can easily make it by hand if you buy almond flour and grate the chocolate into the mix. Like most desserts, this isn't exactly the healthiest thing in the world but it's absolutely gorgeous. Just make sure you enjoy it as it's meant to be enjoyed – a special treat every now and then.

serves 10

7 ounces good-quality bittersweet chocolate (60% cocoa solids), or 1 heaped cup of chips
¾ cup butter, plus extra for greasing
⅔ cup packed soft brown sugar
⅔ cup skinned almonds

2 tablespoons unsweetened cocoa powder
a pinch of salt
4 large eggs, preferably free-range or organic
1⅓ cups self-rising flour
¼ pound soft fudge
crème fraîche, vanilla ice cream, or heavy cream

To make your cake
Preheat the oven to 325°F • Break up the chocolate, put it into a food processor with the butter, sugar, almonds, 1 tablespoon of the cocoa powder, and the salt, and whiz until smooth • Crack your eggs, one at a time, into the food processor and add the flour • Whiz again until smooth

To bake your cake
Get a deep baking pan roughly 10 x 10 inches in size • Butter the dish really well and sprinkle the remaining tablespoon of cocoa powder over it • Shake it around a bit so it lightly coats the whole surface of the pan • Pour the cake batter into the pan, using a spatula to scrape it all out of the processor • Break the fudge into pieces and sprinkle these over the top of the cake batter, pushing any larger pieces down into the batter • Pop the baking pan into the preheated oven and cook for 18 to 20 minutes • Take the cake out of the oven and stick a fork into the middle of it • If there's a little bit of cake mixture on the fork when you pull it out, that's okay – you want the cake to still be a little moist inside so that it's nice and squidgy • However, if it seems a bit wobbly, pop it back into the oven for another 3 to 5 minutes to firm up a bit

To serve your cake
Let your cake cool slightly and serve it warm and gooey • Lovely with a dollop of crème fraîche, a scoop of vanilla ice cream, or a bit of heavy cream

CHEAT'S SPONGE CAKE WITH SUMMER BERRIES AND CREAM

If you need to make a cake fast, this is definitely the recipe for you, as there is no baking involved! Italian panettone cakes can be bought from most grocery stores and delis, and they usually come boxed up really nicely. If you end up with any leftover panettone, just wrap it in plastic wrap and toast it next morning for breakfast – totally delicious.

serves 10–12

1 cup sliced almonds

Vin Santo or sweet dessert wine

2½ cups heavy cream

2 tablespoons superfine sugar

1 vanilla bean or 1 tablespoon vanilla extract

1 × 16-ounce container of strawberries

1 medium or large panettone

1 × 6-ounce container of raspberries

1 x 4-ounce bar of good-quality dark chocolate

To prepare your cake

Put a small dry frying pan on a low heat and add the almonds • Shake the pan around every now and then to toast the nuts, making sure they don't burn • Once they start to turn darker, take the pan off the heat and put them aside to cool • Pour about ⅓ cup of Vin Santo or sweet dessert wine into a wineglass • Pour the cream into a mixing bowl and add the sugar • If using the vanilla bean, halve it lengthways and drag the blade of your knife along the inside of the bean to scrape all the vanilla seeds out • Add the seeds or the vanilla extract to the bowl, and whisk until the cream is thick and forms peaks • Slice the strawberries, removing any stalks

To make your cake

Peel any paper off your panettone and carefully cut it across into 3 round slices, each about ¾ inch thick • Put a slice on a serving plate and spoon a few tablespoons of the Vin Santo or sweet dessert wine over it (there's no need to soak the panettone; you just need enough to flavor it) • Spoon a good dollop of the cream on to the panettone slice and smooth it out to the edges, using a metal spatula or similar • Lay over half your sliced strawberries and top with a second slice of panettone • Repeat the wine, cream, and berry steps until you get to the top layer • Pat this down gently, spoon over the remaining wine, and top it off with the rest of the cream, smoothing it over the top and sides of the cake so it's completely covered – don't worry about getting it all perfect, as it can look messy and still taste delicious! • Squeeze a handful of your toasted nuts to crumble them up, then gently pat them against the side of the cake until all the sides are covered

To serve your cake

Pile the raspberries on top of the cake and sprinkle with some chocolate shavings (simply use a vegetable peeler or a knife and drag it across the bar of chocolate)

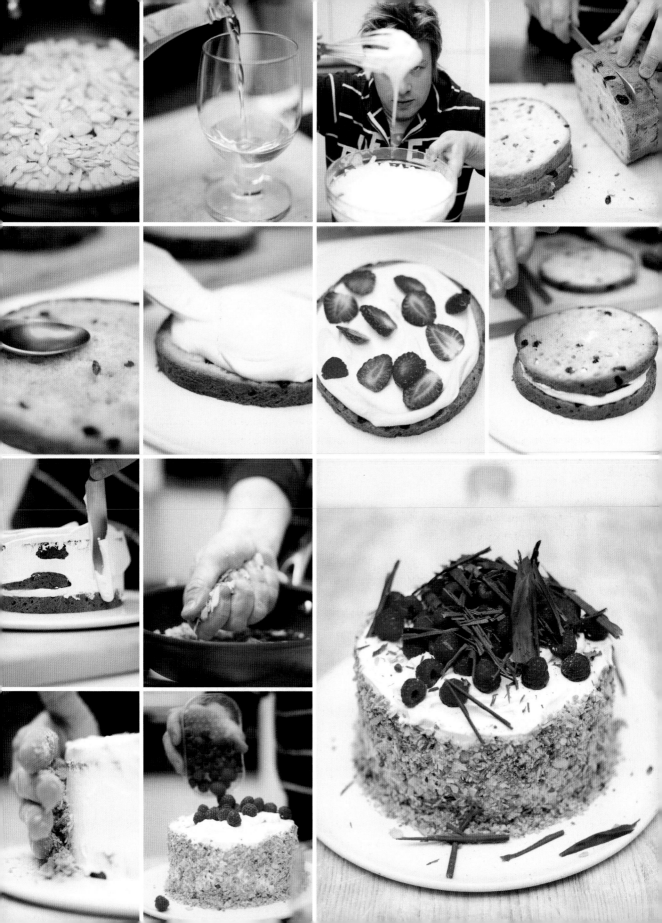

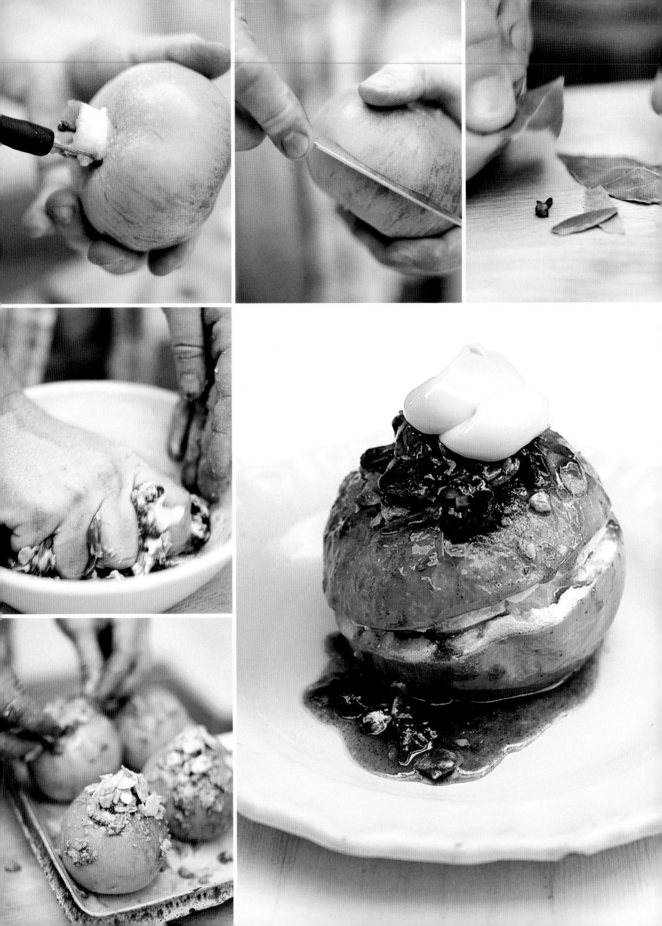

BAKED APPLES

This is an absolutely classic dessert – it's so simple, and a great way to use up cooking apples. Kids and adults love these, they're great eaten all year round, and they're cheap as chips.

serves 4

¼ cup unsalted butter

4 large Macintosh or Granny Smith apples

2 bay leaves, dried or fresh

2 whole cloves

½ cup sliced almonds

1 orange

1 lemon

½ cup packed, soft light brown sugar

½ cup raisins

1 heaped teaspoon mixed spice

1 shot of brandy or whisky

To prepare your apples

Take your butter out of the refrigerator about 15 to 30 minutes before you start making your baked apples so it has time to soften a bit first • Preheat the oven to 350°F • Use an apple corer to remove the cores from your apples, then carefully score around the middle of each one, using a knife • Place the apples in a baking pan • If using dried bay leaves, crumble them into little pieces; if using fresh leaves, you will need to finely chop them • Place into a pestle and mortar with the cloves and bash up • Put into a large bowl with most of the almonds and grate in the zest of the orange and lemon • Add the rest of the ingredients • Using your hands, mix well, squeezing all the flavors into the butter • Stuff this mixture into the hole in each apple (where you removed the core) and rub the outside of each fruit with some of the mixture • Toss the remaining almonds in the bowl so they become lightly coated in any leftover juices, then sprinkle over the top of the apples

To bake your apples

Place in the preheated oven for 35 to 40 minutes, until golden and soft • Remove from the oven and leave to cool down for about 5 minutes before serving • Put each apple into a small bowl and spoon over the lovely caramelized juices from the pan • These apples are absolutely cracking with a dollop of good vanilla ice cream or custard

CHOCOLATE FRUIT AND NUT TART

This is a great tart, because you can add so many different things to the filling, like quick cook oats, or unsweetened shredded coconut, or any other type of nuts – if you want to give your kids a treat, this is the tart for them! Buy good-quality bittersweet chocolate with a minimum 60% cocoa solids. And for those of you who'd like a new challenge, why not make your own pastry (see page 346).

serves 6

all purpose plain flour, for dusting

14 ounces sweet shortcrust pastry (½ of recipe on p. 346)

2 x 3½-ounce bars of good-quality bittersweet chocolate (minimum 60% cocoa solids), or 1¼ cups chips

1¼ cups heavy cream

2 heaped tablespoons superfine sugar

2 tablespoons butter

sea salt

½ cup hazelnuts

⅓ cup raisins

To make your pastry case

Preheat your oven to 350°F • Dust a clean work surface and your rolling pin with flour • Roll the pastry out into a rectangle just under ½ inch thick, dusting with flour as you go • Drape the pastry over your rolling pin and carefully lay it on a jelly roll pan • Pinch the edges with your thumb and forefinger to crimp them up, creating a sort of lip • Using a fork, prick all over the base of the pastry case • Pop it into the freezer until hard, then place in the preheated oven • Cook for 15 minutes until golden

To make the filling

Bash up your chocolate • Put the cream and sugar into a pan and simmer on a low heat for about 5 minutes • Remove from the heat and add the chocolate and butter • Add a pinch of salt and stir slowly until the chocolate and butter have melted • Toast your hazelnuts in a hot, dry pan for a few minutes until golden • Scatter the nuts and raisins over the pastry base • Pour over the melted chocolate and smooth it out evenly to all four sides • Allow to cool before popping into the fridge for 20 minutes, then cut into squares and get stuck in!

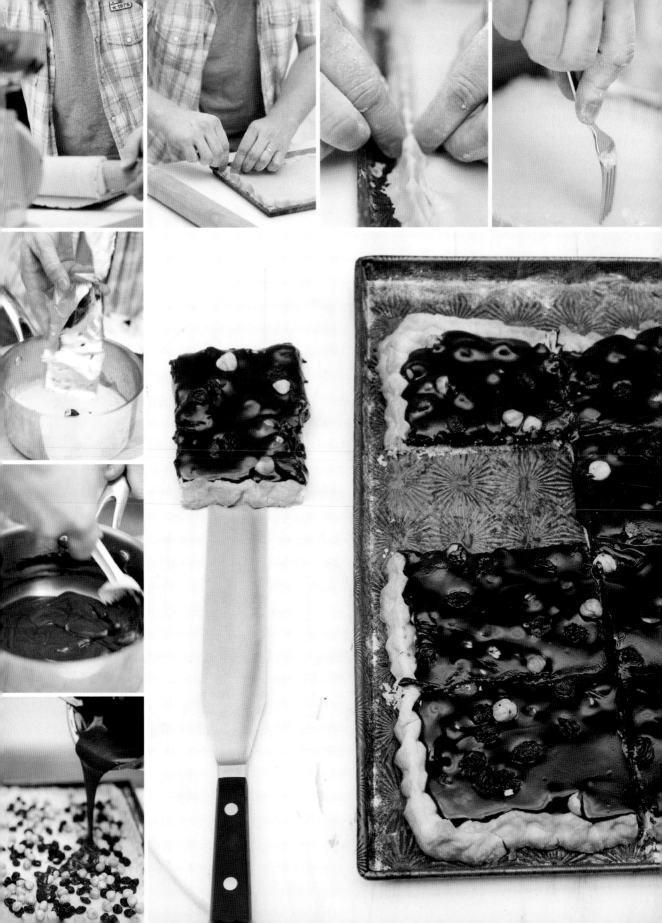

SWEET SHORTCRUST PASTRY

Even if you've never made pastry before, as long as you stick to the correct measurements for the ingredients and you follow this method exactly, you'll be laughing. Try to be confident and bring the pastry together as quickly as you can – don't knead it too much or the heat from your hands will melt the butter. A good tip is to hold your hands under cold running water beforehand to make them as cold as possible. That way you'll end up with a delicate, flaky pastry every time.

To make a savory shortcrust pastry, simply remove the confectioners' sugar from the recipe and mix ½ cup of grated Cheddar cheese into your butter and flour mixture with a generous pinch of sea salt. Replace the lemon zest with a small handful of thyme or chopped rosemary leaves to add flavor.

These quantities will make more pastry than you usually need for the recipe, but it's easy to freeze the extra, well wrapped in plastic wrap, to use another time.

makes 2 pounds of dough

1 cup good-quality cold butter
2 large eggs, preferably free-range or organic
a splash of milk

4¼ cups all-purpose flour, plus extra for dusting
1 cup confectioners' sugar
optional: 1 lemon

Cut your cold butter into small cubes • Crack your eggs into a bowl with a splash of milk and beat together with a fork • Sift the flour from a height on to a clean work surface • Sift the confectioners' sugar over the flour • Using your hands, gently work the cubes of butter into the flour and sugar by rubbing your thumbs against your fingers until you end up with a fine, crumbly mixture • Zest your lemon over the mixture (or add your other chosen flavoring) • Gradually add the eggs and milk and gently work everything together until you get a ball of dough • If your dough feels a little dry and doesn't come together, then add an extra splash of milk • Sprinkle a little flour over the ball • Sprinkle the ball and the work surface with some more flour and place the ball on top • Remember not to work the pastry too much at this stage or it will become elastic and chewy, not crumbly and short • Pat the ball until you have a flat round • Sprinkle it with a little bit more flour, then wrap it in plastic wrap and put it into the refrigerator to rest (or "prove") for about 30 minutes

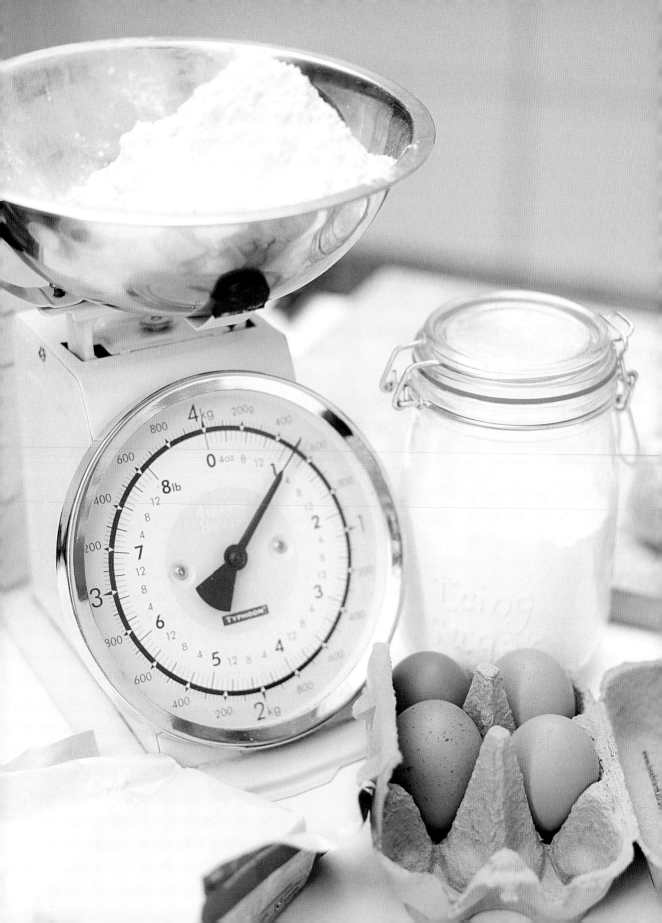

Thanks

A massive thank you to all the wonderful people who have helped me not only with this book but also with the Ministry of Food project in Rotherham. I'm probably going to forget someone's name along the way and, if I do, please accept my sincere apologies. There are so many people involved these days that remembering everyone is a bit of a nightmare – but I'll do my best!

First and foremost to 'Class A' and all the contributors in Rotherham: you guys have been utterly brilliant and brave for throwing yourselves into this project. Thanks for letting me into your homes, for turning up every week to the classes, and for letting me include your lovely selves (and a few of your families!) in the beautiful chapter portraits: Julie Critchlow, Claire Hallam, Debbie Dennis, Natasha Whiteman, Geoff Blackburn, Tracey Fearn, Andy Pickersgill, Robert Tindle, Beccy Hill, Dan Carter, Simon Atkinson, Mick Trueman, Matthew Borrington, William Shepard, and Malcolm Doane. You've all made **pass it on** really come alive for me. You've been an absolute inspiration and a pleasure to get to know.

Big thanks to John Lambert, the Head Teacher at Rawmarsh Community School, and the staff there. You allowed me to take over your home economics rooms on a weekly basis for my lessons, so cheers for putting up with me and for helping **pass it on** to get started!

To Roger Stone and the rest of the gang at Rotherham Council: Steve Pearson, Paul Woodcock, Julie Roberts, Bernadette Rushton, Pete Tomlin, and Stuart Carr. Thanks so much for your help and enthusiasm. Having worked with a few councils before, I can honestly say you're a fantastic, forward-thinking bunch and I've enjoyed working with you.

Nick Crofts-Smith and Alison Norcliffe at the Rotherham College of Arts and Technology were absolutely brilliant. All the support you gave me and my crew on all those bloody crazy projects we did in Rotherham over the past year was crucial. Nice one!

To the wonderfully helpful Fiona Gately, you've done a brilliant job of getting this project up and running, thank you. And big thanks as well to the lovely Lisa Taylor and Jane Pond, who are running my Ministry of Food in Rotherham. I've got to say love and respect to the fantastically generous kitchen company Atrium, who kitted us out with a brand new kitchen for the Ministry of Food for free – essentially for the greater good of the community. If anyone wants a great kitchen, go to www.atriumuk.com! Thanks also to RBT (Connect Ltd) for their kind donation of a computer and printer for the center, and to AMV and Sainsbury's for their help with statistics.

Shout out to Rotherham United FC and, most importantly, thanks to the people of Rotherham. I had an inspiring seven months in your town, met brilliant people, and had lots of laughs. You've got a great community up there – thanks so much for making me feel welcome.

Big love to my dear food and editorial teams. Thanks so much for all of your ridiculously hard work in making this an incredible book. You give me great support and I love you all. On the food side of things: the brilliant and inspirational Peter Begg, the absolutely wonderful Ginny Rolfe, lovely ladies Anna Jones, Georgie Socratous, Abigail Fawcett, and Christina "Scarabouchi" McCloskey. Respect and love to the brilliant Claire Postans, Bobby Sebire, and Helen Martin, who keep it all ticking along like a well-oiled machine! Shout-outs to Kate McCoullough and Jackson Berg for their hard work and support. And of course to the constantly inspiring Gennaro Contaldo for his love and passion. To my girls on words: the lovely Katie Bosher and new girl in the mix Rebecca Walker; and to the old crew, Sophia "Know-it-all" Brown and Suzanna de Jong, thanks for all your hard work.

As ever, a massive thank you to Lord David Loftus and Chris Terry for their incredible photos, hard work, and loyalty – bless your hearts.

Thanks as well to all the TV production team. Although you weren't involved in the making of this book, filming the project and campaign in Rotherham was an incredible inspiration. This production was a bloody nightmare to put together, so the people I mention below are the absolute rocks that made the TV series happen. As ever to my two sidekicks at Fresh One Productions, Zoë Collins and Jo Ralling – love ya! To Dan Reed, the executive producer, for believing in the project, nice one mate, appreciate it; lovely Eve Kay, for running it so well as series producer; Lana Salah, Emily Jones, Emma Palmer-Watts, Emily Taylor, Sarah Rubin, and Helen Crampton, and all the rest of the crew. Thank you all so much. It was a tough one but it was worth it, wasn't it?

To my brilliant personal team, who put up with me and keep my crazy life in order: the lovely Louise Holland, Liz McMullan, Holly Adams, Beth Richardson, and Paul Rutherford. How on earth you allowed me to spend so much time up in Rotherham getting this off the ground when I had so much other stuff on the go I don't know, but good juggling! Love you, guys!

I have a hugely talented, clever bunch of people working for me. So to each one of you in the office, massive love and thanks for all the hard work you put in day after day on my behalf – it's much appreciated.

To all the people in the Penguin Posse: Tom Weldon, my wonderful editor Lindsey Evans, my mate John Hamilton, Keith Taylor, Juliette Butler, Chantal Noel, Kate Brotherhood, Rob Williams, Elizabeth Smith, Tora Orde-Powlett, Naomi Fidler, Clare Pollock, Anna Rafferty, and the rest of their teams. You've been your usual fantastic selves and done a bloody good job once again. These books are tough, so big love for all of your incredible hard work and support. Massive thanks as well again to the lovely Annie Lee and Chris Callard for their hard work on yet another one of my books.

A big thank you to my many brilliant suppliers, and a special thanks to David Mellor for loaning us some of the beautiful plates and kitchenware you see in this book.

And last but most absolutely, definitely not least, thanks to my beautiful wife Jools for putting up with me disappearing every week to Rotherham and looking after the family as brilliantly as she does every single day – love you very much!

Index

Page references in **bold** indicate an illustration

v indicates a vegetarian recipe

q

r

raisins

v   chocolate fruit and nut tart 344, **345**

v   rum and raisins with vanilla ice cream
        326, **327**

raspberries

v   cheat's sponge cake with summer berries
        and cream 340, **341**

v   fresh raspberry sauce with vanilla ice cream
        326, **327**

v   vanilla cheesecake with a raspberry topping
        324, 325

red wine: lamb and red wine stew 180

rice 95

v   basic **94**, 95

     chicken and leek stroganoff 34, **35**

v   cilantro and lime rice 96, **96–7**

v   garlic and nutmeg rice 96, **96–7**

     kedgeree 288, **289**

     leftover curry biriani 78, **79**

v   lemon, ginger and turmeric rice 96, **96–7**

     my sweet and sour pork **64**, 65

     paella 292, **293**

v   rice salad **124**, 125, **125**

     sizzling beef with spring onions and black
        bean sauce 68, 69

v   spicy chile rice 96, **96–7**

rice noodles

     Asian chicken noodle broth **36**, 37

     hardly-any-prep shrimp stir-fry 66, **67**

v   rigatoni: baked Camembert pasta 44, **45**

roast dinners

     a consistently good gravy **204**, 205

     delicious sage and onion stuffing 206, **207**

     perfect roast beef 192, **193**

     perfect roast chicken 196, **197**

     perfect roast lamb 200, **201**

     perfect roast pork **194**, 195

v   roasted potatoes, parsnips, and carrots 202,
        203

v   sauces 210, **211**

v   Yorkshire puddings **208**, 209

rogan josh

     lamb rogan josh **80**, 81

v   paste **98**, 99

rosemary: baked cod wrapped in bacon with
        rosemary 256, **257**

v   rum and raisins with vanilla ice cream 326, **327**

s

sage: delicious sage and onion stuffing
        206, **207**

salads

v   dressed green salad 102, **103**

v   everyday green chopped salad 120, **121**

v   evolution carrot salad 116, **117**

v   evolution cucumber salad 114, **115**

     evolution green salad 108, **109**

     evolution potato salad **110**, 111

     evolution tomato salad **112**, 113

v   jam jar dressings 106, 107, **107**

v   Mediterranean chopped salad 123, **123**

v   pick-and-mix style 118, **118**, **119**

     posh chopped salad 122, **122**

v   rice salad **124**, 125, **125**

salmon

     Asian-style steamed salmon 250, **251**

     fish pie **284**, 285

     posh chopped salad 122, **122**

     quick salmon tikka with cucumber yogurt
        28, **29**

     salmon baked in a foil parcel with green
        beans and pesto 248, **249**

     salmon en croûte **290**, 291

     salmon fish cakes 280, **281**

     super-quick salmon stir-fry 70, **71**

salsas

v   black olive, sun-dried tomato, and celery
        salsa 275, **275**

     chicken fajitas 38, **39**

v   chopped pesto salsa 274, **274**

     griddled lamb chops with chunky salsa
        244, **245**

v   mango, cucumber, and chile salsa 272, **272**

v   tomato salsa 273, **273**

sauces

v   applesauce 210, **211**

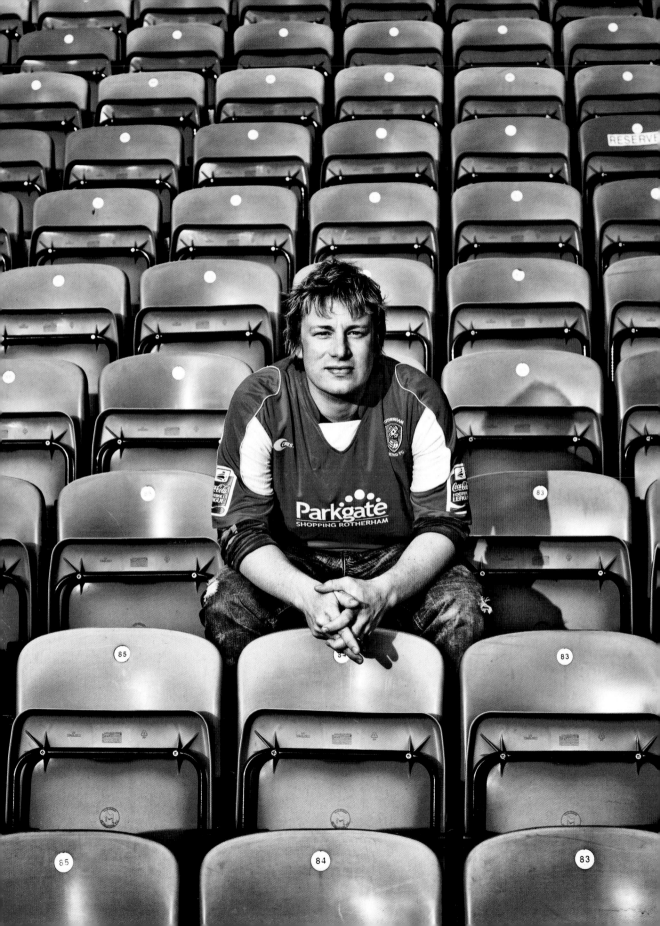